MEDICAL TERMINOLOGY FOR HEALTH PROFESSIONS

Ann Ehrlich

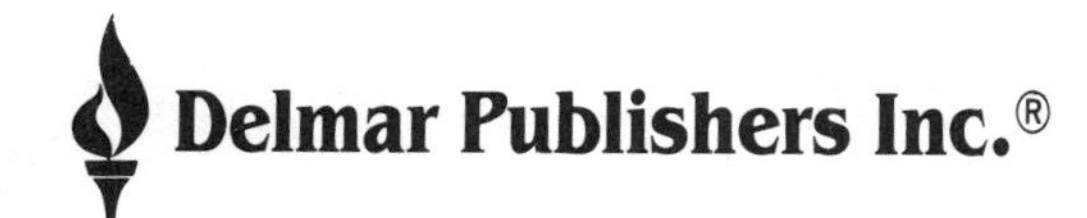

NOTICE TO THE READER

Delmar Staff
Administrative Editor: Leslie Boyer
Developmental Editor: Marjorie A. Bruce
Managing Editor: Barbara A. Christie
Production Editor: Ruth East
Publications Coordinator: Karen Seebald
Design Coordinator: Susan C. Mathews

For information, address Delmar Publishers Inc.
2 Computer Drive West, Box 15-015
Albany, New York 12212

Printed in the United States of America
Published simultaneously in Canada
by Nelson Canada,
a Division of International Thomson Limited

10 9 8 7 6 5 4 3 2

Library of Congress Cataloging-in-Publication Data

Ehrlich, Ann B. (Ann Beard)
Medical terminology for health professions.

Includes index.
1. Medicine–Terminology–Programmed instruction.
I. Title. [DNLM: 1. Nomenclature–programmed instruction. W 18 E33m]
R123.E47 1988 610'.14 87–33216
ISBN 0–8273–3036–7 (textbook)
ISBN 0–8273–3042–1 (Apple diskette)
ISBN 0–8273–3037–5 (instructor's guide)
ISBN 0–8273–3041–3 (IBM diskette)
ISBN 0–8273–3038–3 (audiotapes)

CONTENTS

PREFACE

The range of career options open in the health care professions is diverse and almost limitless. On every level there are opportunities to be part of a caring profession, helping people and fully expressing your own special talents and abilities. However, entering a health care field is somewhat like going to a foreign country. Before you can understand what is going on — you need to learn the language.

In some ways learning medical terminology is like learning a foreign language. There are many words that sound strange and don't make sense. Happily, learning medical terminology is really much easier than starting from scratch with a whole new vocabulary.

As you get into medical terminology you'll soon become aware that many of the words are already familiar. And the new terms will be easier to learn when you discover that many of them are made up of interchangeable parts that are used over and over again in different combinations. To make learning easier, important word parts are highlighted in color and defined.

Once you've mastered this, you will be well on your way to being able to "translate" even complete terms that you've never seen before —and your medical vocabulary and comprehension will increase much more quickly.

This text, and the accompanying teaching materials, are all carefully designed to help you learn medical terminology. You'll want to take advantage of these features: **exercises** at the end of each chapter; **flashcards** to use to study the major combining forms; an appendix of **word parts** and their definitions; an appendix of medical **abbreviations,** and a comprehensive **index** that includes all of the terms defined in this text. There are also **audiotapes** and **computer exercises** for use as teaching aids.

Chapters 1 and 2 introduce medical terminology and the body as a whole, and these chapters should be studied first. The remaining chapters are organized by body systems and may be completed in the order that best suits your course of study. Throughout the book, important terms are printed in boldface and followed by a "see and say" pronunciation. We think you'll like this pronunciation method because it is the same system that radio and television announcers use to enable them to learn how to say complex foreign names and words.

Writing this book and developing the teaching materials has been a particularly interesting and exciting challenge for me. One goal was to include those words you are most likely to encounter in the real world of medicine today. Achieving this goal required research involving many of the latest texts and reference books available in medicine — plus exploring more medical dictionaries than I ever imagined existed. It is my hope that you will find these materials will help you toward a long and rewarding career in the health care profession of your choice.

Special Thanks

I want to offer special thanks to Donald J. Jacobsen and Lacrecia B. Taylor who assisted with the extensive research and work that have gone into developing this text. Without their efforts this would all still be a dream of what might be.

Acknowledgements

Art is an important part of this text and I wish to thank the following authors for their gracious permission to reprint illustrations from these texts.

- Fong, Ferris and Skelley, *Body Structures and Functions,* 6th edition. Delmar Publishers, Inc. 1984.
- Keir, Wise, and Kreb-Shannon, *Medical Assisting: Clinical and Administrative Competencies,* Delmar Publishers, Inc. 1986.
- Walters, Estridge and Reynolds, *Basic Medical Laboratory Techniques,* Delmar Publishers, Inc. 1986.

I am particularly grateful to the reviewers who were such a valuable resource in evaluating the book as it evolved. Their attention to detail, insights, comments, suggestions and encouragement were very important in making certain that this book is "on target" for health careers students.

- **Jane P. Eades, CMA-C,** Department of Medical Services Technology, Eastern Kentucky University, Richmond, KY 40475.
- **Lucille Keir, CMA-A,** Formerly a teacher in the public school system of Columbus, OH.
- **Mary M. Rahr, RN, MS,** Medical Assistant Instructor, Northeast Wisconsin Technical Institute, Green Bay, WI 54307.
- **Lucille Sanders, Director** Florida College of Business, Miami, FL 33147.
- **Carol-Lee Smith, BSHS, Ph.D.,** Coordinator, Medical Assisting, Shasta College, Redding, CA 96003.
- **Diana Bennett, BSN, MAT,** Program Chairman, Medical Assisting, Indiana Vocational Technical College, Indianapolis, IN 46206.
- **Barbara Capone,** Mabel Dean Bacon Vocational High School, Health Career Department, New York, NY 10010.

1

INTRODUCTION TO MEDICAL TERMINOLOGY

LEARNING GOALS

In this chapter you will learn to:

- identify the role of the root words, prefixes, suffixes, and combining forms used in constructing medical terms.
- use your knowledge of word parts to analyze and understand medical terms.
- work with the "sounds like" pronunciation system to correctly pronounce medical terms.
- recognize the importance of always spelling medical terms correctly.
- define prefix, root word, combining form and suffix.
- identify at least forty of the most commonly used word parts (prefixes, combining forms and suffixes.)
- identify the body systems plus the components and major functions of each.

PRONUNCIATION

A new medical term is much easier to understand and remember when you know how to pronounce it properly. To help you do this, each new term in the text is identified in **bold type**, followed (in parentheses) by a commonly accepted pronunciation, and then the definition.

In this "sounds like" pronunciation system, the word is respelled using standard English letters to create sounds that are familiar. To pronounce a new word, just say it as it is spelled in the parentheses.

The part of the word that receives the primary (most) emphasis when you say it, is in capital letters and bold type. For example, **edema** (eh-**DEE**-mah) means excess fluid in body tissues, causing swelling.

The part of the word that receives the secondary emphasis when you say it, is in lower case letters and bold type. For example, **appendicitis** (ah-**pen**-dih-**SIGH**-tis) means an inflammation of the appendix.

A Word of Caution

There are different ways to pronounce some medical terms. The pronunciation shown is one that is commonly accepted; however, your instructor may prefer a different pronunciation. Usually both are correct and it is simply a matter of personal preference.

SPELLING IS IMPORTANT

Although there may be more than one acceptable way to pronounce a medical term, there is only one acceptable spelling — and accuracy is extremely important!

Changing just one or two letters can completely change the meaning of a word — and this difference could literally be a matter of life or death for the patient.

For example, the words prostate and prostrate look and sound almost the same. There is only a one-letter difference in their spelling, but there is a big difference in their meanings!

Prostate (**PROS**-tayt) means a gland surrounding the neck of the bladder and urethra in the male. **Prostrate** (**PROS**-trayt) means to collapse or be overcome with exhaustion.

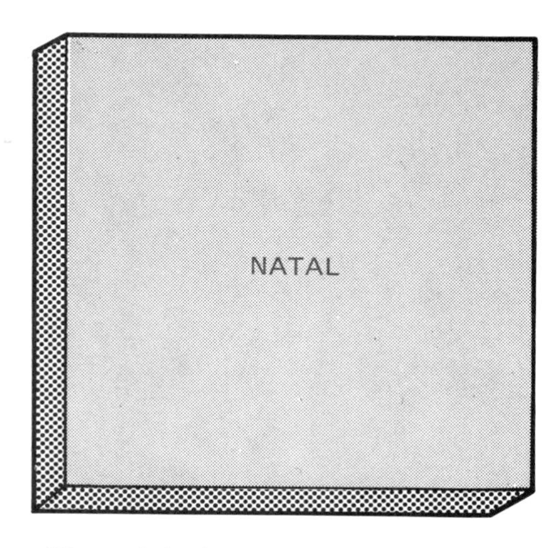

Figure 1-1 A root word stands alone.

WORD PARTS

Learning medical terminology is much easier once you understand how the word parts work together to form new words.

Medical terms are made up of a combination of three basic types of word parts or elements. These are prefixes, suffixes, and root words (or combining forms) which can be joined together to create more complex medical terms.

To help you be aware of these parts (and to learn their meanings) when a prefix, suffix, or combining form appears by itself in the text it is in *ITALICS* and in color.

For example, the combining form *MYEL/O* refers to the spinal cord or bone marrow and the suffix *-PATHY* means disease. The resulting word is **myelopathy** (my-eh-**LOP**-ah-thee) which is any pathological change or disease in the spinal cord or bone marrow.

The combining form *MY/O* refers to the muscles. This, combined with the suffix *-PATHY,* forms **myopathy** (my-**OP**-ah-thee) which is any pathological change or disease of muscle tissue.

Notice how similar these two combining forms are! It is important that you pay close attention to each letter in the word part.

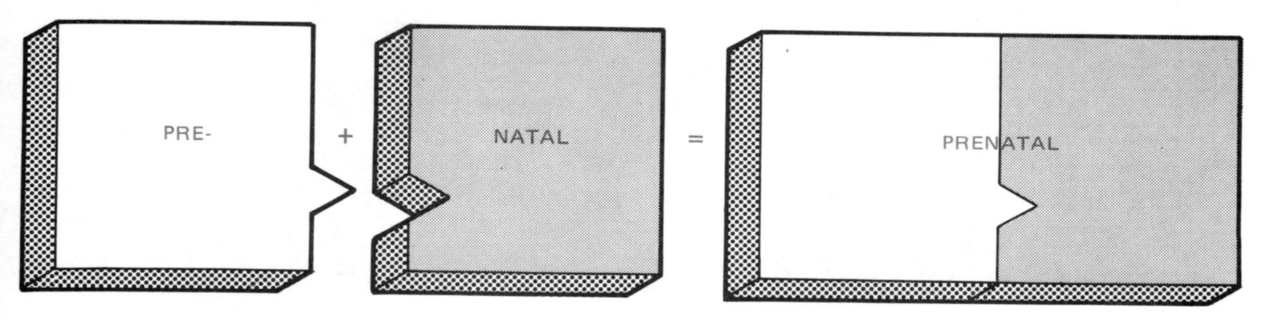

Figure 1-2 **A prefix added to a root word changes the meaning of that term.**

Prefixes

A prefix consists of one or more syllables that are added to the beginning of a root word to change the meaning of that word. Prefixes usually, but not always, indicate location or number.

The prefix *PRE-* means before or in front of. Knowing this will help you remember that prefixes are added to the beginning of the root word.

For example, the root word **natal** (**NAY**-tal) means birth. The prefix *PRE-* means before, therefore **prenatal** (pre-**NAY**-tal) means the time before birth.

The prefix *PERI-* means around. **Perinatal** (**per**-ih-**NAY**-tal) refers to the time around birth. This is the time just before and just after birth.

The prefix *POST-* means after. **Postnatal** (pohst-**NAY**-tal) means the time after birth.

Suffixes

A suffix is a syllable or syllables added to the end of a root word to change the meaning of the word. Suffixes usually, but not always, indicate the procedure, condition, disorder, or disease.

For example, the root word **tonsil** (**TON**-sil) describes a small mass of lymphoid tissue.When the mouth is wide open, it can be seen at the back of the throat.

The combining form of tonsil is *TONSILL/O*. The suffix *-ITIS* means inflammation (indicating the condition). **Tonsillitis** (**ton**-sil-**LYE**-tis) means an inflammation of the tonsils.

The suffix *-ECTOMY* means surgical removal (indicating the procedure). **Tonsillectomy** (**ton**-sih-**LECK**-toh-me) means the surgical removal of the tonsils.

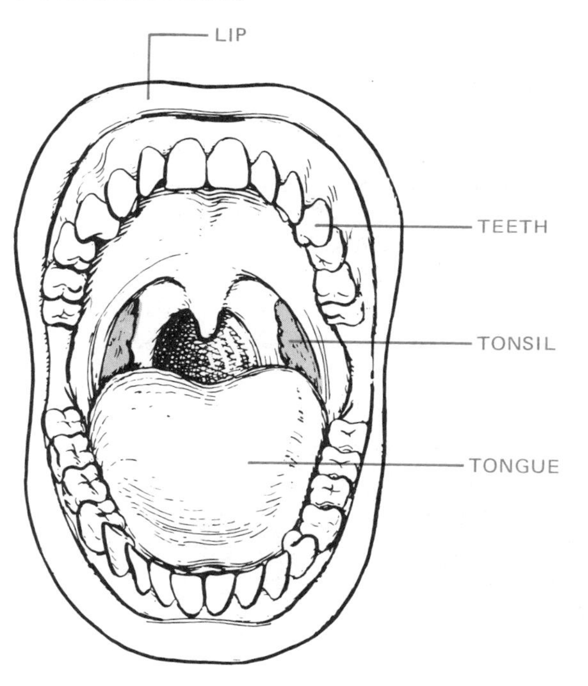

Figure 1-3 **An inflammation of the tonsils is called tonsillitis.**

FORMING TERMS FROM WORD ELEMENTS

When the word element begins with a consonant, the combining vowel is used.	When the word element begins with a vowel, the combining vowel is usually dropped.
The combining form *ERYTHR/O* means red and the root word **derma** refers to the skin. Combined they form **erythroderma** (eh-**rith**-roh-**DER**-mah), which means red skin.	The combining form *HEPAT/O* means liver and the suffix *-ITIS* means inflammation. Combined they form **hepatitis** (**hep**-ah-**TYE**-tis), which means inflammation of the liver.
When the suffix begins with a consonant, the combining form with the "o" is used.	**When the suffix begins with a vowel, the "o" of the combining form is not used.**
The combining form *ARTHR/O* means joint and the suffix *-SCOPY* means to see. Combined they form **arthroscopy** (ar-**THROS**-koh-pee) which is the visual examination of a joint using an instrument called an arthroscope.	The combining form *HYSTER/O* means uterus and the suffix *-ECTOMY* means surgical removal. Combined they form **hysterectomy** (**his**-teh-**RECK**-toh-me) which is the surgical removal of the uterus.

Root Words and Combining Forms

A root word may be used alone and it usually, but not always, describes the part of the body that is involved.

A combining form is a root word with a vowel (usually the letter "o") added to it. The combining form is used with prefixes, suffixes and even other root words to form new words.

The vowel is used with the combining form to modify the spelling so that the new word is easier to pronounce. For example look at the combining form *NEUR/O* which means nerve.

When *NEUR/O* is joined with the suffix *-ITIS,* which means inflammation, they form **neuritis** (new-**RYE**-tis). Neuritis is an inflammation of a nerve or nerves. (Notice the combining "o" was not used.)

When *NEUR/O* is joined with the suffix *-PLASTY,* which means surgical repair, they form **neuroplasty** (**NEW**-row- **plas**-tee). Neuroplasty is the surgical repair of a nerve. (Notice the combining "o" was used here.)

COMBINING ROOT WORDS

When one root word is added to another root word, the combining form of the first root word, complete with the combining "o", is used to join the parts.

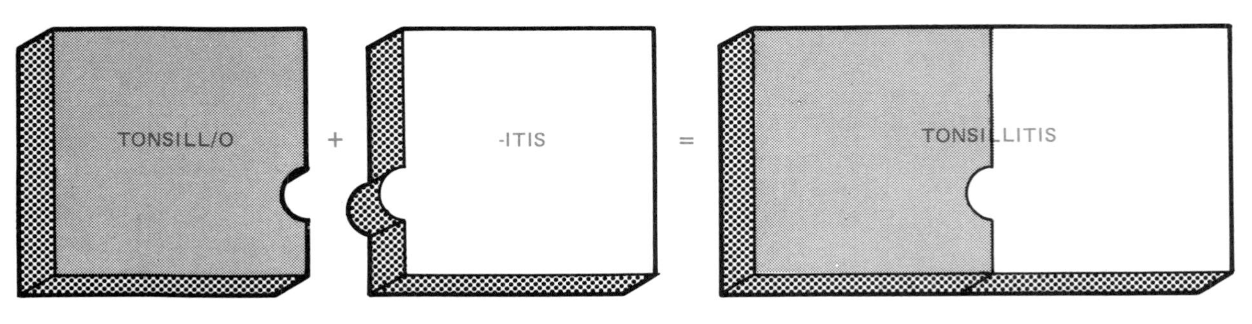

Figure 1-4 A combining form plus a suffix forms a new term.

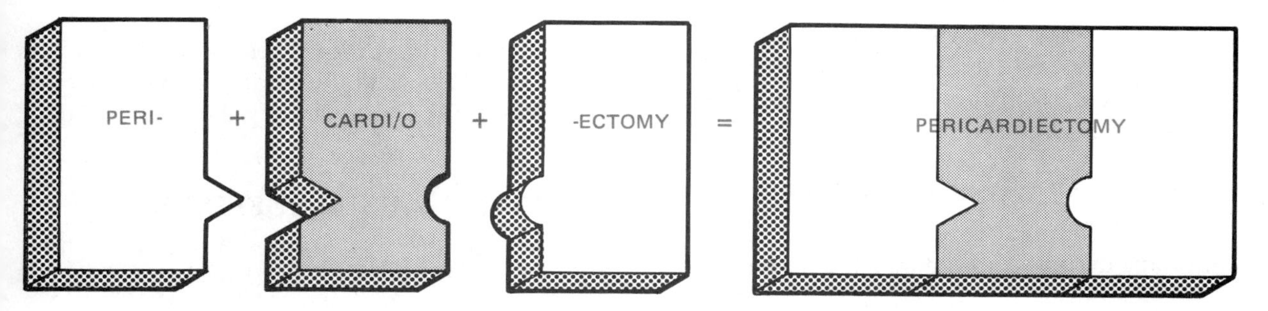

Figure 1-5 A prefix added to a combing form, plus a suffix, forms a new term.

For example, **otorhinolaryngology (oh-toh-rye-no-lar-in-GOL-oh-jee)** is a combination of several root words. The combining form *OT/O* means ear, *RHIN/O* means nose and *LARYNG/O* means larynx.

Notice that the combining "o" was used with *OT/O* and with *RHIN/O*. However, it was dropped when *LARYNG/O* was added to the suffix *-OLOGY,* which begins with a vowel.

The resulting term means the study of the ears, nose, and throat. It is such a long word, that specialists in this field commonly refer to their specialty as ENT (Ear Nose and Throat)!

SINGULAR AND PLURAL ENDINGS

Most of the medical terms for the body's organs originated from Latin words, and most of the terms describing diseases that affect these organs originated from Greek words.

As a result of these different origins, there are unusual rules for changing a singular word into a plural form. In addition to this, English endings have been adopted for some commonly used terms.

Throughout the text, when a term with an unusual singular or plural form is introduced, both the singular and plural forms are included. For example, a **phalanx (FAY-lanks)** is one bone of the fingers or toes. (Plural, **phalanges.**)

DETERMINING WORD MEANINGS

To determine the definition of a new word, you must understand the meaning of each word part. For example, look at the word pericardiectomy.

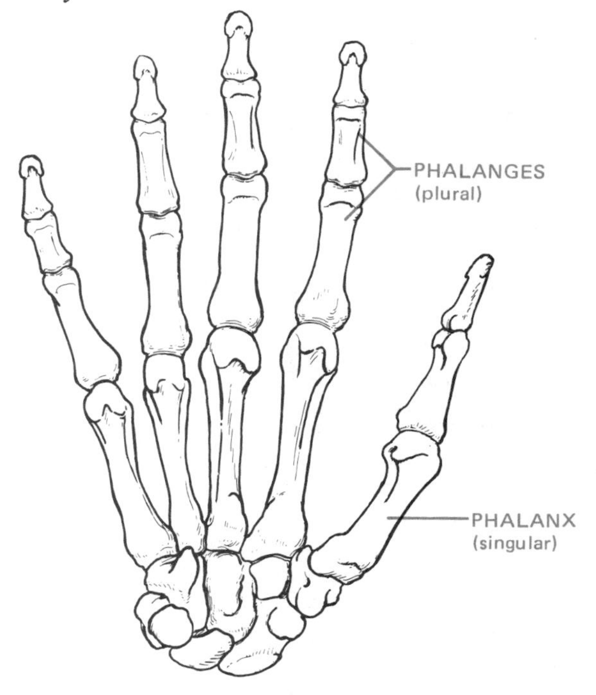

Figure 1-6 A phalanx is one finger (or toe) bone. Two or more of these bones are phalanges.

The prefix *PERI-* means around, the combining form *CARDI/O* means heart and the suffix *-ECTOMY* means surgical removal.

The resulting word is **pericardiectomy** (**per**-ih-**kar**-dee-**ECK**-toh-me) and it means the surgical removal of a portion of the pericardium. (The **pericardium** (per-ih-**KAR**-dee-um) is the sac which surrounds the heart.)

COMMONLY USED PREFIXES

The following prefixes are used to change the meaning of root words and medical terms.

- *A-* means away from, negative, and without. For example, **febrile** means pertaining to fever. **Afebrile** (ay-**FEB**-ril) means without fever. (The combining form *FEBR/I* means fever.)
- *AB-* means away from. For example, **abnormal** means away from normal.
- *AD-* means toward or in the direction of. For example, **addiction** means toward a strong dependence on a drug or substance.
- *DYS-* means difficult, painful or bad. For example, **dysmenorrhea** (**dis**-men-oh-**REE**-ah) means painful menstruation. (**Menorrhea** (**men**-oh-**REE**-ah) refers to the menstrual flow.)
- *HYPER-* means over, above or increased. For example, **hypertension** (**high**-per-**TEN**-shun) is higher than normal blood pressure.
- *HYPO-* means below, under or decreased. For example, **hypotension** (**high**-poh-**TEN**-shun) is lower than normal blood pressure.
- *INTER-* means between or among. For example, **interstitial** (**in**-ter-**STISH**-al) means between, but not within, the parts of a tissue.
- *INTRA-* means within or inside. For example, **intramuscular** (**in**-trah-**MUS**-kyou-lar) means within the muscle.
- *SUB-* means under, less or below. For example, the root word **costal** means pertaining to the ribs. **Subcostal** (sub-**KOS**-tal) means below a rib or ribs.
- *SUPER-* and *SUPRA-* both mean above, excessive or beyond. For example, **supracostal** (**sue**-prah-**KOS**-tal) means above or outside the ribs.

COMMONLY USED SUFFIXES

It is particularly important that you learn the meanings of the following suffixes because they are used in many medical terms.

- *-ALGIA* means pain and suffering. The combining form *NEUR/O* means nerve. **Neuralgia** (new-**RAL**-jee-ah) means nerve pain.
- *-CENTESIS* means surgical puncture to remove fluid. The combining form *AMNI/O* means the fluid surrounding the fetus (unborn child) in the uterus. **Amniocentesis** (**am**-nee-oh-sen-**TEE**-sis) is the removal of amniotic fluid for diagnostic purposes.
- *-ECTOMY* means surgical removal. The combining forms *APPEND/O* and *APPENDIC/O* mean appendix. **Appendectomy** (**ap**-en-**DECK**-toh-me) is the surgical removal of the appendix.
- *-EMIA* means blood or blood condition. The prefix *AN-* means without or less then. **Anemia** (ah-**NEE**-me-ah) means less than the normal number of red blood cells.
- *-GRAPHY* is the process of recording a picture or record. The combining form *ANGI/O* means blood or lymph vessels. **Angiography** (**an**-jee-**OG**-rah-fee) is the process of producing an angiogram which is a special x-ray of the blood vessels.
- *-ITIS* means inflammation. The combining form *OT/O* means ear and **media** means middle. **Otitis media** (oh-**TYE**-tis **ME**-dee-ah) is an inflammation of the middle ear.

- *-MALACIA* means abnormal softening. The combining form *OSTE/O* means bone. **Osteomalacia (oss**-tee-oh-mah-**LAY**-she-ah) is the abnormal softening of the bones.

- *-OLOGY* means the study of. The combining form *PATH/O* means disease. **Pathology** is the study of the changes to the body caused by disease.

- *-OMA* means tumor or neoplasm. The combining form *LYMPH/O* means lymphatic tissue. A **lymphoma** (lim-**FOH**-mah) is a tumor made up of lymphatic tissue.

- *-OSIS* means an abnormal condition. The combining form *PSYCH/O* means mind. A **psychosis** (sigh-**KOH**-sis) is a disorder or abnormal condition of the mind.

- *-OSTOMY* means to surgically create a mouth or opening. The combining form *COL/O* means colon. A **colostomy** (koh-**LAHS**-toh-me) is surgically creating an opening between the colon and the body surface.

- *-OTOMY* means cutting or a surgical incision. The combining form *GASTR/O* means stomach. A **gastrotomy** (gas-**TROT**-oh-me) is a surgical incision into the stomach.

- *-PATHY* means disease or suffering. The combining form *OSTE/O* means bone. **Osteopathy (oss**-tee-**OP**-ah-thee) is a disease that involves bone.

- *-PLASTY* means surgical repair. The combining form *MY/O* means muscle. **Myoplasty (my**-oh-**PLAS**-tee) is the surgical repair of a muscle.

- *-RRHAGE* means bursting forth. The combing form *HEM/O* means relating to blood. **Hemorrhage (HEM**-or-idj) is the escape or bursting forth of blood from the vessels. (This suffix is sometimes spelled *-RHAGE.)*

- *-RRHAPHY* means to suture or stitch. The combining form *NEUR/O* means nerve. **Neurorrhaphy** (new-**ROAR**-ah-fee) means to suture or stitch a divided nerve. (This suffix is sometimes spelled *-RHAPHY.)*

- *-RRHEA* means flow or discharge. The prefix *DIA-* means through. **Diarrhea (dye**-ah-**REE**-ah) means the frequent flow of watery stools. (This suffix is sometimes spelled *-RHEA.)*

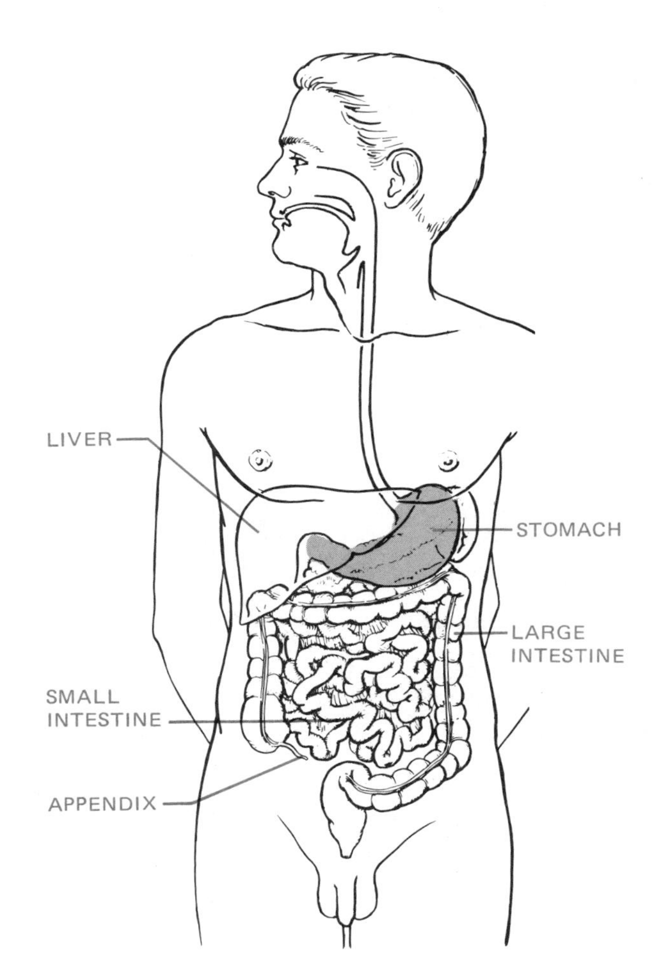

Figure 1-7 The major organs of the digestive system.

MAJOR BODY SYSTEMS

BODY SYSTEM	COMPONENTS	MAJOR FUNCTIONS
Skeletal System	206 bones	Support and shape Protective, Hematopoietic
Muscular System	Striated muscle Smooth muscle Cardiac muscle	Locomotion Holding body erect Movement of body fluids
Cardiovascular System	Heart Blood vessels Blood	Respiratory Nutritive Excretory
Lymphatic and Immune Systems	White blood cells Lymph fluid Lymph vessels and nodes Spleen	Defense against disease Conserve plasma proteins and fluid Lipid absorption Hemolytic action
Digestive System	Mouth, pharynx, esophagus, stomach, intestines and accessory organs	Digestion of ingested food Absorption of digested food Elimination of solid wastes
Urinary System	Kidneys, ureters, bladder and urethra	Elimination of urine Maintenance of homeostasis
Respiratory System	Nose, paranasal sinuses, pharynx, epiglottis, larynx, trachea, bronchi and lungs	Oxygen to the cells Excretion of carbon dioxide Excretion of some water wastes
Nervous System	Central nervous system Peripheral nervous system Special sense organs	Coordinating mechanism Reception of stimuli Transmission of messages
Integumentary System	Skin, hair, nails, sweat and sebaceous glands	Protection of body Temperature and water regulation
Endocrine System	Adrenals (2), gonads (2), pancreas (1), parathyroids (4), pineal (1), pituitary (1), thymus (1) and thyroid (1)	Integrating body functions Homeostatic Growth
Reproductive System	*Male:* testes, ducts, penis *Female:* ovaries, fallopian tubes, uterus, vagina, external genitalia	Production of new life

- *-RRHEXIS* means rupture. The combining form *CARDI/O* means heart. **Cardiorrhexis** (**kar**-dee-oh-**RECK**-sis) means the rupture of the heart. (This suffix is sometimes spelled *-RHEXIS.)*
- *-SCLEROSIS* means abnormal hardening. The prefix *ARTERI/O* means artery. **Arteriosclerosis** (ar-**tee**-ree-oh-skleh-**ROH**-sis) is a group of disorders characterized by abnormal hardening of the arteries.
- *-SCOPY* means to see or a visual examination. The prefix *ENDO-* means within. **Endoscopy** (en-**DOS**-koh-pee) is to examine internally by means of an endoscope.
- *-SPASM* means a sudden involuntary contraction. The combining form *LARYNG/O* means larynx or vocal cords. A **laryngospasm** (lah-**RING**-goh-spazm) is a sudden spasmodic closure of the larynx.
- *-STASIS* means stopping or controlling. The combining form *HEM/O* means blood. **Hemostasis** (**he**-moh-**STAY**-sis) means to control bleeding.

USING THIS BOOK

Body Systems

The tissues and organs of the body are organized into systems that perform specialized functions. These systems are outlined in the table "Major Body Systems" on page 8.

To make your study of medical terminology easier, this text is also organized according to body systems. There is one chapter per system and each chapter stands alone so that you may study them in the sequence (order).

There are also audio tapes available for use with each chapter to help you learn to pronounce the words correctly.

Appendix A

Appendix A contains an extensive list of prefixes, suffixes and combining forms and their definitions. You can use this resource to look up a word part that is unfamiliar.

Appendix B

Appendix B contains an extensive list of abbreviations. Because many medical terms are long and complex, abbreviations are often used as a form of shorthand. For example, it is much easier to say or write "AIDS" instead of spelling out **"Acquired Immune Deficiency Syndrome."**

However, when you look at the abbreviations listed in Appendix B you will notice that many abbreviations have more than one meaning.

Because abbreviations are not used in the same way by everyone, this can lead to confusion or errors. Therefore, it is important that you be very careful when using or translating an abbreviation.

Flash Cards

One of the secrets to mastering medical terminology is to learn the word parts — and this takes practice! To help you with this we've included flash cards at the end of this book. To use them just remove these pages (very carefully) and cut the cards apart.

These cards are a great way to practice and review until you've learned the separate parts. Also, by combining cards you can create more complex medical terms. When you do this, always check in the text or a medical dictionary for the correct spelling and full definition.

IMPORTANT TERMS: INTRODUCTION TO MEDICAL TERMINOLOGY

This list will help you identify and review the major terms from this chapter.

When you work with the audio tape for this chapter, listen to the word, repeat it and then place a ✓ next to it on the list below.

- □ **Afebrile** (ay-**FEB**-ril)
- □ **Amniocentesis** (**am**-nee-oh-sen-**TEE**-sis)
- □ **Anemia** (ah-**NEE**-me-ah)
- □ **Angiography** (**an**-jee-**OG**-rah-fee)
- □ **Appendectomy** (**ap**-en-**DECK**-toh-me)
- □ **Appendicitis** (ah-**pen**-dih-**SIGH**-tis)
- □ **Arteriosclerosis** (ar-**tee**-ree-oh-skleh-**ROH**-sis)
- □ **Arthroscopy** (ar-**THROS**-koh-pee)
- □ **Cardiorrhexis** (**kar**-dee-oh-**RECK**-sis)
- □ **Colostomy** (koh-**LAHS**-toh-me)
- □ **Diarrhea** (**dye**-ah-**REE**-ah)
- □ **Dysmenorrhea** (**dis**-men-oh-**REE**-ah)
- □ **Edema** (eh-**DEE**-mah)
- □ **Endoscopy** (en-**DOS**-koh-pee)
- □ **Erythroderma** (eh-**rith**-roh- **DER**-mah)
- □ **Gastrotomy** (gas-**TROT**-oh-me)
- □ **Hemorrhage** (**HEM**-or-idj)
- □ **Hemostasis** (**he**-moh-**STAY**-sis)
- □ **Hepatitis** (**hep**-ah-**TYE**-tis)
- □ **Hysterectomy** (**his**-teh- **RECK**-toh-me)
- □ **Interstitial** (**in**-ter-**STISH**-al)
- □ **Intramuscular** (**in**-trah-**MUS**-kyou-lar)
- □ **Laryngospasm** (lah-**RING**-goh-spazm)
- □ **Lymphoma** (lim-**FOH**-mah)
- □ **Myelopathy** (my-eh-**LOP**-ah-thee)
- □ **Myopathy** (my-**OP**-ah-thee)
- □ **Myoplasty** (**my**-oh-**PLAS**-tee)
- □ **Neuralgia** (new-**RAL**-jee-ah)
- □ **Neuritis** (new-**RYE**-tis)
- □ **Neuroplasty** (**NEW**-row-**plas**-tee)
- □ **Neurorrhaphy** (new-**ROAR**-ah-fee)
- □ **Osteomalacia** (**oss**-tee-oh-mah-**LAY**-she-ah)
- □ **Osteopathy** (**oss**-tee-**OP**-ah-thee)
- □ **Otitis media** (oh-**TYE**-tis **ME**-dee-ah)
- □ **Otorhinolaryngology** (**oh**-toh-**rye**-no-**lar**-in-**GOL**-oh-jee)
- □ **Pericardium** (per-ih-**KAR**-dee-um)
- □ **Pericardiectomy** (**per**-ih-**kar**-dee-**ECK**-toh-me)
- □ **Perinatal** (**per**-ih-**NAY**-tal)
- □ **Phalanx** (**FAY**-lanks)
- □ **Postnatal** (pohst-**NAY**-tal)
- □ **Prostate** (**PROS**-tayt)
- □ **Prostrate** (**PROS**-trayt)
- □ **Psychosis** (sigh-**KOH**-sis)
- □ **Subcostal** (sub-**KOS**-tal)
- □ **Supracostal** (**sue**-prah-**KOS**-tal)
- □ **Tonsillectomy** (**ton**-sih-**LECK**-toh-me)
- □ **Tonsillitis** (**ton**-sil-**LYE**-tis)

EXERCISES

DEFINING WORD PARTS

Write the definition for each of these word parts.
(As necessary, use Appendix A to find these definitions.)

1. *A-* ____________________
2. *AB-* ____________________
3. *AD-* ____________________
4. *-ALGIA* ____________________
5. *APPEND/O, APPENDIC/O* ____________________
6. *ARTERI/O* ____________________
7. *ARTHR/O* ____________________
8. *CARCIN/O* ____________________
9. *CARDI/O* ____________________
10. *-CENTESIS* ____________________
11. *COL/O* ____________________
12. *DYS-* ____________________
13. *-ECTOMY* ____________________
14. *-EMIA* ____________________
15. *ENDO-* ____________________

16. *ERYTHR/O* ______________________

17. *-ESTHESIA* ______________________

18. *GASTR/O* ______________________

19. *-GRAPHY* ______________________

20. *HEM/O* ______________________

21. *HEPAT/O* ______________________

22. *HYSTER/O* ______________________

23. *-ITIS* ______________________

24. *LARYNG/O* ______________________

25. *LYMPH/O* ______________________

26. *-MALACIA* ______________________

27. *MYEL/O* ______________________

28. *MY/O* ______________________

29. *NEPHR/O* ______________________

30. *NEUR/O* ______________________

31. *-OLOGY* ______________________

32. *-OMA* ______________________

33. *-OSIS* ______________________

34. *OSTE/O* ______________________

35. *-OSTOMY* ______________________

36. *OT/O* ______________________

37. *-OTOMY* ______________________

38. *-PATHY* ______________________

39. *PERI-* ______________________

40. *-PLASTY* ______________________

41. *PSYCH/O* ______________________

42. *-RRHAGE* ______________________

43. *-RRHAPHY* ______________________

44. *-RRHEA* ______________________

45. *-RRHEXIS* ____________________

46. *-SCLEROSIS* ____________________

47. *-SCOPY* ____________________

48. *-SPASM* ____________________

49. *-STASIS* ____________________

50. *TONSILL/O* ____________________

SPELLCHECK

Select the correct spelling and write it on the line.

1. ____________________ means to suture or stitch a divided nerve.
   Neurorrhaphy
   Neurraphy
   Neworrhapy

2. In the male, the ____________________ gland surrounds the bladder and urethra.
   postate
   prostate
   prostrate

3. The removal of amnionic fluid for diagnostic purposes is called
   ____
   amniocentesis.
   amniocentosis.
   amnionicentesis.

4. ____________________ is a group of disorders characterized by abnormal hardening of the arteries.
   Angiosclerosis
   Arteriosclerosis
   Atheriosclerosis

5. ____________________ means the rupture of the heart.
   Cardiorrhage
   Cardiorrhea
   Cardiorrhexis

6. A ____________________ is the surgical removal of the tonsils.
   tonsilectomy
   tonsillectomy
   tonsilloectomy

7. ________________________ means the sudden bursting forth of blood.
Hemaorrhage
Hemeorrhage
Hemorrhage

8. An ________________________ is the surgical removal of the appendix.
appendectomy
appendixectomy
appendoectomy

9. ________________________ means to control bleeding.
Hemastasis
Hemeostasis
Hemostasis

10. ________________________ means within the muscle.
Intermuscular
Intramuscular
Intromuscular

WORD BUILDING

Write the correct word or word part on the line. (These terms are defined in this chapter.)

1. Inflammation of the liver
   a) The combining form ________________________ means liver.
   b) The suffix ________________________ means inflammation.
   c) The term ________________________ means inflammation of the liver.
2. Visual examination of an internal structure of the body
   a) The combining form ________________________ means within.
   b) The suffix ________________________ means visual examination.
   c) The term ________________________ means visual examination of an internal structure of the body.
3. Less than the normal number of red blood cells
   a) The prefix ________________________ means without or less then.
   b) The suffix ________________________ means blood or blood condition.
   c) The term ________________________ means less than the normal number of red blood cells.
4. Surgically creating an opening between the colon and the body surface
   a) The combining form ________________________ means colon.
   b) The suffix ________________________ means to surgically create an opening.
   c) The term ________________________ means surgically creating an opening between the colon and the body surface.

5. Recording an x-ray study of blood or lymph vessels
   a) The combining form ______________________ means blood or lymph vessels.
   b) The suffix ______________________ means the process of recording a record.
   c) The term ______________________ means the process of recording a special x-ray study of blood or lymph vessels.

6. The study of disease
   a) The combining form ______________________ means disease.
   b) The suffix ______________________ means study of.
   c) The term ______________________ means the study of the changes to the body caused by disease.

7. Surgical repair of a muscle
   a) The combining form ______________________ means muscle.
   b) The suffix ______________________ means surgical repair.
   c) The term ______________________ means the surgical repair of a muscle.

8. Abnormal condition of the mind
   a) The combining form ______________________ means mind.
   b) The suffix ______________________ means abnormal condition.
   c) The term ______________________ means an abnormal condition of the mind.

9. Inflammation of the appendix
   a) The combining form ______________________ means appendix.
   b) The suffix ______________________ means inflammation.
   c) The term ______________________ means inflammation of the appendix.

10. Nerve pain
    a) The combining form ______________________ means nerve.
    b) The suffix ______________________ means pain.
    c) The term ______________________ means nerve pain.

11. To control bleeding
    a) The combining form ______________________ means blood.
    b) The suffix ______________________ means to stop or control.
    c) The term ______________________ means to control bleeding.

12. Surgical removal of the uterus
    a) The combining form ______________________ means uterus.
    b) The suffix ______________________ means surgical removal.
    c) The term ______________________ means surgical removal of the uterus.

13. Inflammation of the middle ear
    a) The combining form ______________________ means ear.
    b) The suffix ______________________ means inflammation.
    c) The word ______________________ means middle.
    d) The term ______________________ means inflammation of the middle ear.

14. Before birth
    a) The prefix ______________________ means before.
    b) The root word ______________________ means birth.
    c) The term ______________________ means before birth.

15. Frequent flow of watery stool
    a) The prefix ______________________ means through.
    b) The suffix ______________________ means frequent flow.
    c) The term means frequent flow of watery stool.

CASE STUDIES

1. Andrew Weller suffers from a severe disorder of the mind. The diagnosis is that he suffers from a ______________________.

2. Beverly Gaston suffers from ______________________ which is higher than normal blood pressure.

3. After his fever went down, and his temperature was back to normal, Carlos LaPinta was described as being ______________________.

4. During her pregnancy Mrs. Tillson had ______________________ (the removal of anmionic fluid) performed for diagnostic purposes.

5. Elderly Mr. Gusterson suffers from ______________________ which is characterized by abnormal hardening of the arteries.

CHALLENGE WORD BUILDING

Write the correct word or word part on the line. (These terms are not defined in this chapter; however, all of their word parts were introduced. Also, these terms are defined elsewhere in the text so you can look them up to verify your answers.)

1. Visual examination of the larynx
    a) The combining form ______________________ means larynx.
    b) The suffix ______________________ means visual examination.
    c) The term ______________________ means visual examination of the larynx.

2. Surgical repair of the nose
   a) The combining form ______________________ means nose.
   b) The suffix ______________________ means surgical repair.
   c) The term ______________________ means surgical repair of the nose.

3. The removal of fluid from a joint
   a) The combining form ______________________ means joint.
   b) The suffix ______________________ means surgical puncture to remove fluid.
   c) The term ______________________ means the surgical puncture of a joint to remove fluid.

4. Abnormal softening of muscle
   a) The combining form ______________________ means muscle.
   b) The suffix ______________________ means abnormal softening.
   c) The term ______________________ means abnormal softening of muscle.

5. Surgical repair of blood or lymph vessels
   a) The combining form ______________________ means blood or lymph vessels.
   b) The suffix ______________________ means surgical repair.
   c) The term ______________________ means the surgical repair of blood or lymph vessels.

6. Inflammation of the stomach
   a) The combining form ______________________ means stomach.
   b) The suffix ______________________ means inflammation.
   c) The term ______________________ means inflammation of the stomach.

7. Visual examination of the stomach
   a) The combining form ______________________ means stomach.
   b) The suffix ______________________ means visual examination.
   c) The term ______________________ means visual examination of the stomach.

8. Inflammation of the colon
   a) The combining form ______________________ means colon.
   b) The suffix ______________________ means inflammation.
   c) The term ______________________ means inflammation of the colon.

9. Muscle pain
   a) The combining form ______________________ means muscle.
   b) The suffix ______________________ means pain and suffering.
   c) The term ______________________ means the pain or tenderness of muscle.

10. The surgical repair of bones
    a) The combining form ______________________________ means bone.
    b) The suffix ______________________________ means surgical repair.
    c) The term ______________________________ means surgical repair of the bones.

LABELING EXERCISES

Identify the numbered items on this diagram.

1. ______________________________
2. ______________________________
3. ______________________________
4. ______________________________
5. ______________________________

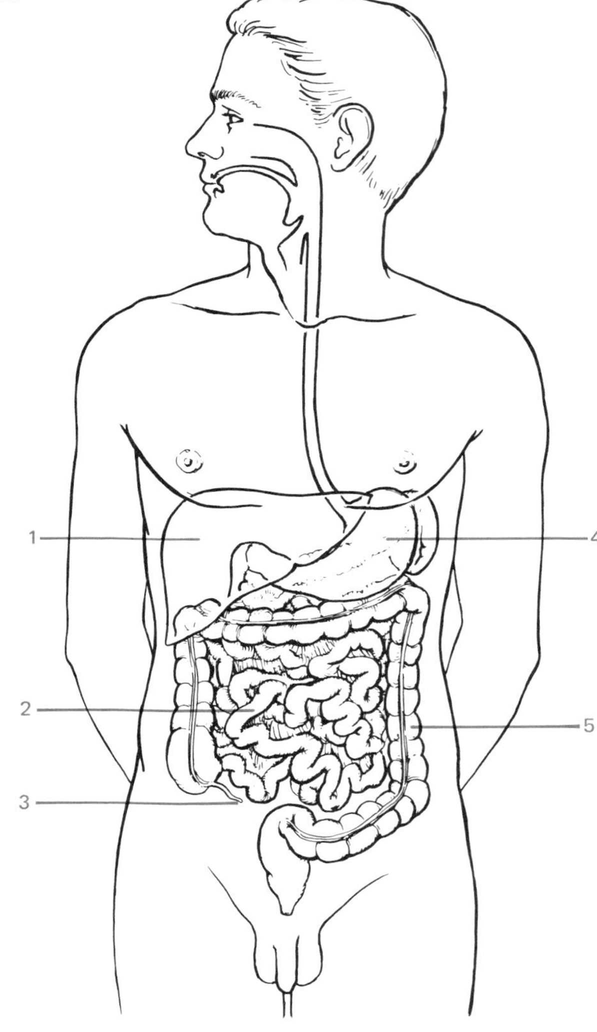

2

THE STRUCTURE OF THE HUMAN BODY

LEARNING GOALS

In this chapter you will learn to:

- differentiate between the terms anatomy and physiology.
- define the terms used in the major anatomical reference systems to describe directions, body planes and cavities.
- identify the terms used to describe the structure of cells and tissues.
- recognize and define the terms related to pathology of tissue formation.
- recognize and define the terms related to oncology.
- describe the major medical specialties.

ANATOMICAL REFERENCE SYSTEMS

Anatomy (ah-**NAT**-oh-me) is the study of the structure of the body. **Physiology** (**fiz-ee-OL**-oh-jee) is the study of the processes and functions of the human body.

Anatomical reference systems are used in order to make it easier to describe the body parts and their functions. The basic reference systems are: body planes, body directions, body cavities and structural units.

BODY PLANES

Planes are imaginary lines used to divide the body into sections. The use of these planes makes it easier to describe the location of an organ or problem.

The Midline

The midline, also known as the midsagittal plane (mid-**SADJ**-ih-tal), is a vertical plane that divides the body, from top to bottom, into left and right halves. (A **vertical plane** is an up and down line at a right angle to the horizon.)

A sagittal plane (**SADJ**-ih-tal) is any vertical plane parallel to the midsagittal line that divides the body into left and right portions.

The Coronal Plane

The coronal plane (koh-**ROH**-nal), also known as the **frontal plane,** is any vertical plane, at right angles to the sagittal plane, that divides the body into anterior (front) and posterior (back) portions.

The Transverse Plane

The transverse plane (trans-**VERSE**), also known as the **horizontal plane** divides the body into superior (upper) and inferior (lower) portions. (The prefix *TRANS-* means across.)

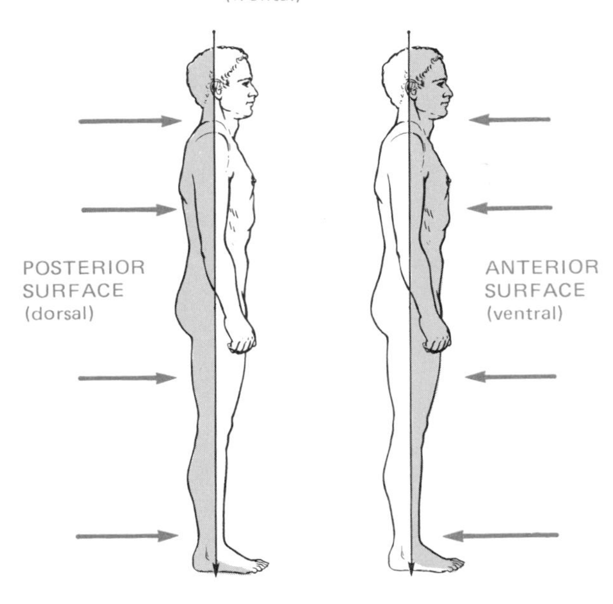

Figure 2-1 Anterior versus posterior.

BODY DIRECTIONS

The following terms are used to describe directions in relation to the whole body.

Ventral and Dorsal

Ventral (**VEN**-tral) refers to the front or belly side of the body. (The combining form *VENTR/O* means front or belly side.)

Dorsal (**DOOR**-sal) refers to the back of the body. (The combining form *DORS/O* means back of the body.)

Anterior and Posterior

Anterior (an-**TEER**-ee-or) means situated in the front, or on the forward part of an organ. The term is also used in reference to the ventral surface of the body. (The combing form *ANTER/O* means front.)

Posterior (pos-**TEER**-ee-or) means situated in the back, or on the back part of an organ. This term is also used in reference to the dorsal surface of the body. (The combining form *POSTER/O* means back.)

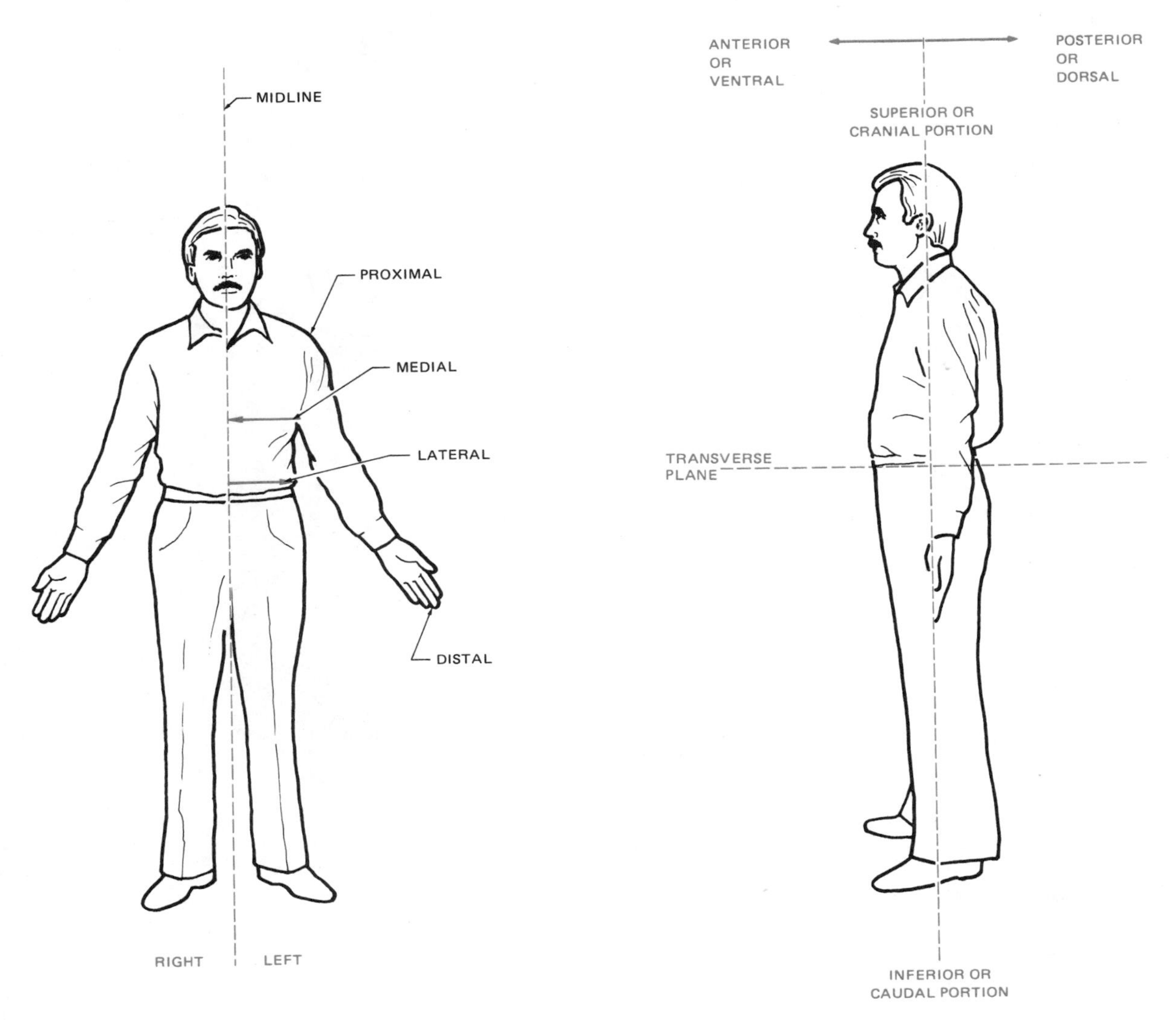

Figure 2-2 Anterior and lateral views with directional references.

Superior and Inferior

Superior means uppermost, above or toward the head. For example, the lungs are located superior to (above) the diaphragm. (The combining form *SUPER/O* means above or higher than.)

This direction is also known as **cephalic** (seh-**FAL**-ick), which means toward the head. (The combining form *CEPHAL/O* means head.)

Inferior means lowermost, below or toward the feet. For example, the stomach is located inferior to (below) the diaphragm. (The combining form *INFER/O* means beneath or below.)

This direction is also known as **caudal** (**KAW**-dal), which means toward the tail or lower part of the body. (The combining form *CAUD/O* means tail.)

Proximal and Distal

Proximal (**PROCK**-sih-mal) means near the midline or the beginning of a body structure. For example, the proximal end of the humerus (the bone of the upper arm) forms part of the shoulder. (The combining form *PROXIM/O* means near.)

Distal (**DIS**-tal) means away from the midline or the beginning of a body structure. For example, the distal end of the humerus (the bone of the upper arm) forms part of the elbow. (The combining form *DIST/O* means far.)

Lateral and Medial

Lateral means toward the side or away from the midline of the body or structure. **Bilateral** means having two sides or pertaining to both sides. (The prefix *BI-* means two.) **Ambilateral** means pertaining to both sides. (The prefix *AMBI-* means both or both sides.)

Medial means pertaining to the middle or toward the midline. (The combining form *MEDI/O* means middle.)

Afferent and Efferent

Afferent (**AF**-er-ent) means conducting toward a center or a particular structure. (The prefix *AF-* means toward.) For example, afferent nerves carry impulses toward the brain.

Efferent (**EF**-er-ent) means conducting away from a center or a particular structure. (The prefix *EF-* means away from.) For example, efferent nerves carry impulses away from the brain.

THE MAJOR BODY CAVITIES

A body cavity is a space within the body that contains internal organs.

Dorsal Cavity

The dorsal cavity contains the structures of the nervous system that coordinate the bodily functions.

The dorsal cavity is divided into the **cranial cavity,** which contains the brain, and the **spinal cavity,** which contains the spinal cord.

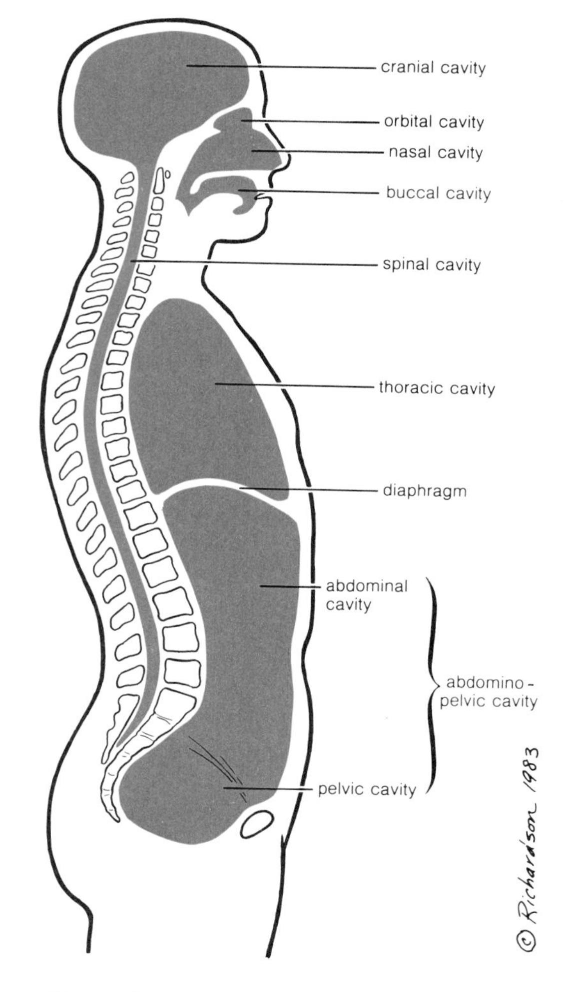

Figure 2-3 Major body cavities.

Ventral Cavity

The ventral cavity contains the body organs that maintain homeostasis. (**Homeostasis** (**hoh**-me-oh-**STAY**-sis) means maintaining a constant internal environment.) The ventral cavity is divided into three parts

The **thoracic cavity** (thoh-**RAS**-ick) contains the heart and the lungs. (The combining form *THORAC/O* means chest.)

The **diaphragm** separates the thoracic cavity and abdominal cavities.

The **abdominal cavity** (ab-**DOM**-ih-nal), also known as the abdomen (ab-**DOH**-men) or the belly, contains primarily the major organs of digestion. (The combining form *ABDOMIN/O* means abdominal.)

The **pelvic cavity** (**PEL**-vick) is the space formed by the pelvic bones. It contains primarily the organs of the reproductive and excretory systems. (The combining form *PELV/O* means pelvic cavity.)

The abdominal and pelvic cavities may be referred to together as the **abdominopelvic cavity** (ab-**dom**-ih-no-**PEL**-vick).

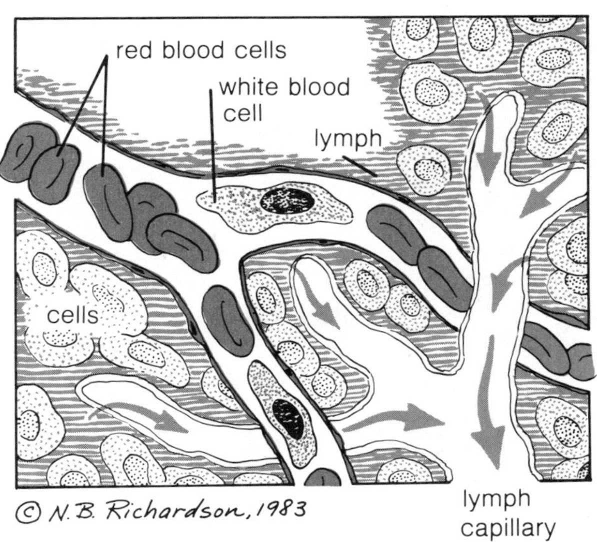

Figure 2-5 Red and white blood cells in capillary circulation.

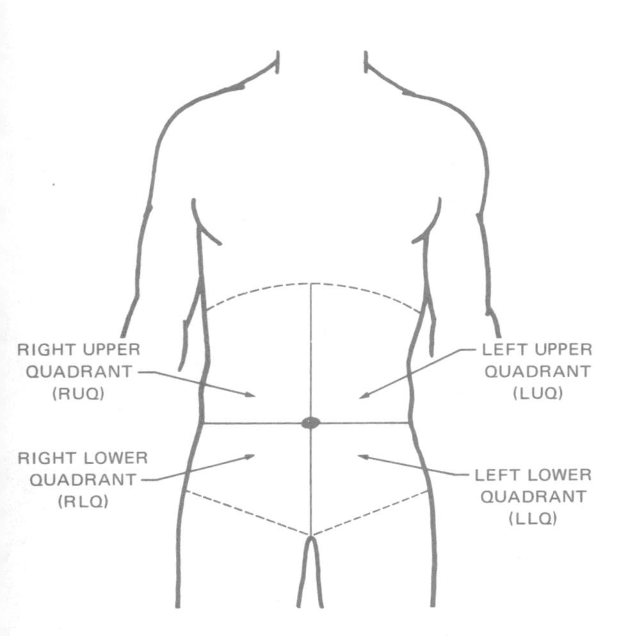

Figure 2-4 Abdominal quadrants.

Abdominal Quadrants

Several systems are used to make it easier to describe where an organ (or a pain) is located in the abdomen. The method used most frequently is to divide the abdomen into imaginary quadrants as shown in figure 2-4.

CELLS

Cells are the basic structural units of the body. They are specialized and grouped together to form the tissues and organs of the body. **Cytology** (sigh-**TOL**-oh-jee) is the study of cells, their origin, structure, function and pathology. (The combining form *CYT/O* means cell.)

Protoplasm

Protoplasm (**PROH**-toh-plazm) is all the material that makes up the cell. This includes the cytoplasm, the nucleoplasm and the cell membrane. (The combining form *PROT/O* means first and the suffix *-PLASM* means formative substance.)

The **cell membrane** is the structure surrounding and protecting the cell. (A **membrane** (**MEM**-brain) is a thin layer of tissue that covers a surface, lines a cavity or divides a space or organ.)

Cytoplasm (**SIGH**-toh-plazm) is the protoplasm that is within the cell membrane, but outside of the nucleus.

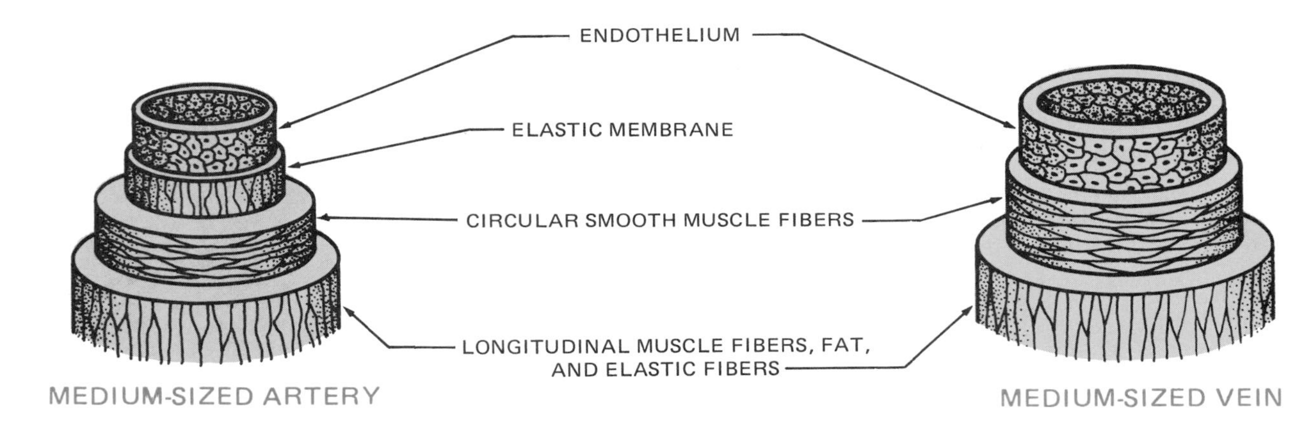

Figure 2-6 Different types of tissues arranged to form veins and arteries.

The Nucleus

The **nucleus** (NEW-klee-us) is a structure within the cell which contains nucleoplasm and chromosomes. (The combining form *NUCLE/O* means nucleus.) (Plural, **nuclei.**)

Chromosomes (**KROH**-moh-sohmes), also known as **genes,** contain genetic material and information. **DNA** (deoxyribonucleic acid) is the chemical within the chromosomes which determines hereditary characteristics.

Nucleoplasm (**NEW**-klee-oh-**plazm**) is the protoplasm within the nucleus of the cell.

Karyoplasm (**CARE**-ee-oh-plazm) is another term meaning nucleoplasm. (The combining form *KARY/O* also means nucleus.)

TISSUES

A tissue is a group or layer of similarly specialized cells which join together to perform certain specific functions.

Histology (his-**TOL**-oh-jee) is the study of the structure, composition and function of tissues. (The combining form *HIST/O* means tissue.)

Epithelial Tissue

Epithelial tissue (**ep**-ih-**THEE**-lee-al) covers both the internal and external surfaces of the body. It is divided into two types.

Epithelium (**ep**-ih-**THEE**-lee-um) is the specialized form of epithelial tissue that covers the external surfaces of the body as the outer layer of the skin. (The prefix *EPI-* means upon or above.)

Endothelium (**en**-doh-**THEE**-lee-um) is the specialized form of epithelial tissue that forms the lining of all of the internal organs including the blood vessels. (The combining form *ENDO-* means within or inside.)

Connective Tissue

Connective tissue holds the organs in place and binds all parts of the body together.

Bones and cartilage are one kind of connective tissue. (See Chapter 3.)

Adipose tissue (**AD**-ih-pohs), also known as fat, is another form of connective tissue. (The combining form *ADIP/O* means fat.)

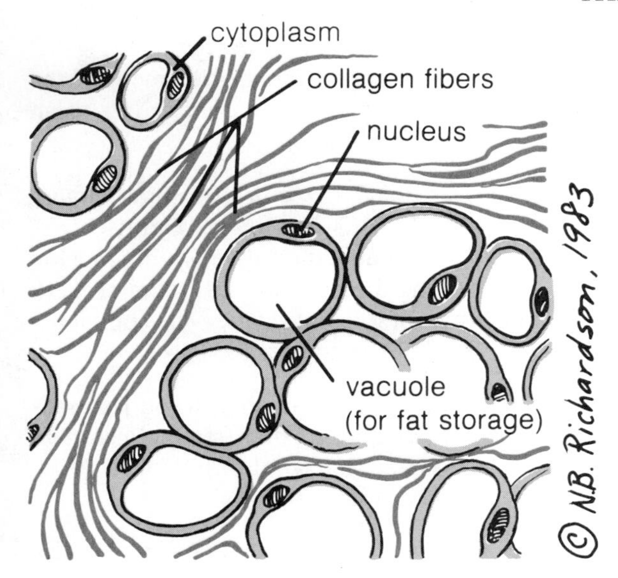

Figure 2-7 Adipose connective tissue.

Pathology of Tissue Formation

The suffix *-PLASIA* means formation, development and growth of tissue and cells. Combined with different prefixes it is used to describe problems of tissue formation.

- **Aplasia** (ah-**PLAY**-zee-ah) means the lack of development of an organ or tissue. (The prefix *A-* means without.)
- **Hypoplasia (high**-poh-**PLAY**-zee-ah) is the incomplete development of an organ or tissue, but it is less severe in degree than aplasia. (The prefix *HYPO-* means decreased or deficient.)
- **Hyperplasia (high**-per-**PLAY**-zee-ah) is an abnormal increase in the number of normal cells in normal arrangement in a tissue. (The prefix *HYPER-* means increased or excessive.)
- **Anaplasia (an**-ah-**PLAY**-zee-ah) is a change in the structure of cells and in their orientation to each other. These are abnormal cells and anaplasia is characteristic of malignancy. (The prefix *ANA-* means without.)

ONCOLOGY

Oncology (ong-**KOL**-oh-jee) is the study of cancerous tumors. **Cancer** is a neoplasm characterized by the uncontrolled growth of abnormal cells that tend to invade surrounding tissue and to metastasize to distant body sites.

A **neoplasm,** also known as a **tumor,** is any abnormal growth of new tissue, benign or malignant. (The combining form *NE/O* means new or strange.)

A **benign neoplasm** is not malignant, is not recurring and has a favorable chance for recovery.

A **malignant neoplasm** tends to get progressively worse, spreads and is life-threatening.

Metastasis (meh-**TAS**-tah-sis) is the process by which tumor cells are spread to distant parts of the body. (The prefix *META-* means both beyond and change.) (Plural, **metastases.**)

Sarcomas

A **sarcoma** (sar-**KOH**-mah) is a malignant neoplasm of the soft tissues arising from supportive and connective tissue such as bone, fat, muscle, bone marrow and lymphatic tissue. (The combining form *SARC/O* means flesh.) (Plural, **sarcomas** or **sarcomata.**)

Carcinomas

A **carcinoma (kar**-sih-**NO**-mah) is a malignant epithelial neoplasm that tends to invade surrounding tissue and to metastasize to distant regions of the body. (Epithelial tissues form the internal and external covering of the body.) (The combining form *CARCIN/O* means cancer.)

Epithelial Tumors

Benign tumors of epithelial origin are usually named by using the suffix *-OMA.* Malignant tumors of epithelial origin are named by adding the suffix *-CARCINOMA* to the type of tissue in which the tumor occurs. (Note that these rules hold only for tumors arising from epithelial tissues.)

For example, an **adenoma (ad-eh-NO-mah)** is a benign tumor of glandular epithelium in which the cells of the tumor are arranged in a recognizable glandular structure. (The combining form *ADEN/O* means gland.) (Plural, **adenomas** or **adenomata.**)

An **adenocarcinoma (ad-eh-no-kar-sih-NO-mah)** is any one of a large group of malignant, epithelial cell tumors of the glands.

THE MAJOR MEDICAL SPECIALTIES

Medical practice is divided into many specialties and sub-specialties. The following are the names and descriptions of the more common specialties.

- A specialist in **adolescent medicine** treats the special needs of patients between puberty and the completion of physical growth (roughly from 11 to 19 years of age).
- An **allergist (AL-er-jist)** specializes in diagnosing and treating conditions of altered immunological reactivity (allergic reactions).
- An **anesthesiologist (an-es-thee-zee-OL-oh-jist)** specializes in administering anesthetic agents prior to and during surgery. (The prefix *AN-* means without and the combining form *ESTHESI/O* means feeling or sensation.)
- An **anesthetist** (ah-**NES**-theh-tist) is a person who is trained in administering anesthesia but who is not necessarily a physician. For example, a nurse anesthetist.
- A **cardiologist (kar-dee-OL-oh-jist)** specializes in diagnosing and treating abnormalities, diseases, and disorders of the heart. (The combining form *CARDI/O* means heart.)
- A **chiropractor (KIGH-roh-prack-tor)** holds a Doctor of Chiropractic (DC) degree and specializes in manipulative treatment of disorders originating from misalignment of the spinal vertebrae. (The combining form *CHIR/O* means hand.)
- A **dentist** holds a Doctor of Dental Surgery (DDS) or Doctor of Medical Dentistry degree (DMD) and specializes in diagnosing and treating diseases and disorders of teeth and tissues of the oral cavity. (The combining form *DENT/O* means tooth.)
- A **dermatologist (der-mah-TOL-oh-jist)** specializes in diagnosing and treating disorders of the skin. (The combining form *DERMAT/O* means skin.)
- An **endocrinologist (en-doh-krih-NOL-oh-jist)** specializes in diagnosing and treating diseases and malfunctions of the glands of internal secretion. (The prefix *ENDO-*means within and the combining form *CRIN/O* means to secrete.)
- An **epidemiologist (ep-ih-dee-me-OL-oh-jist)** specializes in **epidemiology** which is the study of sudden outbreaks of disease within a population group. (The prefix *EPI-*means upon or above and the combining form *DEM/O* means people.)
- A **family practitioner** treats patients of all ages and centers around family units. (Also known as **family medicine.**)
- A **gastroenterologist (gas-troh-en-ter-OL-oh-jist)** specializes in diagnosing and treating diseases and disorders of the stomach and intestines. (The combining form *GASTR/O* means stomach and the combining form *ENTER/O* means intestine.)
- A **gerontologist (jer-on-TOL-oh-jist)** specializes in diagnosing and treating diseases, disorders, and problems associated with aging. (The combining form *GERONT/O* means old age.)

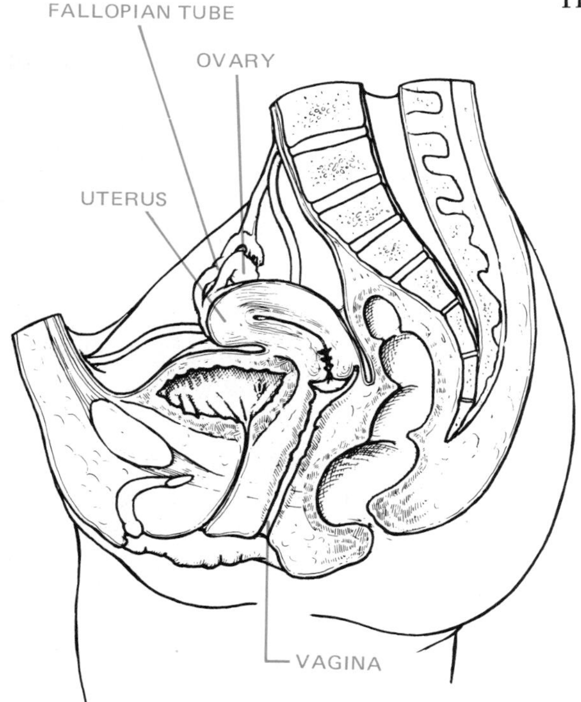

Figure 2-8 The female reproductive system.

- A **gynecologist (guy-**neh-**KOL-**oh-jist) specializes in diagnosing and treating diseases and disorders of the female reproductive system. (The combining form *GYNEC/O* means female.)
- A **hematologist (hem-**ah-**TOL-**oh-jist) specializes in diagnosing and treating diseases and disorders of the blood and blood-forming tissues. (The combining form *HEMAT/O* means blood.)
- An **immunologist (im-**you-**NOL-**oh-jist) specializes in the study of the immune system. (The combining form *IMMUN/O* means protected.)
- An **infertility specialist** diagnoses and treats problems association with conception and maintaining pregnancy.
- An **internist** specializes in diagnosing and treating diseases and disorders of the internal organs.
- A **neonatologist (nee-**oh-nay-**TOL-**oh-jist) specializes in diagnosing and treating disorders of the newborn. (The prefix *NEO-* means new and the combining form *NAT/I* means birth.)
- A **nephrologist** (neh-**FROL-**oh-jist) specializes in diagnosing and treating diseases and disorders of the kidneys. (The combining form *NEPHR/O* means kidney.)
- A **neurologist** (new-**ROL-**oh-jist) specializes in diagnosing and treating diseases and disorders of the central nervous system. (The combining form *NEUR/O* means nerve.)
- An **obstetrician (ob-**steh-**TRISH-**un) specializes in providing medical care to women during pregnancy, childbirth, and immediately thereafter. (The combining form *OBSTETR/O* means midwife or one who stands to receive.)
- An **occupational medicine specialist** diagnoses, treats and tries to prevent diseases or conditions arising from occupational hazards. (Also known as **industrial medicine.**)
- An **oncologist** (ong-**KOL-**oh-jist) specializes in diagnosing and treating malignant disorders such as tumors and cancer. (The combining form *ONC/O* means tumor.)
- An **ophthalmologist** (ahf-thal-**MOL-**oh-jist) specializes in diagnosing and treating diseases and disorders of the eye. (The combining form *OPHTHALM/O* means eye.)
- An **optometrist** (op-**TOM-**eh-trist) holds a Doctor of Optometry (OD) degree and specializes in measuring the accuracy of vision to determine if corrective lenses or eyeglasses are needed. (The combining form *OPT/O* means eye or vision.)

- An **orthopedist (or**-thoh-**PEE**-dist) specializes in diagnosing and treating diseases and disorders involving the bones, joints and muscles. (Also known as an **orthopedic surgeon.**) (The combining form *ORTH/O* means straight or normal.)
- **Osteopathic physicians** (oss-tee-oh-**PATH**-ick) hold a Doctor of Osteopathy (DO) degree and specialize in treating health problems by manipulation (changing the positions of the bones). They may also use traditional forms of medical treatment. (The combining form *OSTE/O* means bone.)
- An **otorhinolaryngologist (oh**-toh-**rye-no-lar**-in-**GOL**-oh-jist) specializes in diagnosing and treating diseases and disorders of the ear, nose, and throat. (Also known as an ENT Specialist.) (The combining form *OT/O* means ear, *RHIN/O* means nose, and *LARYNG/O* means larynx or throat.)
- A **pathologist** specializes in the analysis of tissue samples to confirm diagnosis and in performing autopsies. (An **autopsy** is an examination in order to determine the cause of death.) (The combining form *PATH/O* means disease or suffering.)
- A **pediatrician (pee**-dee-ah-**TRISH**-un) specializes in diagnosing, treating and preventing disorders and diseases of children. (The combining forms *PED/O* and *PEDI/A* mean child.)
- A **physical medicine specialist** treats disorders and diseases with physical agents such as physical therapy.
- A **plastic surgeon** specializes in the surgical restoration and reconstruction of body structures.
- A **podiatrist** (poh-**DYE**-ah-trist) holds a Doctor of Podiatry (DP) degree and specializes in diagnosing, treating and correcting disorders of the foot. (The combining forms *POD/O* and *PED/I* mean foot.)
- A **proctologist** (prock-**TOL**-oh-jist) specializes in disorders of the rectum and anus. (The combining form *PROCT/O* means anus and rectum.)
- A **psychiatrist** (sigh-**KYE**-ah-trist) specializes in diagnosing and treating chemical dependencies, emotional problems and mental illness. (The combing form *PSYCH/O* means mind.)
- A **psychologist** (sigh-**KOL**-oh-jist) holds a Doctor of Philosophy (PhD), or lesser degree, and specializes in evaluating and treating emotional problems.
- A **radiologist (ray**-dee-**OL**-oh-jist) specializes in diagnosing and treating diseases and disorders with x-rays and other forms of radiant energy.
- A **sports medicine specialist** diagnoses, treats and tries to prevent injuries sustained in athletic events.
- A **surgeon** specializes in diagnosing and treating diseases, injuries, and deformities by operative methods. There are many subspecialties of surgery.
- A specialist in **trauma medicine** diagnoses and treats acute illnesses and injuries. **(Trauma (TRAW**-mah) means wound or injury.) (Also known as **emergency medicine.)**
- A **urologist** (you-**ROL**-oh-jist) specializes in diagnosing and treating diseases and disorders of the urinary system of females and the genitourinary system of males. (The combining form *UR/O* means relating to urine or the urinary organs.)

IMPORTANT TERMS: THE STRUCTURE OF THE HUMAN BODY

This list will help you identify and review the major terms from this chapter.

When you work with the audio tape for this chapter, listen to the word, repeat it and then place a ✓ next to it on the list below.

- ☐ **Abdomen** (ab-**DOH**-men)
- ☐ **Abdominal** (ab-**DOM**-ih-nal)
- ☐ **Abdominopelvic** (ab-**dom**-ih-no-**PEL**-vick)
- ☐ **Adenocarcinoma** (**ad**-eh-no-**kar**-sih-**NO**-mah)
- ☐ **Adenoma** (**ad**-eh-**NO**-mah)
- ☐ **Adipose** (**AD**-ih-pohs)
- ☐ **Afferent** (**AF**-er-ent)
- ☐ **Allergist** (**AL**-er-jist)
- ☐ **Anaplasia** (**an**-ah-**PLAY**-zee-ah)
- ☐ **Anatomy** (ah-**NAT**-oh-me)
- ☐ **Anesthesiologist** (**an**-es-**thee**-zee-**OL**-oh-jist)
- ☐ **Anesthetist** (ah-**NES**-theh-tist)
- ☐ **Anterior** (an-**TEER**-ee-or)
- ☐ **Aplasia** (ah-**PLAY**-zee-ah)
- ☐ **Carcinoma** (**kar**-sih-**NO**-mah)
- ☐ **Cardiologist** (**kar**-dee-**OL**-oh-jist)
- ☐ **Caudal** (**KAW**-dal)
- ☐ **Cephalic** (seh-**FAL**-ick)
- ☐ **Chiropractor** (**KIGH**-roh-**prack**-tor)
- ☐ **Chromosomes** (**KROH**-moh-sohmes)
- ☐ **Coronal** (koh-**ROH**-nal)
- ☐ **Cytology** (sigh-**TOL**-oh-jee)
- ☐ **Cytoplasm** (**SIGH**-toh-plazm)
- ☐ **Dermatologist** (**der**-mah-**TOL**-oh-jist)
- ☐ **Distal** (**DIS**-tal)
- ☐ **Dorsal** (**DOOR**-sal)
- ☐ **Efferent** (**EF**-er-ent)
- ☐ **Endocrinologist** (**en**-doh-krih-**NOL**-oh-jist)
- ☐ **Endothelium** (**en**-doh-**THEE**-lee-um)
- ☐ **Epidemiologist** (**ep**-ih-dee-me-**OL**-oh-jist)
- ☐ **Epithelial** (**ep**-ih-**THEE**-lee-al)
- ☐ **Epithelium** (**ep**-ih-**THEE**-lee-um)
- ☐ **Gastroenterologist** (**gas**-troh-**en**-ter-**OL**-oh-jist)
- ☐ **Gerontologist** (**jer**-on-**TOL**-oh-jist)
- ☐ **Gynecologist** (**guy**-neh-**KOL**-oh-jist)
- ☐ **Hematologist** (**hem**-ah-**TOL**-oh-jist)
- ☐ **Histology** (his-**TOL**-oh-jee)
- ☐ **Homeostasis** (**hoh**-me-oh-**STAY**-sis)
- ☐ **Hyperplasia** (**high**-per-**PLAY**-zee-ah)
- ☐ **Hypoplasia** (**high**-poh-**PLAY**-zee-ah)
- ☐ **Immunologist** (**im**-you-**NOL**-oh-jist)
- ☐ **Karyoplasm** (**CARE**-ee-oh-plazm)
- ☐ **Membrane** (**MEM**-brain)
- ☐ **Metastasis** (meh-**TAS**-tah-sis)
- ☐ **Midsagittal** (mid-**SADJ**-ih-tal)
- ☐ **Neonatologist** (**nee**-oh-nay-**TOL**-oh-jist)
- ☐ **Nephrologist** (neh-**FROL**-oh-jist)
- ☐ **Neurologist** (new-**ROL**-oh-jist)
- ☐ **Nucleoplasm** (**NEW**-klee-oh-**plazm**)
- ☐ **Nucleus** (**NEW**-klee-us)

- ☐ **Obstetrician (ob**-steh-**TRISH**-un)
- ☐ **Oncologist** (ong-**KOL**-oh-jist)
- ☐ **Oncology** (ong-**KOL**-oh-jee)
- ☐ **Ophthalmologist** (ahf-thal-**MOL**-oh-jist)
- ☐ **Optometrist** (op-**TOM**-eh-trist)
- ☐ **Orthopedist (or**-thoh-**PEE**-dist)
- ☐ **Osteopathic (oss**-tee-oh-**PATH**-ick)
- ☐ **Otorhinolaryngologist** (**oh**-toh-**rye**-no-**lar**-in-**GOL**-oh-jist)
- ☐ **Pediatrician (pee**-dee-ah-**TRISH**-un)
- ☐ **Pelvic (PEL**-vick)
- ☐ **Physiology (fiz**-ee-**OL**-oh-jee)
- ☐ **Podiatrist** (poh-**DYE**-ah-trist)
- ☐ **Posterior** (pos-**TEER**-ee-or)
- ☐ **Proctologist** (prock-**TOL**-oh-jist)
- ☐ **Protoplasm (PROH**-toh-plazm)
- ☐ **Proximal (PROCK**-sih-mal)
- ☐ **Psychiatrist** (sigh-**KYE**-ah-trist)
- ☐ **Psychologist** (sigh-**KOL**-oh-jist)
- ☐ **Radiologist (ray**-dee-**OL**-oh-jist)
- ☐ **Sagittal (SADJ**-ih-tal)
- ☐ **Sarcoma** (sar-**KOH**-mah)
- ☐ **Thoracic** (thoh-**RAS**-ick)
- ☐ **Transverse** (trans-**VERSE**)
- ☐ **Trauma (TRAW**-mah)
- ☐ **Urologist** (you-**ROL**-oh-jist)
- ☐ **Ventral (VEN**-tral)

EXERCISES

DEFINING WORD PARTS

Write the definition for each of these word parts.

1. *ADIP/O* ______
2. *CAUD/O* ______
3. *CEPHAL/O* ______
4. *CYT/O* ______
5. *DORS/O* ______
6. *ENTER/O* ______
7. *GERONT/O* ______
8. *GYNEC/O* ______
9. *HEMAT/O* ______
10. *HIST/O* ______
11. *KARY/O* ______
12. *NE/O* ______
13. *NUCLE/O* ______
14. *ONC/O* ______
15. *OPT/O* ______
16. *PED/O, PEDI/A* ______

17. *PELV/O* ____________________

18. *POD/O, PED/I* ____________________

19. *THORAC/O* ____________________

20. *VENTR/O* ____________________

DEFINITIONS

Circle the letter next to the correct answer.

1. Afferent means ____________
   a) above the midline.
   b) away from the center of a structure.
   c) below the midline.
   d) toward the center of a structure.

2. An endocrinologist specializes in diagnosing and treating diseases and malfunction of the ____________
   a) glands of internal secretion.
   b) internal organs.
   c) reproductive organs.
   d) stomach and intestines.

3. A/an ____________, also known as a tumor, is any abnormal growth of new tissue, benign or malignant.
   a) anaplasia
   b) cancer
   c) keratoplasm
   d) neoplasm

4. A gerontologist specializes in diagnosing and treating diseases ____________
   a) and disorders of the blood and blood forming tissues.
   b) and disorders of the stomach and intestines.
   c) and disorders and problems associated with aging.
   d) with the use of radionuclides.

5. The dorsal cavity contains the ____________
   a) heart and lungs.
   b) major organs of digestion.
   c) organs that maintain a constant internal environment.
   d) structures of the nervous system.

6. Lateral means _______________
   a) near the beginning of the structure.
   b) near the front of the body.
   c) toward the midline.
   d) toward the side.

7. _______________ tissue covers both the internal and external surfaces of the body.
   a) Adipose
   b) Cytoplasm
   c) Endothelial
   d) Epithelial

8. _______________ is the process by which tumor cells are spread to distant parts of the body.
   a) Hypoplasia
   b) Malignancy
   c) Metastasis
   d) Oncology

9. The midsagittal plane divides the body into _______________
   a) anterior and posterior portions.
   b) cephalic and caudal halves.
   c) left and right halves.
   d) upper and lower sections.

10. _______________ means away from the midline or the beginning of a body structure.
   a) Caudal
   b) Distal
   c) Lateral
   d) Medial

MISSING WORDS

Write the missing word on the line.

1. _______________________ means near the midline or beginning of a body structure.
2. _______________________ nerves carry impulses away from the brain.
3. _______________________ means maintaining a constant internal environment.
4. _______________________ is the protoplasm of the nucleus of the cell.
5. A/an _______________________ is a person trained to administer anesthesia, but not necessarily a physician.
6. _______________________ tissue holds organs in place and binds all parts of the body together.
7. _______________________ means toward the anterior or belly side of the body.

8. ______________________ means toward the posterior or back of the body.

9. ______________________ is the study of cancerous tumors.

10. A/an ______________________ is the basic structural unit of the body.

11. ______________________ means the lack of development of an organ or tissue.

12. The ______________________ cavity contains the heart and lungs.

13. A/an ______________________ specializes in diagnosing and treating abnormalities, diseases and disorders of the heart.

14. A ______________________ is a malignant neoplasm of the soft tissues arising from supportive and connective tissue.

15. A ______________________ neoplasm tends to get progressively worse, spreads and is life-threatening.

SPELLCHECK

Select the correct spelling and write it on the line.

1. A specialist in ______________________ medicine diagnoses and treats acute illnesses and injuries.
   traoma
   trauma
   trawma

2. _______________ contain genetic material commonly known as genes.
   Chramasones
   Chromosomes
   Cromosomes

3. _______________ tissue forms the lining of all the internal organs.
   Epathelial
   Epithelial
   Epothelial

4. A _______________ specializes in diagnosing and treating diseases and disorders of the blood and blood-forming tissues.
   hematologist
   hemitologist
   hemotologist

5. A _______________ specializes in diagnosing and treating diseases and disorders of the central nervous system.
   neuralogist
   neurologist
   nurologist

6. _______________ refers to the head.
   Caphalic
   Cephalic
   Cephelic

7. A _______________ is a malignant epithelial neoplasm that tends to invade the surrounding tissue and to metastasize to distant regions of the body.
   carcanoma
   carcenoma
   carcinoma

8. The _______________ cavity contains the brain.
   cranial
   craniel
   craniol

9. A specialist in _______________ medicine treats the special needs of patients between puberty and the completion of physical growth.
   adilescent
   adolescent
   adolesent

10. The _______________ cavity contains primarily the major organs of digestion.
    abdominal
    abominal
    adbominal

11. An _______________ specialist diagnoses and treats problems associated with conception and maintaining pregnancy.
    enfertility
    infertility
    inferotility

12. A _______________ specializes in diagnosing and treating diseases and disorders of the urinary system.
    uralogist
    uriologist
    urologist

13. A _______________ specializes in diagnosing, treating and preventing disorders and diseases of children.
    pedatrician
    pediatrican
    pediatrician

14. An _______________ specializes in diagnosing and treating conditions of altered immunological reactivity.
    allergist
    allerogist
    allirgist

15. An _______________ specializes in diagnosing and treating malignant disorders.
    onchiologist
    oncologist
    onkologist

CASE STUDIES

Write the correct answer on the line.

1. Rita Haynes has ______________________ which is an abnormal increase in the number of normal cells in normal arrangement in a tissue.

2. Gerald Farmer has severe acne. He is being treated by a/an ______________________ who specializes in diagnosing and treating disorders of the skin.

3. Brenda Carlson has a serious blood disorder. She was referred to a/an ______________________ who specializes in diagnosing and treating diseases and disorders of the blood and blood-forming tissues.

4. Wally Foster has a kidney disease. He was treated by a/an ______________________ who specializes in diagnosing and treating diseases and disorders of the kidneys.

5. Mr. Reynolds had a pain in his neck. He went to a/an ______________________ who specializes in manipulative treatment of disorders originating from misalignment of the spine.

6. When Ralph Jenkins broke his ankle in a skiing accident he sought the services of a/an ______________________ who specializes in diagnosing and treating diseases and disorders involving the bones, joints and muscles.

7. Dr. Ames specializes in measuring the accuracy of vision to determine if corrective lenses or eyeglasses are needed. She is a/an ______________________.

8. For her regular pap test, Carmella Ortega seeks the services of a/an ______________________ who specializes in diagnosing and treating diseases and disorders of the female reproductive system.

9. Because Melissa Vaughn has been severely depressed, she sought the services of a/an ______________________ who specializes in evaluating and treating emotional problems.

10. For his annual physical Stephen Wong went to Dr. Adams, a/an ______________________ who specializes in diagnosing and treating diseases and disorders of the internal organs.

11. The newborn son of Mr. and Mrs. Larson is very sick. The baby is being treated by a/an ______________________.

12. Phyllis Durkin has foot trouble. She seeks the help of a/an ______________________.

13. After Mr. Wilkins died the autopsy was performed by a/an ______________________.

14. Mrs. Brewster's x-rays were interpreted by a/an ______________________.

15. The cause of the sudden outbreak of measles in the city was studied by a/an ______________.

WORD BUILDING

Write the correct word or word part on the line.

1. Incomplete tissue development
   a) The prefix ______________________ means decreased or deficient.
   b) The suffix ______________________ means development or growth of tissue.
   c) The term ______________________ means the incomplete development of an organ or tissue.

2. Cell structure
   a) The combining form ______________________ means first.
   b) The suffix ______________________ means formative substance.
   c) The term ______________________ means all of the material that makes up the cell.

3. A body cavity
   a) The combining form ______________________ means abdomen.
   b) The combining form ______________________ means pelvic.
   c) Together these two are referred to as the ______________________ cavity.

4. Cells
   a) The combining form ______________________ means cell.
   b) The suffix ______________________ means the study of.
   c) The term ______________________ means the study of cells.

5. Fleshy tumors
   a) The combining form ______________________ means flesh.
   b) The suffix ______________________ means tumor.
   c) The term ______________________ means malignant tumors of the soft tissues.

LABELING EXERCISES

Identify the numbered items on these diagrams.

1. ______________________ or ______________________ surface
2. ______________________ or ______________________ surface
3. ______________________ or midsagittal line
4. ______________________ or cephalic direction
5. ______________________ or caudal direction

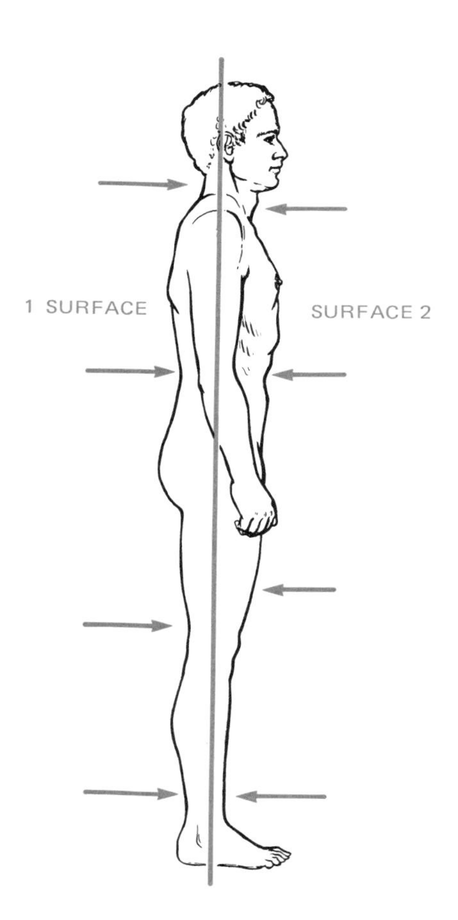

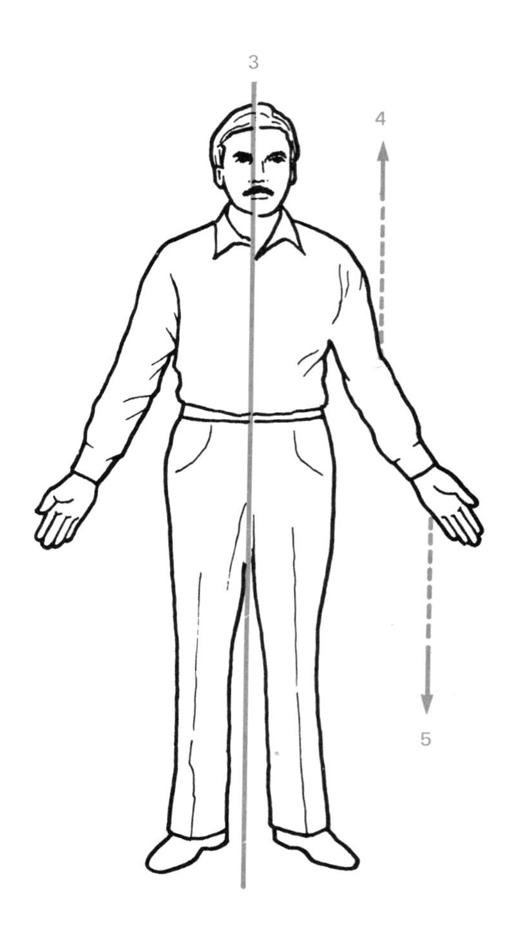

3

THE SKELETAL SYSTEM

LEARNING GOALS

In this chapter you will learn to:

- define the major anatomical terms related to the structure and function of the bones and joints of the skeletal system.
- name the major groups of bones of the body.
- use combining forms to build and analyze terms related to the skeletal system.
- recognize and define terms related to the diagnosis, pathology and treatment of diseases of the skeletal system.

THE STRUCTURE OF BONE

Bone is one of the hardest tissues in the human body; only the enamel of the teeth is harder. However, throughout life normal bone goes through an ongoing process of building up and tearing down, and is capable of healing and repair. (The combining forms *OSTE/O, OSS/E* and *OSS/I* all mean bone or bony.)

Periosteum

The periosteum (**per**-ee-**OSS**-tee-um) is the tough and fibrous outermost covering of bone. (The prefix *PERI-* means around or surrounding.)

The Kinds of Bone

There are two kinds of bone: compact bone and cancellous bone.

Compact bone, also known as **cortical bone,** is hard, dense and very strong. It forms the outer layer of the bones. Compact bone is found just under the periosteum.

Cancellous bone, (**KAN**-sell-us) also known as **spongy bone,** is lighter in weight but not as strong as compact bone. Cancellous bone is commonly found in long bones such as the femur.

Bone Marrow

Bone marrow is located within the cancellous bone. (The combining form *MYEL/O* means both bone marrow and the spinal cord.)

Red bone marrow is hematopoietic and manufactures red blood cells and hemoglobin, as well as white blood cells and thrombocytes.

Hematopoietic (**hem**-ah-toh-poi-**ET**-ick) means pertaining to the formation of blood cells. (The combining form *HEMAT/O* means blood and the suffix *-POIETIC* means pertaining to formation.)

Yellow bone marrow is composed chiefly of fat cells.

Cartilage

Cartilage (**KAR**-tih-lidj) is more elastic than bone and makes up parts of the skeleton such as the flexible portion of the tip of the nose. (The combining form *CHONDR/O* means cartilage.)

An important function of cartilage is to cover the joint surfaces of bones. Here it is known as **articular cartilage.**

The **meniscus** (meh-**NIS**-kus) is the curved fibrous cartilage found in some joints, such as the knee.

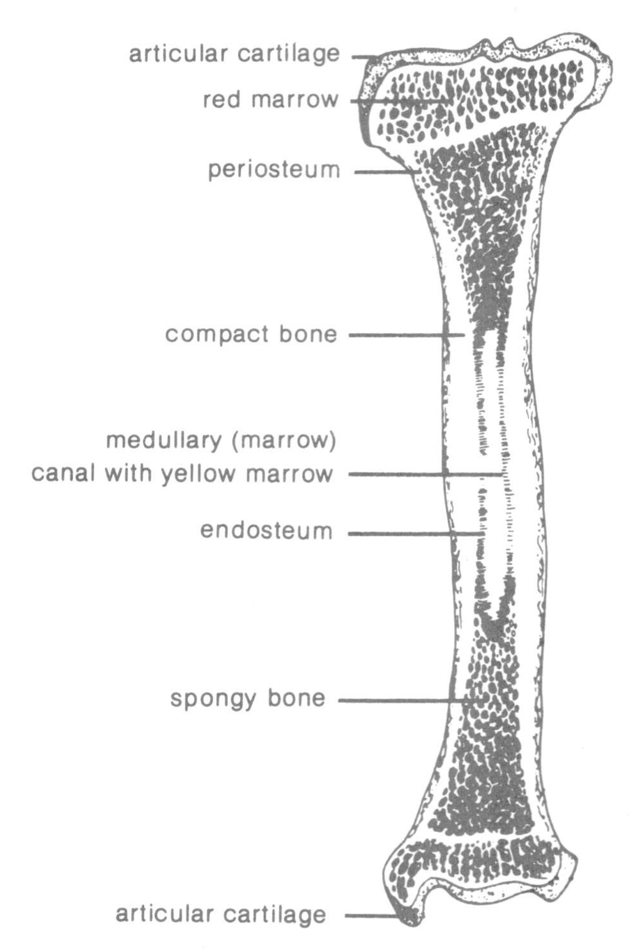

Figure 3-1 Internal structure of a long bone.

JOINTS

Joints, known as **articulations,** are connections between bones. (The combining form *ARTHR/O* means joint.)

Articulate (ar-**TICK**-you-late) means to join or to come together.

TYPES OF JOINTS
Fibrous joints, such as the sutures of the skull, do not move. A **suture** is the jagged line where the bones articulate and form a joint that does not move.
Cartilaginous joints hold the bones firmly together. Normally they move only very slightly. This type of joint is also known as a **symphysis** (**SIM**-fih-sis).
Synovial joints (sih-**NOH**-vee-al) are the movable joints of the body. **Ball and socket joints,** such are the hips and shoulders, are synovial joints that allow a wide range of movement. **Hinge joints,** such as the knees and elbows, are synovial joints that allow movement in one direction or plane.

Ligaments

Ligaments are fibrous, connective tissue bands that join together the articulating ends of bones. (The combining form *LIGAMENT/O* means ligament.)

Be careful not to confuse ligaments and tendons. **Tendons** are narrow bands of fibrous tissue that attach muscles to bone. (Tendons are discussed in Chapter 4.)

The Bursa

A **bursa** (**BER**-sah) is a fibrous sac between certain tendons and the bones beneath them. (The combining form *BURS/O* means bursa.) (Plural, **bursae.)**

The bursa is also lined with synovial membrane and filled with synovial fluid. The function of the bursa is to act as a cushion to ease movement.

Synovial Membrane and Fluid

The synovial membrane secretes synovial fluid. This fluid acts as a lubricant to make the smooth movement of the joint possible. (The combining form *SYNOVI/O* refers to both the synovial membrane and lubricating fluid.)

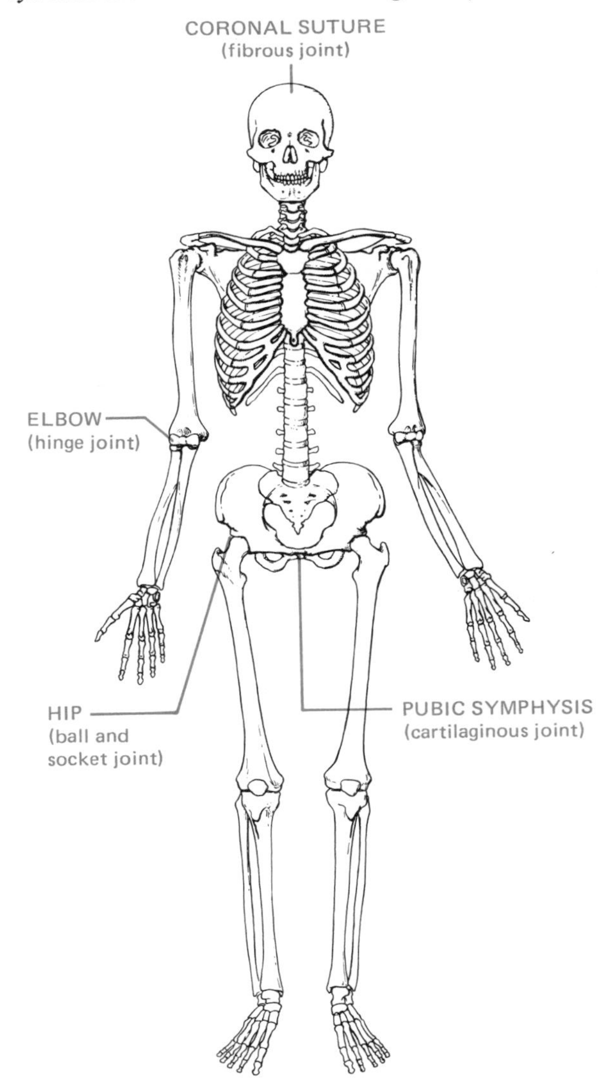

Figure 3-2 Types of joints.

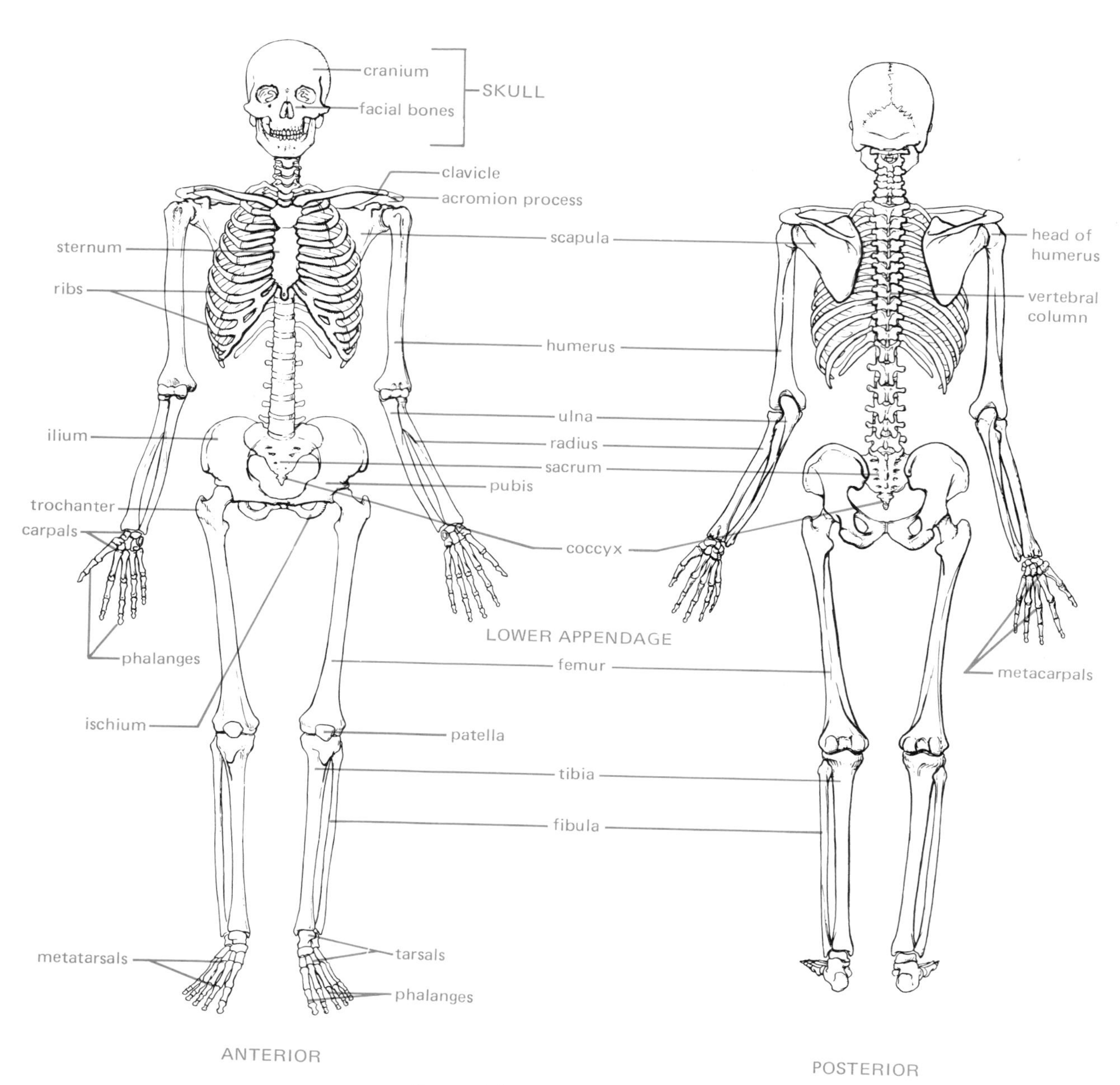

Figure 3-3 The bones of the body.

INTRODUCTION TO THE SKELETAL SYSTEM

There are 206 bones in the human body and, for descriptive purposes, the skeleton is divided into the axial and appendicular skeletal systems.

In figure 3-3 the bones of the axial skeleton are shaded. The bones of the appendicular skeleton are not.

The Axial Skeleton

The axial skeleton (80 bones) consists of the skull, spinal column, ribs and sternum. It protects the major organs of the nervous, respiratory and circulatory systems.

The Appendicular Skeleton

The appendicular skeleton (126 bones) consists of the upper extremities and shoulder girdle plus the lower extremities and pelvic girdle. It makes body movement possible and also protects the organs of digestion, excretion and reproduction.

THE BONES OF THE SKULL

The Bones of the Cranium

The **cranium (KRAY-nee-um)** is the portion of the skull which encloses the brain. (The combining form *CRANI/O* means skull.) The cranium is made up of the following bones.

- The **frontal bone** forms the forehead and contains the **frontal sinuses.** (A **sinus** is an air-filled cavity within a bone.)

- The **parietal bones** (pah-**RYE**-eh-tal) form most of the roof and upper sides of the cranium.

  In a baby the **fontanelle (fon**-tah-**NELL)** is the soft spot where the sutures between the frontal and parietal bones have not yet closed. This disappears as the child grows and the sutures close. (This is also spelled **fontanel.)**

- The **occipital bone** (ock-**SIP**-ih-tal) forms the posterior floor and walls of the cranium. The spinal cord passes through the **foramen magnum** of the occipital bone.

  A **foramen** (foh-**RAY**-men) is an opening in a bone through which blood vessels, nerves and ligaments pass. (Plural, **foramina.)**

- The **temporal bones** form the sides and base of the cranium.

  The temporal bones contain the **external auditory meatus** which is the bony passage of the outer ear. (A **meatus** (me-**AY**-tus) is the external opening of a canal.)

  The **mastoid process** is a projection on the temporal bone located just behind the ear. (A **process** is a prominence or projection on a bone.)

- The **sphenoid bone** (**SFEE**-noid) forms part of the base of the skull, and parts of the floor and sides of the orbit.

  The **orbit** is the bony socket surrounding and protecting the eye. The sphenoid bone also contains the **sphenoid sinuses.**

  The **sella turcica** (**SELL**-ah **TUR**-sih-kah) is a depression in the superior surface of the sphenoid bone that protects the pituitary gland.

- The **ethmoid bone** (**ETH**-moid) forms part of the nose, the orbit and the floor of the cranium. It contains the **ethmoid sinuses.**

The Auditory Ossicles

These are the bones of the middle ear. (**Auditory** refers to hearing and **ossicle** (**OS**-sih-kul) means small bone.)

The auditory ossicles include the: **malleus** (**MAL**-ee-us), **incus** (**ING**-kus) and **stapes** (**STAY**-peez).

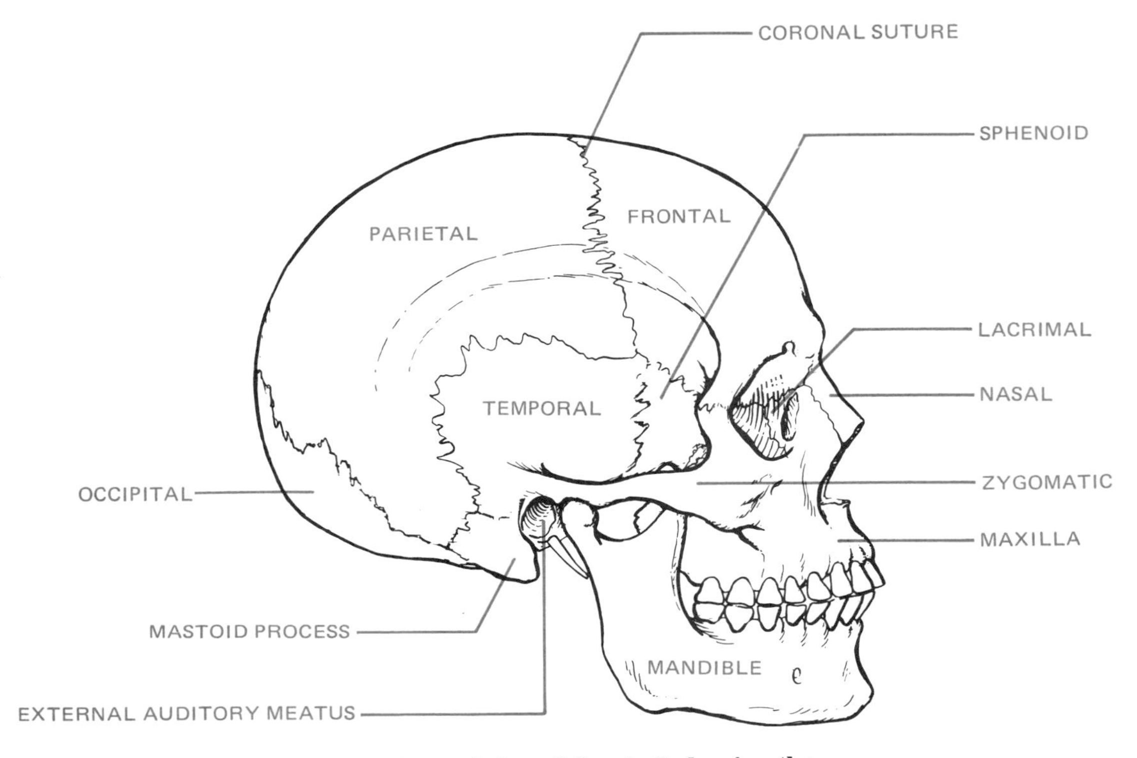

Figure 3-4 Lateral view of the skull showing the major bones and anatomical landmarks.

The Bones of the Face

- The **zygomatic bones** (**zye**-goh-**MAT**-ick), also known as the **cheekbones,** articulate with the frontal bones.
- The **maxillary bones** (**MACK**-sih-**ler**-ee) form most of the upper jaw. They contain the **maxillary sinuses.** (Singular, **maxilla.**)
- The **palatine bones** (**PAL**-ah-tine) form part of the hard palate of the mouth and the floor of the nose.
- The **lacrimal bones** (**LACK**-rih-mal) make up part of the orbit at the inner angle of the eye.
- The **inferior conchae** (**KONG**-kee) are the thin, scroll-like bones that form part of the interior of the nose. (Singular, **concha.**)
- The **vomer bone** (**VOH**-mer) forms the base for the nasal septum. (The **nasal septum** is the cartilage structure that divides the two nasal cavities and forms the tip of the nose.)
- The **mandible** (**MAN**-dih-bul), also known as the lower jaw bone, is the only movable bone of the skull.

  The upper portion of the mandible forms a condyle that articulates with a fossa in the temporal bones to form the **temporomandibular joint** (**tem**-poh-roh-man-**DIB**-you-lar) (TMJ).

  A **condyle** (**KON**-dial) is a rounded knuckle-like projection on a bone and is usually found where one bone articulates with another bone.

  A **fossa** is a hollow or depressed area in a bone. (Plural, **fossae.**)

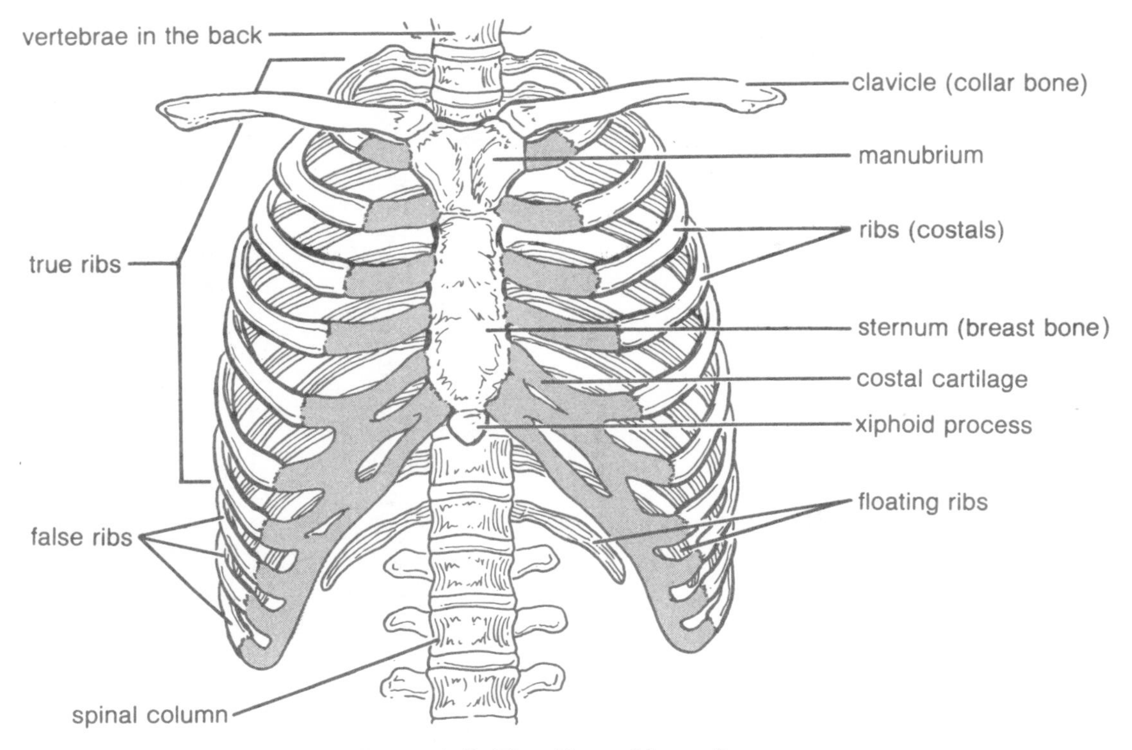

Figure 3-5 The ribs and breastbone.

- The **hyoid bone** (**HIGH**-oid) is unique because it does not articulate with any other bone. Instead it is suspended between the mandible and the larynx.

THE RIBS AND SPINAL COLUMN

The Ribs and Sternum

The ribs, sternum and thoracic vertebrae make up the rib cage that encloses the thoracic cavity. The thoracic cavity protects the heart and lungs. (The combining form *THORAC/O* means chest.)

The **sternum** (**STER**-num), also known as the breastbone, is the long flat bone in the middle of the front of the rib cage.

The **manubrium** (mah-**NEW**-bree-um) is the upper portion of the sternum. The lower portion, which is made of cartilage, is called the **xiphoid process** (**ZIF**-oid).

There are 12 pairs of ribs, also called **costals,** which attach posteriorly to the thoracic vertebrae. (The combining form *COST/O* means rib.)

- The first 7 pairs of ribs are attached anteriorly to the sternum. These are also called **true ribs.**
- The next 3 pairs of ribs are attached anteriorly to cartilage which joins with the sternum. These are also called **false ribs.**
- The last 2 pairs of ribs are not attached anteriorly and are called **floating ribs.**

The Spinal Column

The spinal column, which is also known as the **vertebral column** (**VER**-teh-bral), supports the head and body and provides bony protection for the spinal cord.

(The combining form *MYEL/O* means the spinal column and bone marrow. The combining form *SPONDYL/O* means vertebra or vertebral column.)

The spinal column consists of 26 **vertebrae (VER**-teh-bree). (The combining form *VERTEBR/O* refers to the vertebrae.) (Singular, **vertebra.)**

The vertebrae are separated and cushioned from each other by **intervertebral discs** which are made of cartilage.

The **lamina (LAM**-ih-nah) is the projecting posterior portion of each vertebra. (The combining form *LAMIN/O* means lamina.) (Plural, **laminae.)**

- **Cervical vertebrae. (SER**-vih-kal) The first set of seven vertebrae form the neck and are known as C1 through C7. (**Cervical** means neck.)
- **Thoracic vertebrae.** (thoh-**RASS**-ick) The second set of twelve vertebrae form the outward curve of the spine and are known as T1 through T12. These vertebrae are sometimes referred to as the **dorsal vertebrae** D1 through D12.
- **Lumbar vertebrae. (LUM**-bar) The third set of five vertebrae are known as L1 through L5. They are the largest and strongest of the vertebrae and form the inward curve of the spine.
- **Sacrum. (SAY**-krum) The sacrum is a slightly curved, triangular shaped bone. At birth it is composed of separate sacral bones; however, they fuse together in the young child.
- **Coccyx. (KOCK**-sicks) Also known as the tailbone, it is made up of several small vertebrae fused together.

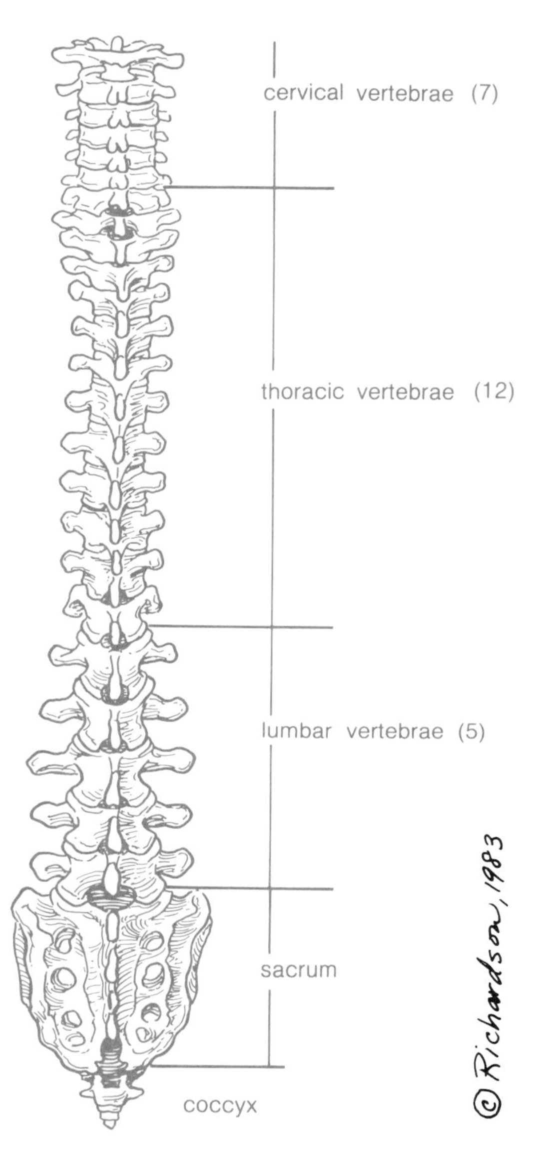

Figure 3-6 Dorsal view of the spine.

THE SHOULDERS, ARMS AND HANDS

The Shoulders

The shoulders form the **pectoral girdle** that supports the arms and hands.

- The **clavicle (KLAV**-ih-kul), also known as the collarbone, is a slender bone that connects the sternum to the scapula.
- The **scapula (SKAP**-you-lah) is also known as the shoulder blade.
- The **acromion** (ah-**KROH**-me-on) is an extension of the scapula that forms the high point of the shoulder.

The Arms, Wrists and Hands

- The **humerus (HEW**-mer-us) is the bone of the upper arm.
- The **ulna (ULL**-nah) is the larger inner bone of the forearm.

  The **olecranon** (oh-**LEK**-rah-non) is a proximal projection on the ulna that forms the point of the elbow.
- The **radius (RAY**-dee-us) is the smaller outer bone of the forearm.
- The **carpals (KAR**-palz) are the bones of the wrist.
- The **metacarpals** (met-ah-**KAR**-palz) are the bones of the hands.
- The **phalanges** (fah-**LAN**-jeez) are the bones of the fingers. (Singular, **phalanx.)**

THE HIPS, LEGS AND FEET

The Hips

The **os coxae (OSS KOCK**-sigh), also known as the hip or pelvic bones, form the **pelvic girdle** which provides structure for the hip area.

The pelvic girdle is made up of three bones fused together:

- The **ilium (ILL**-ee-um) is the upper, blade-shaped part of the hip on each side of the pelvic girdle. (The combining form *ILI/O* means ilium or hip bone.) (Be careful with this word! It is very similar to **ileum** — and that is part of the small intestine.)

  The **sacroiliac (say**-kroh-**ILL**-ee-ack) is the slightly movable articulation between the ilium and the sacrum.
- The **ischium (ISS**-key-um) is the lower and posterior portion of the pelvic girdle.

  The **acetabulum (ass**-eh-**TAB**-you-lum), the large socket in the pelvic bones, forms the hip socket for the head of the femur.
- The **pubis (PEW**-bis) is the anterior portion of the pelvic girdle.

  The two pubic bones fuse together at the **pubic symphysis (PEW**-bick **SIM**-fih-sis).

The Legs and Knees

- The **femur (FEE**-mur) is the upper leg bone.

  The **trochanter** (tro-**KAN**-ter) is the large bony projection on the upper end of the femur.

  The **femoral neck (FEM**-or-al) is the narrow area just below it.
- The **patella** (pah-**TEL**-ah) is the bony portion of the kneecap.
- The **tibia (TIB**-ee-ah), also known as the shin bone, is the larger weight-bearing bone of the lower leg.

  An **epiphysis** (eh-**PIF**-ih-sis) is the wide end of a long bone such as the tibia.
- The **fibula (FIB**-you-lah) is the smaller of the two bones of the lower leg.

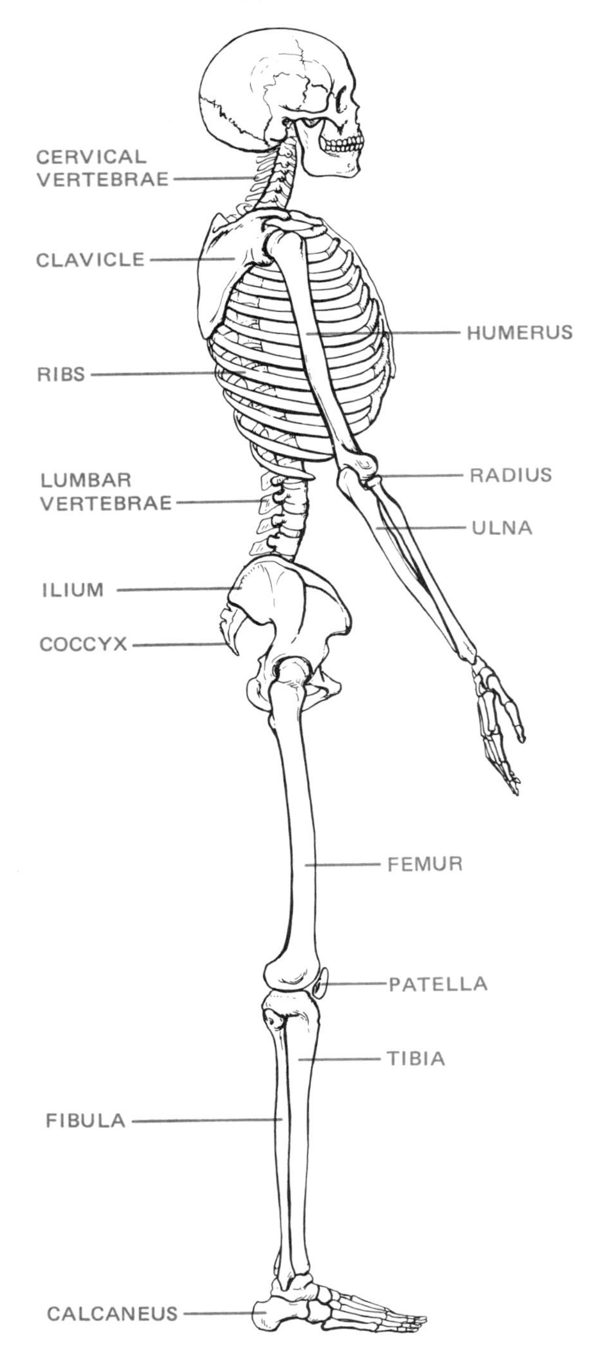

Figure 3-7 Lateral view of the skeleton.

The Ankles, Feet and Toes

- The **tarsals** (**TAHR**-salz) are the bones that make up the ankles.

  The **malleolus** (mal-**LEE**-oh-lus) is the rounded bony protuberance on each side of the ankle. (Plural, **malleoli.**)

  The **calcaneal** (kal-**KAY**-nee-al) or heel bone, is the largest of the tarsal bones.

- The **metatarsals** (**met**-ah-**TAR**-salz) are the bones of the foot.

- The **phalanges** (fah-**LAN**-jeez) are the bones of the toes. (Singular, **phalanx.**)

DIAGNOSTIC PROCEDURES RELATED TO THE SKELETAL SYSTEM

- An **acoustogram** (ah-**KOOS**-toh-gram) is a record of the sounds produced by the motion of a joint. (The combining form *ACOUST/O* means hearing.)

- **Arthrocentesis** (**ar**-throh-sen-**TEE**-sis) is a surgical puncture of the joint space with a needle. Synovial fluid is removed for analysis.

- **Arthroscopy** (ar-**THROS**-koh-pee) is the visual examination of the internal structure of a joint using an **arthroscope.**

Imaging Techniques Applied to the Skeletal System

- **Arthrography** (ar-**THROG**-rah-fee) is the x-ray examination of a joint after the injection of a contrast medium. The resulting film is an **arthrogram.**

- **Myelography** (**my**-eh-**LOG**-rah-fee) is the diagnostic study of the spinal cord after the injection of a contrast medium. The resulting film is a **myelogram.**

PATHOLOGY OF THE SKELETAL SYSTEM

Pathology of the Joints

- **Arthropathy** (ar-**THROP**-ah-thee) is any disease of a joint.
- **Arthralgia** (ar-**THRAL**-jee-ah), also known as **arthrodynia** (**ar**-throh-**DIN**-ee-ah) is pain in a joint.
- **Arthropyosis** (**ar**-throh-pye-**OH**-sis) is the formation of pus in a joint. (The combining form *PY/O* means pus.)
- **Arthritis** (ar-**THRIGH**-tis) is an inflammatory condition of one or more joints. There are many forms of arthritis.

  Rheumatoid arthritis (**ROO**-mah-toyd) is a chronic systemic disease affecting the connective tissues and joints in which the joints are swollen and painful.

  Juvenile rheumatoid arthritis affects children and may cause skin rash, fever, slowed growth, fatigue and swelling in the joints.

  Osteoarthritis (**oss**-tee-oh-ar-**THRIGH**-tis), is a degenerative joint disease and is the form of arthritis most commonly associated with aging.

  Gouty arthritis (**GOW**-tee), also known as **gout,** is a form of arthritis in which uric acid crystals deposit in the joints.

  Lupus erythematosus (**LOO**-pus er-ih-**thee**-mah-**TOH**-sus) is an acute form of arthritis that may cause skin rashes and severely damage joints and organs throughout the body.
- **Ankylosis** (**ang**-kih-**LOH**-sis) is the loss or absence of mobility in a joint because the bones have abnormally fused together. (The combining form *ANKLY/O* means crooked, bent or stiff.)
- **Luxation** (luck-**SAY**-shun), also known as **dislocation,** is the dislocation or displacement of a bone from its joint.
- **Subluxation** (**sub**-luck-**SAY**-shun) is the partial displacement of a bone from its joint.
- **Chondropathy** (kon-**DROP**-ah-thee) is disease of the cartilage.
- **Chondromalacia** (**kon**-droh-mah-**LAY**-she-ah) is abnormal softening of the cartilage.
- **Bursitis** (ber-**SIGH**-tis) is an inflammation of a bursa.

Pathology of the Spinal Column

- **Spondylosis** (**spon**-dih-**LOH**-sis) is any degenerative condition of the spine.
- **Ankylosing spondylitis** is an inflammatory joint disease characterized by progressive stiffening of the spine caused by fusion of the vertebral bodies.
- A **herniated disk** is a rupture of the intervertebral disk that results in pressure on spinal nerve roots. (**Hernia** means rupture, breakthrough or tear.)
- **Lumbago** (lum-**BAY**-go), also known as low back pain, is pain of the lumbar region.
- **Kyphosis** (kigh-**FOH**-sis), also known as humpback, is an abnormal increase in the outward curvature of the thoracic spine as viewed from the side.
- **Lordosis** (lor-**DOH**-sis), also known as swayback, is an abnormal increase in the anterior curvature of the lower or lumbar spine.
- **Scoliosis** (**skoh**-lee-**OH**-sis) is an abnormal lateral (sideways) curvature of the spine.
- **Spina bifida** (**BIF**-ih-dah) is a congenital failure of the spinal canal to close over the spinal cord due to lack of union of the laminae of the vertebrae. (The combining form *BIFID/O* means cleft or split.)

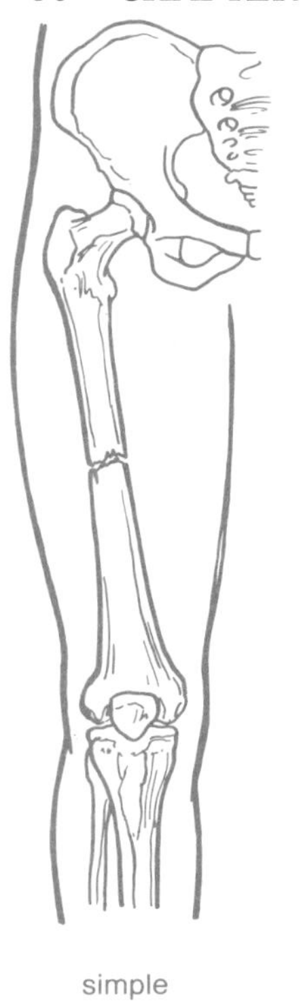

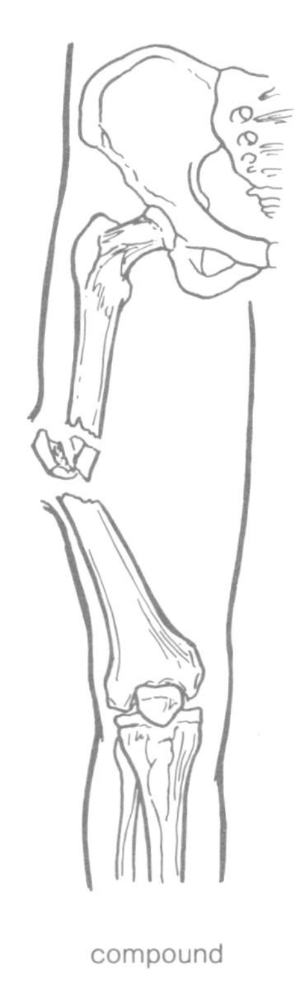

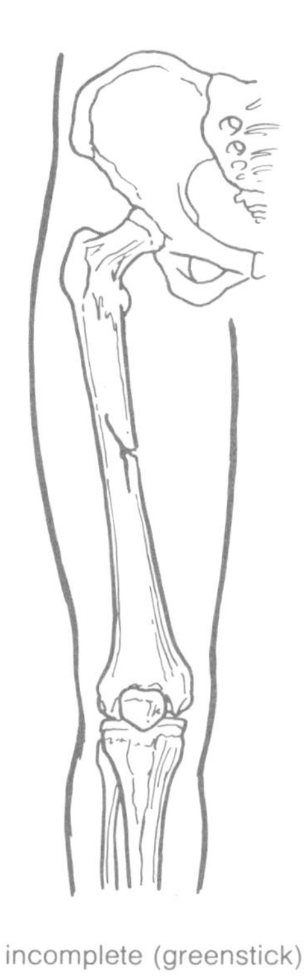

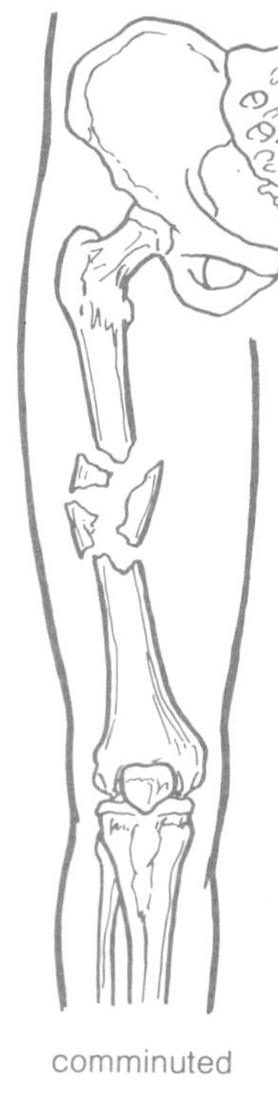

Figure 3-8 Types of fractures.

- **Spondylolisthesis (spon-**dih-loh-**LIS-**thee-sis) is a subluxation of one vertebra over the one below it.

Fractures

- A **fracture** is a broken bone. Fractures are described in terms of their complexity.
- **Crepitation (krep-**ih-**TAY-**shun) is the crackling sensation that is felt and heard when the ends of a broken bone move together.
- A **closed fracture,** also known as a **simple fracture,** is a fracture in which the bone is broken but there is no open wound in the skin.
- An **open fracture,** also known as a **compound fracture,** is a fracture in which the bone is broken and there is an open wound in the skin.
- A **comminuted fracture (KOM-**ih-**newt-**ed) is a fracture in which the bone is splintered or crushed.
- An **impacted fracture** is a fracture in which the ends of the bones are jammed into each other.
- A **compression fracture** occurs when the bone is pressed together (compressed) upon itself.
- A **spiral fracture** occurs as the result of a severe twisting motion.
- A **greenstick fracture,** or **incomplete fracture,** is a fracture in which the bone is only partially broken.

Pathology of Bone

- **Periostitis** (**per**-ee-os-**TYE**-tis) is an inflammation of the periosteum.
- **Osteopathy** (**oss**-tee-**OP**-ah-thee) refers to any bone disease.
- **Ostealgia** (**oss**-tee-**AL**-jee-ah), also called **ostalgia** (os-**TAL**-jee-ah), is any pain that is linked to an abnormal condition within a bone.
- **Osteitis** (**oss**-tee-**EYE**-tis) is an inflammation of bone.
- **Osteomyelitis** (**oss**-tee-oh-**my**-eh-**LYE**-tis) is an inflammation of the bone and bone marrow.
- **Osteonecrosis** (**oss**-tee-oh-nee-**KROH**-sis) is the destruction and necrosis (death) of bone tissue caused by ischemia, infection, malignancy or trauma.

  Ischemia (is-**KEY**-me-ah) is a decreased blood supply.
- A **sequestrum** (see-**KWES**-trum) is a piece of dead bone that is partially or fully detached from the adjacent or surrounding healthy bone.
- **Osteomalacia** (**oss**-tee-oh-mah-**LAY**-she-ah) is the softening of bones due to disease.
- **Osteoporosis** (**oss**-tee-oh-poh-**ROH**-sis) is a marked loss of bone density and increase in bone porosity that may result in bone fractures.
- **Rickets** (**RICK**-ets) is caused by calcium and vitamin D deficiencies in early childhood and results in demineralized bones and related deformities.
- An **exostosis** (**eck**-sos-**TOH**-sis) is a benign growth on the surface of a bone.
- A **myeloma** (**my**-eh-**LOH**-mah) is a malignant tumor made up of cells normally found in the bone marrow. Myelomas are named for the cells they are composed of.
- **Osteogenic sarcoma** (**oss**-tee-oh-**JEN**-ick sar-**KOH**-mah), also known as **osteosarcoma** (**oss**-tee-oh-sar-**KOH**-mah), is a malignant tumor usually involving the upper shaft of long bones, the pelvis, or knee.
- **Paget's disease,** also known as **osteitis deformans** (**oss**-tee-**EYE**-tis dee-**FOR**-manz), is a disease of unknown cause that is characterized by extensive bone destruction followed by abnormal bone repair.

PROCEDURES RELATED TO THE SKELETAL SYSTEM

- A **bursectomy** (ber-**SECK**-toh-me) is the surgical removal of a bursa.
- **Chondroplasty** (**KON**-droh-**plas**-tee) is the surgical repair of cartilage.
- **Synovectomy** (sin-oh-**VECK**-toh-me) is the surgical removal of a synovial membrane from a joint.
- **Periosteotomy** (**per**-ee-**oss**-tee-**OT**-oh-me) is an incision of the periosteum.
- An **arthrectomy** (ar-**THRECK**-toh-me) is the surgical removal of a joint.
- An **amputation** is the removal or all or part of a limb or body part.
- **Arthroplasty** (**AR**-throh-**plas**-tee) is the surgical repair or replacement of a damaged joint.
- A **craniectomy** (**kray**-nee-**EK**-toh-me) is the surgical removal of a portion of the skull.
- **Cranioplasty** (**KRAY**-nee-oh-**plas**-tee) is the surgical repair of the skull.
- A **craniotomy** (**kray**-nee-**OT**-oh-me) is a surgical incision or opening into the skull.

- **Diskectomy** (dis-**KECK**-toh-me) is the surgical removal of an intervertebral disk.
- A **laminectomy** (**lam**-ih-**NECK**-toh-me) is the surgical removal of a spinal lamina.
- **Arthrodesis** (**ar**-throh-**DEE**-sis), also known as **fusion**, is the surgical joining of spinal vertebrae. It also means surgical fusion of a joint. (The suffix *-DESIS* means to bind or tie together.)
- **Osteoclasis** (**oss**-tee-**OCK**-lah-sis) is the intentional surgical fracture of a bone to correct a deformity. (The suffix *-CLASIS* means break.)
- **Ostectomy** (oss-**TECK**-toh-me) is the surgical removal of bone.
- **Osteoplasty** (**OSS**-tee-oh-**plas**-tee) is the surgical repair of the bones.
- **Osteotomy** (**oss**-tee-**OT**-oh-me) is the surgical division or section of a bone.
- **Sequestrectomy** (**see**-kwes-**TRECK**-toh-me) is the surgical removal of a sequestrum.

The Treatment of Fractures

- **Reduction** is the process of pulling the bone pieces back into alignment. **Traction** may be used to reduce the fracture.
- The fractured bone is **immobilized** (not allowed to move) while it heals. This is usually accomplished with a **cast** or **splint.**
- As the bone heals a **callus** forms a bulging deposit around the area of the break. This eventually becomes bone.

IMPORTANT TERMS: THE SKELETAL SYSTEM

This list will help you identify and review the major terms from this chapter.

When you work with the audio tape for this chapter, listen to the word, repeat it and then place a ✓ next to it on the list below.

- ☐ **Acetabulum** (**ass**-eh-**TAB**-you-lum)
- ☐ **Acoustogram** (ah-**KOOS**-toh-gram)
- ☐ **Acromion** (ah-**KROH**-me-on)
- ☐ **Ankylosis** (**ang**-kih-**LOH**-sis)
- ☐ **Arthralgia** (ar-**THRAL**-jee-ah)
- ☐ **Arthrectomy** (ar-**THRECK**-toh-me)
- ☐ **Arthritis** (ar-**THRIGH**-tis)
- ☐ **Arthrocentesis** (**ar**-throh-sen-**TEE**-sis)
- ☐ **Arthrodesis** (**ar**-throh-**DEE**-sis)
- ☐ **Arthrodynia** (**ar**-throh-**DIN**-ee-ah)
- ☐ **Arthrography** (ar-**THROG**-rah-fee)
- ☐ **Arthroplasty** (**AR**-throh-**plas**-tee)
- ☐ **Arthropyosis** (**ar**-throh-pye-**OH**-sis)
- ☐ **Arthropathy** (ar-**THROP**-ah-thee)
- ☐ **Arthroscopy** (ar-**THROS**-koh-pee)
- ☐ **Articulate** (ar-**TICK**-you-late)
- ☐ **Bifida** (**BIF**-ih-dah)
- ☐ **Bursa** (**BER**-sah)
- ☐ **Bursectomy** (ber-**SECK**-toh-me)
- ☐ **Bursitis** (ber-**SIGH**-tis)
- ☐ **Calcaneal** (kal-**KAY**-nee-al)
- ☐ **Cancellous** (**KAN**-sell-us)
- ☐ **Carpals** (**KAR**-palz)

- ☐ **Cartilage (KAR-**tih-lidj)
- ☐ **Cervical (SER-**vih-kal)
- ☐ **Chondropathy** (kon-**DROP-**ah-thee)
- ☐ **Chondroplasty (KON-**droh-**plas-**tee)
- ☐ **Chondromalacia (kon-**droh-mah-**LAY-**she-ah)
- ☐ **Clavicle (KLAV-**ih-kul)
- ☐ **Coccyx (KOCK-**sicks)
- ☐ **Conchae (KONG-**kee)
- ☐ **Condyle (KON-**dial)
- ☐ **Craniectomy (kray-**nee-**EK-**toh-me)
- ☐ **Cranioplasty (KRAY-**nee-oh-**plas-**tee)
- ☐ **Craniotomy (kray-**nee-**OT-**oh-me)
- ☐ **Cranium (KRAY-**nee-um)
- ☐ **Crepitation (krep-**ih-**TAY-**shun)
- ☐ **Diskectomy** (dis-**KECK-**toh-me)
- ☐ **Epiphysis** (eh-**PIF-**ih-sis)
- ☐ **Ethmoid (ETH-**moid)
- ☐ **Exostosis (eck-**sos-**TOH-**sis)
- ☐ **Femoral (FEM-**or-al)
- ☐ **Femur (FEE-**mur)
- ☐ **Fibula (FIB-**you-lah)
- ☐ **Fontanelle (fon-**tah-**NELL)**
- ☐ **Foramen** (foh-**RAY-**men)
- ☐ **Gouty (GOW-**tee)
- ☐ **Hematopoietic (hem-**ah-toh-poi-**ET-**ick)
- ☐ **Humerus (HEW-**mer-us)
- ☐ **Hyoid (HIGH-**oid)
- ☐ **Ilium (ILL-**ee-um)
- ☐ **Incus (ING-**kus)
- ☐ **Ischemia** (is-**KEY-**me-ah)
- ☐ **Ischium (ISS-**key-um)
- ☐ **Kyphosis** (kigh-**FOH-**sis)
- ☐ **Lacrimal (LACK-**rih-mal)
- ☐ **Lamina (LAM-**ih-nah)
- ☐ **Laminectomy (lam-**ih-**NECK-**toh-me)
- ☐ **Lordosis** (lor-**DOH-**sis)
- ☐ **Lumbago** (lum-**BAY-**go)
- ☐ **Lumbar (LUM-**bar)
- ☐ **Lupus erythematosus (LOO-**pus er-ih-**thee-**mah-**TOH-**sus)
- ☐ **Luxation** (luck-**SAY-**shun)
- ☐ **Malleolus** (mal-**LEE-**oh-lus)
- ☐ **Malleus (MAL-**ee-us)
- ☐ **Mandible (MAN-**dih-bul)
- ☐ **Manubrium** (mah-**NEW-**bree-um)
- ☐ **Maxillary** (**MACK-**sih-**ler-**ee)
- ☐ **Meatus** (me-**AY-**tus)
- ☐ **Meniscus** (meh-**NIS-**kus)
- ☐ **Metacarpals** (met-ah-**KAR-**palz)
- ☐ **Metatarsals (met-**ah-**TAR-**salz)
- ☐ **Myelography (my-**eh-**LOG-**rah-fee)
- ☐ **Myeloma (my-**eh-**LOH-**mah)
- ☐ **Occipital** (ock-**SIP-**ih-tal)
- ☐ **Olecranon** (oh-**LEK-**rah-non)
- ☐ **Os coxae (OSS KOCK-**sigh)
- ☐ **Ostalgia** (os-**TAL-**jee-ah)
- ☐ **Ostealgia (oss-**tee-**AL-**jee-ah)

- ☐ **Ostectomy** (oss-**TECK**-toh-me)
- ☐ **Osteitis deformans** (**oss**-tee-**EYE**-tis dee-**FOR**-manz)
- ☐ **Osteoarthritis** (**oss**-tee-oh-ar-**THRIGH**-tis)
- ☐ **Osteoclasis** (**oss**-tee-**OCK**-lah-sis)
- ☐ **Osteogenic** (**oss**-tee-oh-**JEN**-ick)
- ☐ **Osteomalacia** (**oss**-tee-oh-mah-**LAY**-she-ah)
- ☐ **Osteomyelitis** (**oss**-tee-oh-**my**-eh-**LYE**-tis)
- ☐ **Osteonecrosis** (**oss**-tee-oh-nee-**KROH**-sis)
- ☐ **Osteopathy** (**oss**-tee-**OP**-ah-thee)
- ☐ **Osteoplasty** (**OSS**-tee-oh-**plas**-tee)
- ☐ **Osteoporosis** (**oss**-tee-oh-poh-**ROH**-sis)
- ☐ **Osteosarcoma** (**oss**-tee-oh-sar-**KOH**-mah)
- ☐ **Osteotomy** (**oss**-tee-**OT**-oh-me)
- ☐ **Palatine** (**PAL**-ah-tine)
- ☐ **Parietal** (pah-**RYE**-eh-tal)
- ☐ **Patella** (pah-**TEL**-ah)
- ☐ **Periosteotomy** (**per**-ee-**oss**-tee-**OT**-oh-me)
- ☐ **Periostitis** (**per**-ee-os-**TYE**-tis)
- ☐ **Periosteum** (**per**-ee-**OSS**-tee-um)
- ☐ **Phalanges** (fah-**LAN**-jeez)
- ☐ **Pubic symphysis** (**PEW**-bick **SIM**-fih-sis)
- ☐ **Pubis** (**PEW**-bis)
- ☐ **Radius** (**RAY**-dee-us)
- ☐ **Rheumatoid** (**ROO**-mah-toyd)
- ☐ **Rickets** (**RICK**-ets)
- ☐ **Sacroiliac** (say-kroh-**ILL**-ee-ack)
- ☐ **Sacrum** (**SAY**-krum)
- ☐ **Scapula** (**SKAP**-you-lah)
- ☐ **Scoliosis** (**skoh**-lee-**OH**-sis)
- ☐ **Sella turcica** (**SELL**-ah **TUR**-sih-kah)
- ☐ **Sequestrum** (see-**KWES**-trum)
- ☐ **Sequestrectomy** (**see**-kwes-**TRECK**-toh-me)
- ☐ **Sphenoid** (**SFEE**-noid)
- ☐ **Spondylolisthesis** (**spon**-dih-loh-**LIS**-thee-sis)
- ☐ **Spondylosis** (**spon**-dih-**LOH**-sis)
- ☐ **Stapes** (**STAY**-peez)
- ☐ **Sternum** (**STER**-num)
- ☐ **Subluxation** (**sub**-luck-**SAY**-shun)
- ☐ **Synovectomy** (sin-oh-**VECK**-toh-me)
- ☐ **Tarsals** (**TAHR**-salz)
- ☐ **Temporomandibular** (**tem**-poh-roh-man-**DIB**-you-lar)
- ☐ **Thoracic** (thoh-**RASS**-ick)
- ☐ **Tibia** (**TIB**-ee-ah)
- ☐ **Trochanter** (tro-**KAN**-ter)
- ☐ **Ulna** (**ULL**-nah)
- ☐ **Vertebrae** (**VER**-teh-bree)
- ☐ **Vertebral** (**VER**-teh-bral)
- ☐ **Vomer** (**VOH**-mer)
- ☐ **Xiphoid** (**ZIF**-oid)
- ☐ **Zygomatic** (zye-go-**MAT**-ick)

3

EXERCISES

DEFINING WORD PARTS

Write the definition for each of these word parts.

1. *ARTHR/O* ______
2. *BURS/O* ______
3. *CHONDR/O* ______
4. *COST/O* ______
5. *CRANI/O* ______
6. *ILI/O* ______
7. *LAMIN/O* ______
8. *LIGAMENT/O* ______
9. *MYEL/O* ______
10. *OSS/E, OSS/I* ______
11. *OSTE/O* ______
12. *SPONDYL/O* ______
13. *SYNOVI/O* ______
14. *THORAC/O* ______
15. *VERTEBR/O* ______

DEFINITIONS

Circle the letter next to the correct answer.

1. Cancellous bone is also known as _______________ bone.
   a) compact
   b) cortical
   c) periosteal
   d) spongy

2. The tarsals are the bones that make up the _______________
   a) ankles.
   b) fingers.
   c) toes.
   d) wrists.

3. The manubrium is the _______________
   a) lower jaw.
   b) lower portion of the sternum.
   c) thin, scroll-like bone of the nose.
   d) upper portion of the sternum.

4. The _______________ skeleton consists of the skull, spinal column, ribs and sternum.
   a) appendicular
   b) axial
   c) pectoral
   d) ventral

5. The sacrum is _______________
   a) slightly curved.
   b) triangular in shape.
   c) separate bones at birth.
   d) a, b and c.

6. The fontanelle is the _______________
   a) base of the skull.
   b) bone that forms the forehead.
   c) head of the femur.
   d) soft spot on a baby's head.

7. Ligaments are _______________
   a) fibrous connective bands that unite the articulating ends of bones.
   b) joints that move only slightly.
   c) more elastic than bone.
   d) b and c.

8. The acetabulum is the ____________________
   a) extension of the scapula that forms the high point of the shoulder.
   b) knee cap.
   c) large socket in the pelvic bones.
   d) shin bone.

9. The thoracic vertebrae ____________________
   a) are a set of twelve vertebrae.
   b) are also known as the dorsal vertebrae.
   c) form the outward curve of the spine.
   d) a, b and c.

10. The trochanter is the large bony projection of the ____________________
    a) fibula.
    b) lower end of the ilium.
    c) upper end of the femur.
    d) tibia.

MISSING WORDS

Write the missing word on the line.

1. ____________________ is the form of arthritis most commonly associated with aging.
2. The ____________________ is the bony socket surrounding the eye.
3. A/an ____________________ is a fibrous sac between certain tendons and the bones beneath them.
4. A/an ____________________ is the surgical removal of a spinal lamina.
5. ____________________ is the loss or absence of mobility in a joint because the bones have abnormally fused together.
6. A/an ____________________ fracture occurs when the bone is pressed together upon itself.
7. ____________________ joints are the moveable joints of the body.
8. The ____________________ process is the lower portion of the sternum.
9. ____________________ is caused by calcium and vitamin D deficiencies in early childhood.
10. ____________________ is the sound heard when the ends of a broken bone move together.
11. The ____________________ are the bones of the fingers and toes.
12. A/an ____________________ is a harmless growth on the surface of a bone.
13. The ____________________ is the tough and fibrous outermost covering of bone.

14. The spinal column consists of 26 ____________________.

15. As a fractured bone heals, a/an ____________________ forms a bulging deposit around the area of the break.

SPELLCHECK

Select the correct spelling and write it on the line.

1. ____________________ is also known as low back pain.
   Lumbaego
   Lumbago
   Lumbargo

2. The ____________________ is also known as the collar bone.
   clavical
   clavicle
   clavicole

3. The ____________________ is the projecting posterior portion of each vertebra.
   lamina
   laminae
   laminax

4. ____________________ is any degenerative condition of the spine.
   Spondilosis
   Spondolosis
   Spondylosis

5. A ____________________ disk is a rupture of the intervertebral disk that results in pressure on spinal nerve roots.
   hernia
   herneated
   herniated

6. ____________________ is an abnormal lateral curvature of the spine.
   Scoliosis
   Scolliosis
   Scolosis

7. A ____________________ is a piece of dead bone that is partially or fully detached from the surrounding healthy bone.
   sequestrium
   sequestrom
   sequestrum

8. The ______________________ is the bony portion of the kneecap.
   patella
   patilla
   potella

9. In a ______________________ fracture the bone is splintered or crushed.
   cominuted
   comminuted
   commuted

10. ______________________ is the diagnostic study of the spinal cord after the injection of a contrast medium.
    Myalography
    Myelography
    Myography

11. ______________________ is the abnormal softening of the cartilage.
    Chondomalacia
    Chondromalacia
    Chrondromalacia

12. The ______________________ is the rounded bony protuberance on each side of the ankle.
    mallalus
    malleolus
    malleulus

13. The ______________________ is the curved fibrous cartilage found in some joints such as the knee.
    menicus
    meniocus
    meniscus

14. The ______________________ bones form most of the roof and upper sides of the cranium.
    parietal
    parital
    paritel

15. The ______________________ is commonly known as the tailbone.
    coccix
    coccyx
    cocoyx

CASE STUDIES

Write the correct answer on the line.

1. Bobby Jenkins fell out of a tree and broke his arm. Dr. Parker described this as a closed or ________________________ fracture because although the bone was broken there was no open wound of the skin.
2. Eduardo Sanchez has ________________________ which is an inflammation of the bone and bone marrow.
3. Elderly Mrs. Hargreaves broke her hip because of ________________________ which is a marked decrease in bone density.
4. Mr. Morton suffers from ________________________. This condition is also known as humpback.
5. Willard Sorenson has a/an ________________________ which is a tumor made up of cells normally found in the bone marrow.
6. Henry Turner suffers from ________________________ disease, which is also known as osteitis deformans.
7. Doris Horner is being treated for a/an ________________________ sarcoma of the knee.
8. Harold Ewing was born with ________________________ which is a congenital failure of the spinal canal to close over the spinal cord.
9. Because of her back problems, Patricia Gilmer required a/an ________________________ of three spinal vertebrae.
10. As Jack Hansen's fractured fibula began to heal, a bulging deposit called a/an ________________________ formed around the area of the break.
11. Betty Greene has been running for several years; however, now her knees hurt. Dr. Baskin diagnosed that she has ________________________ which is an abnormal softening of the cartilage in these joints.
12. Robert Young has a very sore shoulder. Dr. Wilson diagnosed it as ________________________ or an inflammation of the bursa.
13. As a result of his motorcycle accident, Martin Hagelman required ________________________ to surgically reconstruct his damaged knee.
14. Dr. Jackson performed ________________________ to remove synovial fluid for analysis.
15. Patty Turner (age 7) has ________________________ ________________________ arthritis, which results in swollen and painful joints.

16. When Mrs. Adams fell, she broke the portion of the femoral bone just below the trochanter. This was described on her chart as a fracture of the ______________________ neck.

17. Cindy Pollack, age 4, fell and hurt her leg. Dr. Brown said that she had an incomplete or ______________________ fracture.

18. Because of his back injury, David Newman required a/an ______________________ which is the complete removal of an intervertebral disk.

19. Patricia Chu fell and broke both bones in her lower left arm. Dr. Ross called these bones the ______________________ and the ______________________.

20. The injury to his neck damaged one of Sam Green's ______________________ vertebrae.

WORD BUILDING

Write the correct word or word part on the line.

1. Bone and bone marrow
   a) The combining form ______________________ means bone.
   b) The combining form ______________________ means bone marrow.
   c) The suffix ______________________ means inflammation.
   d) The term ______________________ means an inflammation of the bone and bone marrow.

2. Visual examination of a joint
   a) The combining form ______________________ means joint.
   b) The suffix ______________________ means visual examination.
   c) The term ______________________ means visual examination of a joint.

3. Surgical fusion
   a) The combining form ______________________ means joint.
   b) The suffix ______________________ means to bind or tie together.
   c) The term ______________________ means fusion or surgical joining of a joint (particularly of spinal vertebrae).

4. Abnormal softening of cartilage
   a) The combining form ______________________ means cartilage.
   b) The suffix ______________________ means abnormal softening.
   c) The term ______________________ means abnormal softening of cartilage.

LABELING EXERCISES

Identify the numbered items on these diagrams.

1. ______________________________
2. ______________________________
3. ______________________________
4. ______________________________
5. ______________________________
6. ______________________________
7. ______________________________
8. ______________________________
9. ______________________________
10. ______________________________

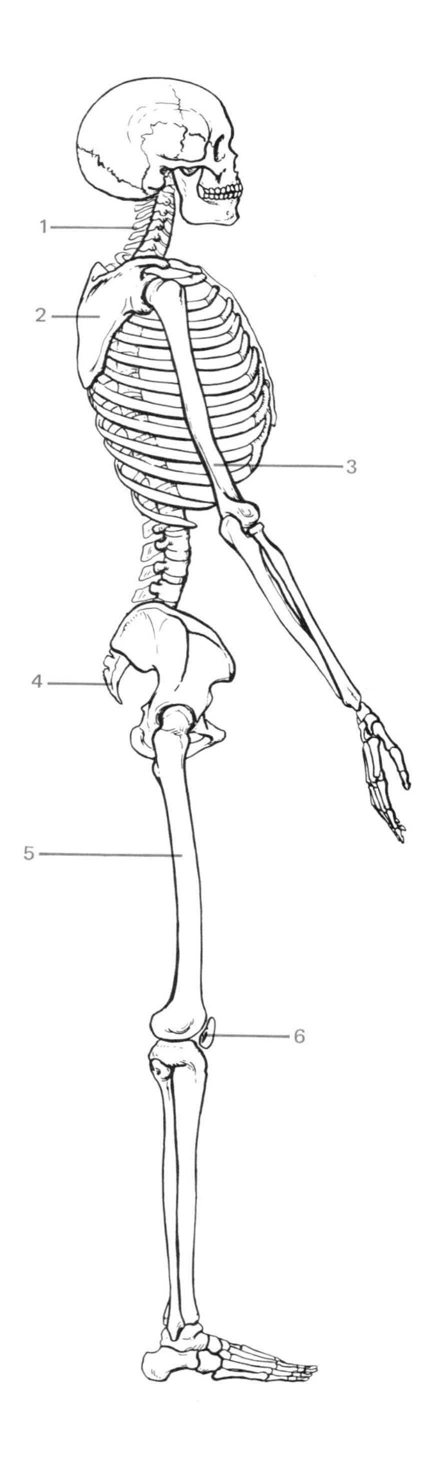

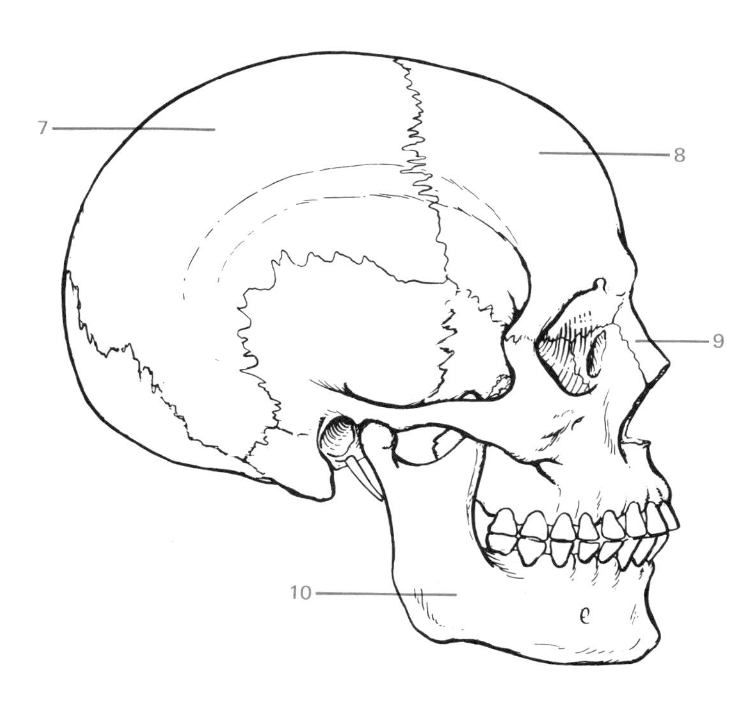

4

THE MUSCULAR SYSTEM

LEARNING GOALS

In this chapter you will learn to:

- describe how muscle fibers are organized and attached to bones.
- name the three types of muscles.
- define the terms related to muscles and to muscle action.
- recognize and define the terms related to the diagnosis, pathology and treatment of disorders of the muscular system.

INTRODUCTION TO THE MUSCULAR SYSTEM

The muscular system makes possible movement and many of the internal functions of the human body. (The combining form *MY/O* means muscle.)

THE STRUCTURE OF MUSCLES

Muscle Fibers

The muscles are composed of long, slender cells known as muscle fibers. Each muscle consists of a group of fibers held together by connective tissue and enclosed in a fibrous sheath. (The combining form *FIBROS/O* means fibrous tissue.)

Fascia

Fascia (**FASH**-ee-ah) is the fibrous sheet of connective tissue that covers, supports, and separates muscles. (The combining form *FASCI/O* means fascia or fibrous band.)

Tendons

A tendon is a narrow band of fibrous tissue that attaches a muscle to bone. (The combing forms *TEN/O, TEND/O,* and *TENDIN/O* all mean tendon.)

Be careful not to confuse tendons with ligaments, which are discussed in Chapter 3.

The **Achilles tendon,** also known as the **tendon calcaneus,** extends from the calf to the heel. The **hamstrings,** which are the tendons of the thigh muscles, flex the leg at the knee.

Aponeurosis

An aponeurosis (**ap**-oh-new-**ROH**-sis) is a broad, flat sheet of fibrous connective tissue.

An aponeurosis serves as a specialized tendon to attach muscles to bone. It may also serve as fascia to bind muscles together. (Plural, **aponeuroses.**)

TYPES OF MUSCLES

There are three types of muscle tissue. These types are described according to their appearance and their function.

Striated Muscle

Striated (**STRY**-ayt-ed) muscles are so named because dark and light bands in the muscle fibers create a striped, or striated, appearance. Striated muscles are also known as the skeletal or voluntary muscles.

- **Skeletal muscles** attach to the bones of the skeleton and make bodily motion possible.
- **Voluntary muscles,** such as the muscles of the face and eyes, are so named because we have conscious (voluntary) control over these muscles.

Smooth Muscle

Smooth muscle fibers move the internal organs such as the digestive tract, blood vessels, and secretory ducts leading from glands.

In contrast to the marked contraction and relaxation of the striated muscles, smooth muscles produce relatively slow contraction.

Smooth muscles are also know as unstriated, involuntary, or visceral muscles.

- **Unstriated muscles** are so named because they do not have the dark and light bands that produce the striped (striated) appearance seen in striated muscles.
- **Involuntary muscles** are so named because they are under the control of the autonomic nervous system and are not controlled voluntarily.
- **Visceral muscles** are so named because they are found in the visceral organs (except the heart) and in hollow structures such as the digestive and urinary tracts.

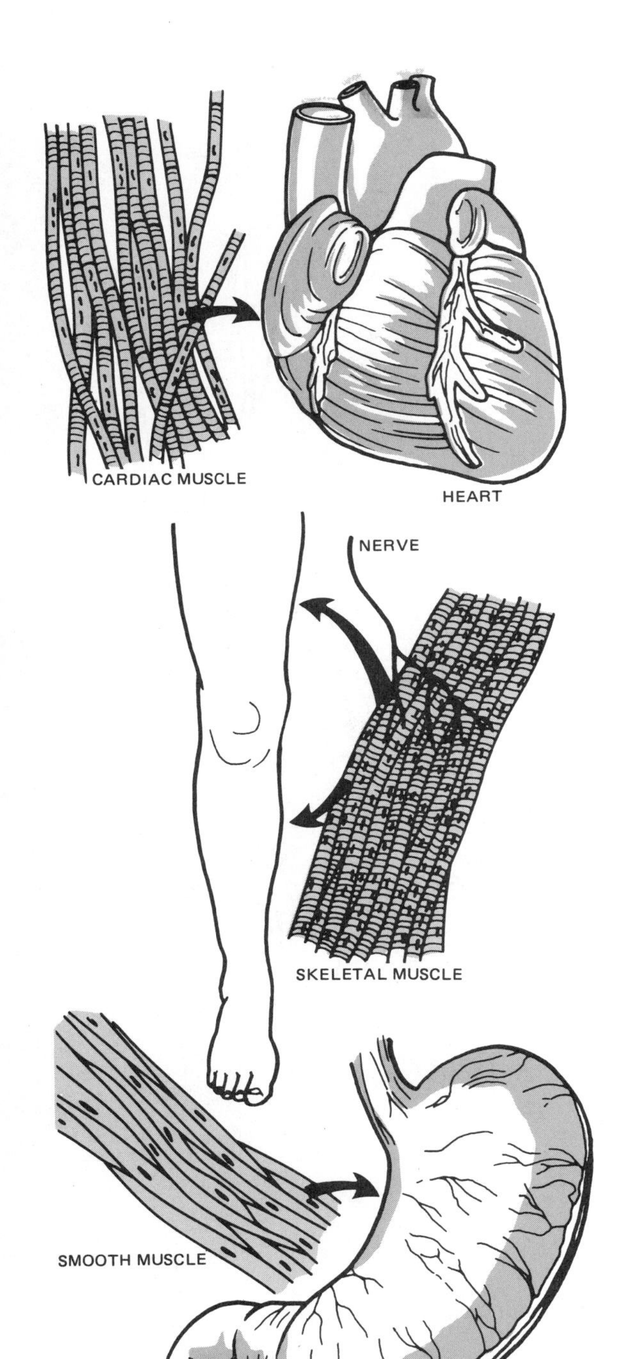

Figure 4-1 Types of muscles.

Cardiac Muscle

Cardiac muscle, also known as **myocardium,** (**my-oh-KAR-**dee-um) is striated in appearance but like smooth muscle in its action. (The combining form *CARDI/O* means heart.)

Cardiac muscle forms most of the wall of the heart. It is the contraction of this muscle that causes the heartbeat.

TYPES OF MUSCLE MOVEMENTS

Flexion and Extension

Flexion (FLECK-shun) means decreasing the angle between two bones or bending a limb at a joint. A **flexor** is a muscle that bends a limb at a joint. **Dorsiflexion** is backward bending as of the hand or foot. (The combining form *DORS/I* means back of the body and *FLEX/O* means bend.)

Extension means increasing the angle between two bones or straightening out a limb. An **extensor** is a muscle that straightens a limb at a joint. (The prefix *EX-* means away from and the combining form *TENS/O* means to stretch out, extend or strain.)

Abduction and Adduction

Abduction is movement away from the midline of the body. (The prefix *AB-* means away from and the combining form *DUCT/O* means to carry or lead.) An **abductor** is a muscle that moves a part away from the midline.

Adduction is movement toward the midline of the body. (The prefix *AD-* means toward.) An **adductor** is a muscle that moves a part toward the midline.

Rotation and Circumduction

Rotation is a circular movement around an axis. A **rotator** is a muscle that rotates a body part on its axis.

For example, when you hold your arm straight out from your body and swing it in a wide circle, you are rotating it.

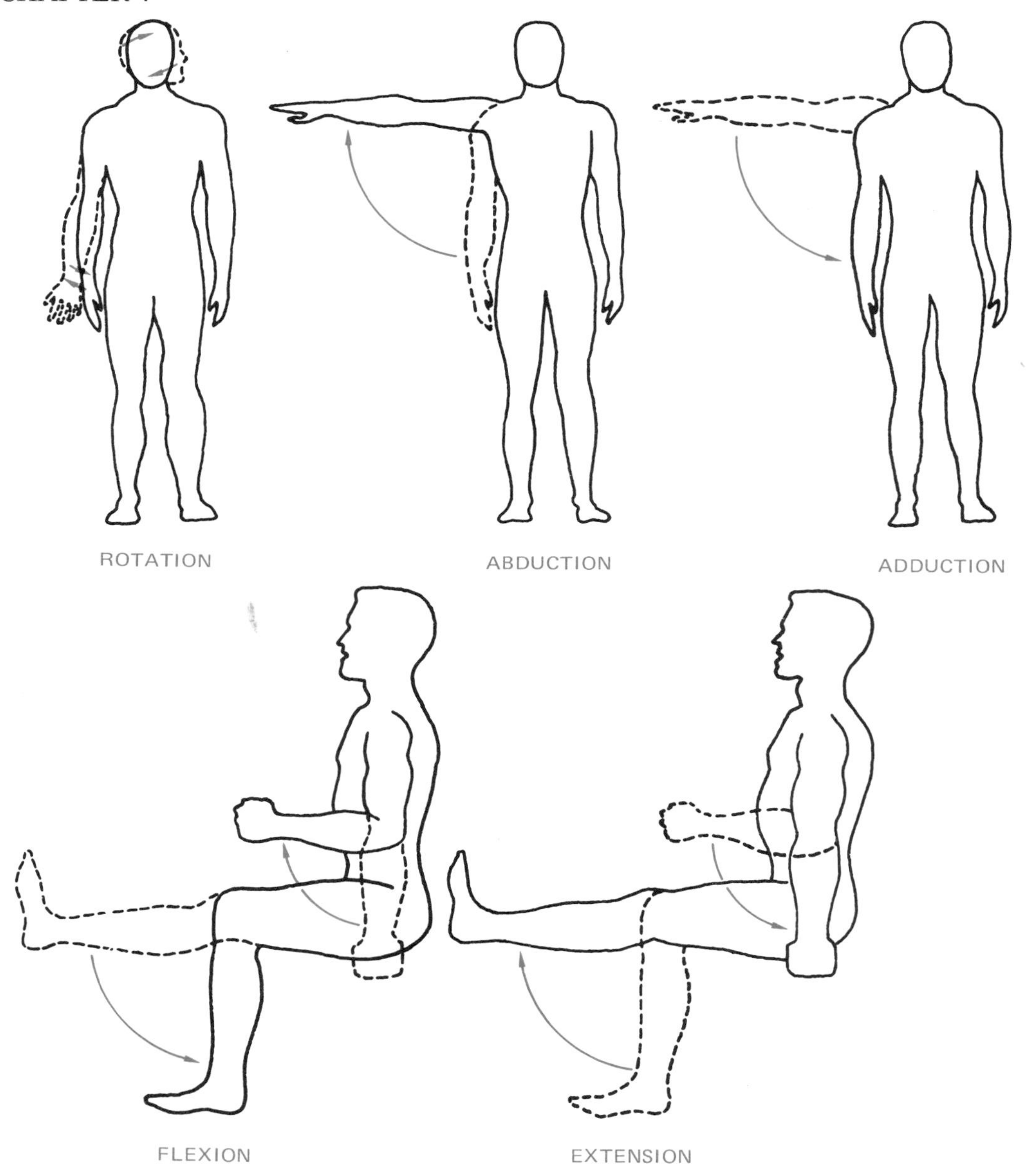

Figure 4-2 Kinds of movements.

Circumduction (**ser**-kum-**DUCK**-shun) is a circular movement of a limb at the far end. It also refers to the movement of a bone within a joint and the circular movement of the eye. (The prefix *CIRCUM-* means around.) For example, the movement of the head of the femur within the hip joint is circumduction.

Pronation and Supination

Pronation (proh-NAY-shun) is a rotating movement in which the forearm turns the hand so that the palm is downward or backward.

Supination (soo-pih-NAY-shun) is a rotating movement in which the forearm turns the hand so that the palm is forward or upward.

Elevation and Depression

Elevation is the act of raising or lifting up a body part such as raising the ribs when breathing in. A **levator** (lee-VAY-tor) is a muscle that raises a body part. (The combining forms *LEV/O* and *LEVAT/O* mean to raise or lift up.)

Depression is the act of lowering a body part such as lowering the ribs when breathing out. A **depressor** is a muscle that lowers a body part. (The combining form *PRESS/O* means to press or draw.)

Contraction and Relaxation

Muscles are the only body tissues with the specialized ability to contract and relax. **Contraction** is the tightening of a muscle, during which it becomes shorter and thicker.

Relaxation occurs when a muscle returns to its original form or shape. It is these contrasting actions that make motion possible.

Kinesiology (kih-nee-see-OL-oh-jee) is the study of muscular activity and the movement of body parts. (The combining form *KINESI/O* and the suffix *-KINESIS* both mean movement or motion.)

Antagonistic Muscle Pairs

The muscles of the body are arranged in antagonistic pairs. One produces movement in a single direction. The other does so in the opposite direction.

For example, the muscles of the upper arm are an antagonist pair. When the biceps (located on the front) contracts and the triceps (located on the back) relaxes, the arm is bent at the elbow. When the triceps contracts and the biceps relaxes, the arm is extended.

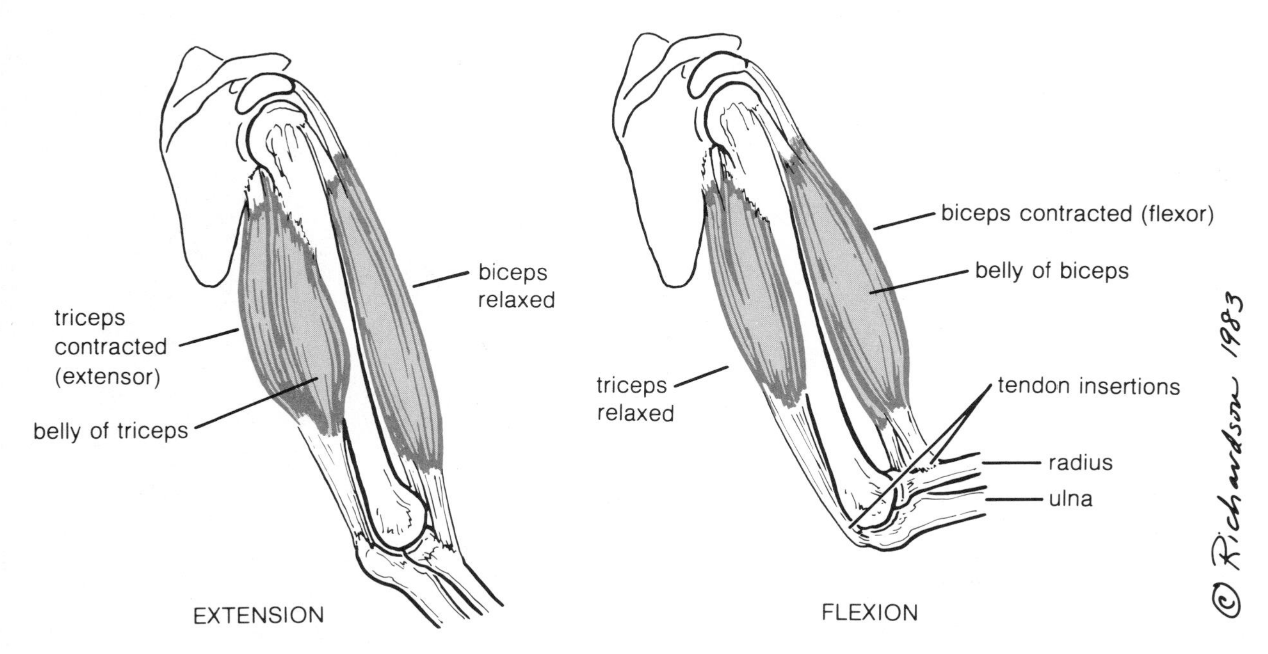

Figure 4-3 Coordination of antagonistic muscles.

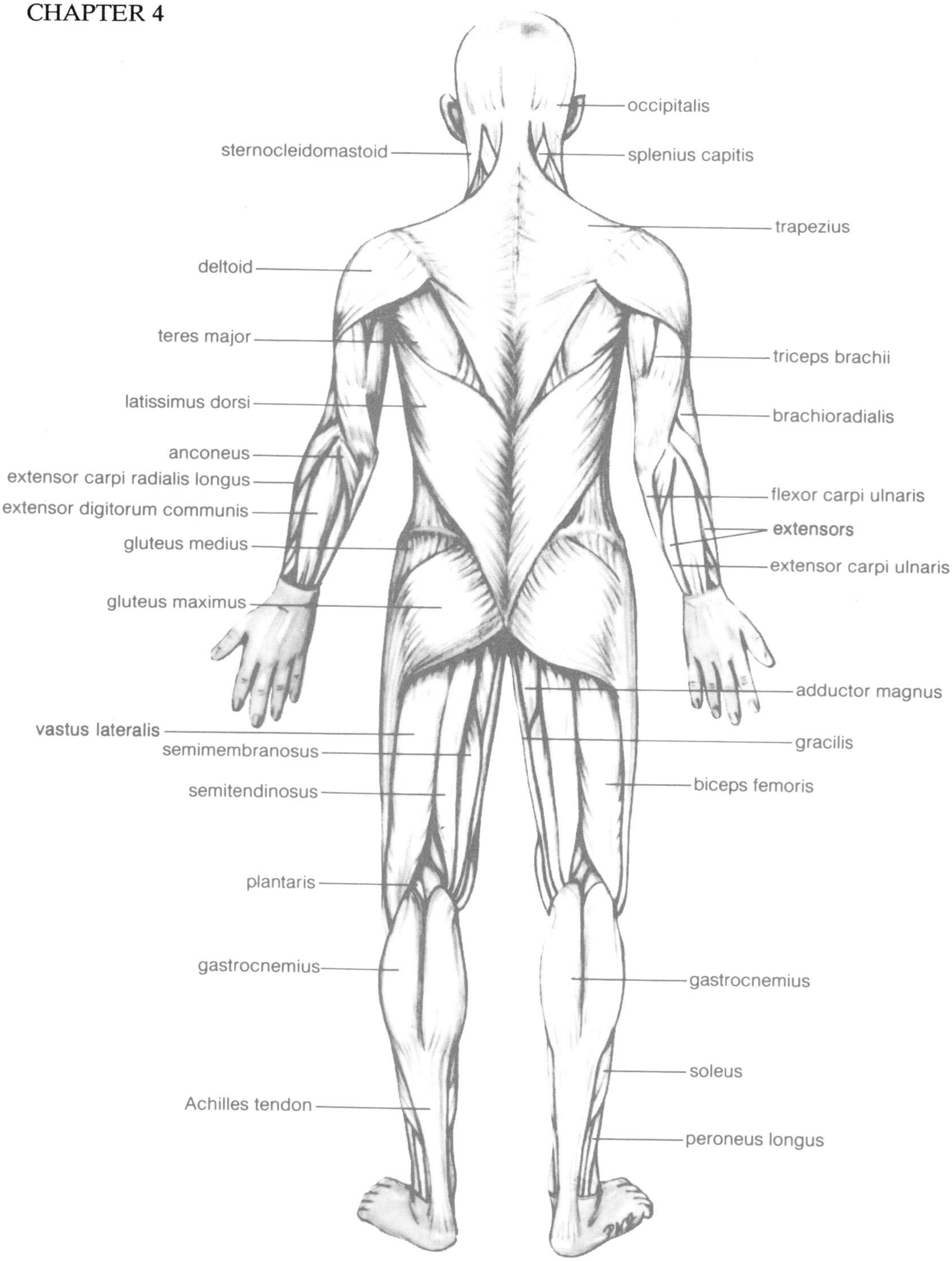

occipitalis
sternocleidomastoid
splenius capitis
trapezius
deltoid
teres major
triceps brachii
latissimus dorsi
brachioradialis
anconeus
extensor carpi radialis longus
flexor carpi ulnaris
extensor digitorum communis
extensors
gluteus medius
extensor carpi ulnaris
gluteus maximus
adductor magnus
vastus lateralis
semimembranosus
gracilis
semitendinosus
biceps femoris
plantaris
gastrocnemius
gastrocnemius
soleus
Achilles tendon
peroneus longus

Figure 4-4 Major muscles of the body (posterior view).

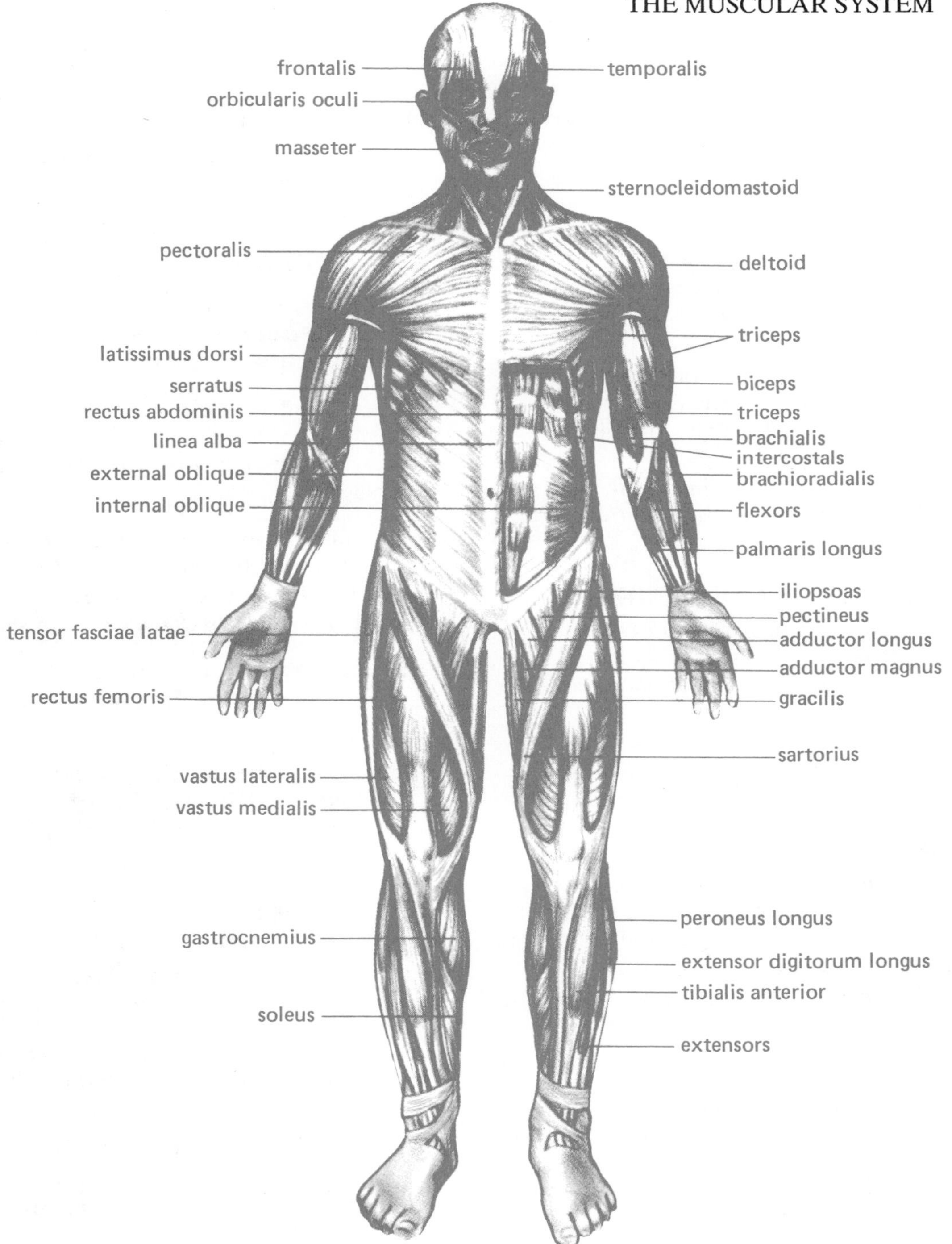

Figure 4-5 Major muscles of the body (anterior view).

Muscle Tone

Muscle tone, also known as **tonus** (**TOH**-nus), is the normal state of balanced tension that is present in the body when one is awake. (The combining form *TON/O* means tone, tension or stretching.)

MUSCLE STIMULATION

All muscle actions, either contraction or relaxation, are stimulated by nerve impulses. These impulses are provided by motor nerves.

A **myoneural junction** (**my-oh-NEW-ral**) is the point at which nerve endings come into contact with muscle cells. (The combining form *NEUR/O* means nerve.)

If the nerve impulse is interrupted, the muscle is paralyzed and cannot either contract or relax.

HOW MUSCLES ARE NAMED

There are more than 600 muscles in the body. Happily it is not necessary to memorize all of their names. However, you will find it helpful to understand how muscles are named.

Origin and Insertion

The names of some muscles are formed by joining the names of the place of origin and the place of insertion.

Muscle origin is the place where the muscle begins (originates). This is the more fixed attachment and/or the end of the muscle that is toward the midline of the body.

Muscle insertion is the place where the muscle ends (inserts). It is the more moveable end and/or the portion of the muscle that is away from the midline of the body.

For example, the **sternocleidomastoid** (**ster-no-kly-doh-MASS-toid**) helps to flex the neck and rotate the head. It originates from the sternum *(STERN/O)* and clavicle *(CLEID/O)* which are both near the midline.

It inserts into the mastoid *(MAST/O)* process of the temporal bone, which is further away from the midline.

Muscles Named for Their Action

Some muscles are named for their action such as lifting, flexing or extending.

For example, **levatores costarum** (**lev-ah-TOH-reez kahs-TAH-rum**) are the lifting muscles of the ribs.

Muscles Named for Fiber Direction

Some muscles are named according to the direction of the muscle fibers such as vertical, horizontal or transverse directions. For example:

- **Rectus abdominis** is the abdominal muscle in a straight alignment with the vertical axis of the body. (**Rectus** (**RECK-tus**) means straight.)
- The **oblique externus abdominis** is an abdominal muscle that slants outward, at an angle, from the midline. (**Oblique** (**oh-BLEEK**) means slanted or at an angle.)
- The **transversus abdominis** is the transverse abdominal muscle. (**Transverse** means in a crosswise direction.)
- The **anal sphincter** closes the rectum. (A **sphincter** (**SFINK-ter**) is a ring-like muscle that tightly constricts the opening of a passageway.)

Muscles Named for the Number of Divisions

Some muscles are named according to the number of divisions forming them. For example:

- The **biceps** is the muscle of the anterior upper arm. It flexes the elbow. It is formed from two divisions.
- The **triceps brachii** (**BRAY-kee-eye**) is the muscle of the posterior upper arm. It extends the elbow and is formed from three divisions.

- The **quadriceps femoris** (**FEM**-or-iss) is the large muscle on the anterior thigh. It assists in extending the leg and is formed from four divisions.

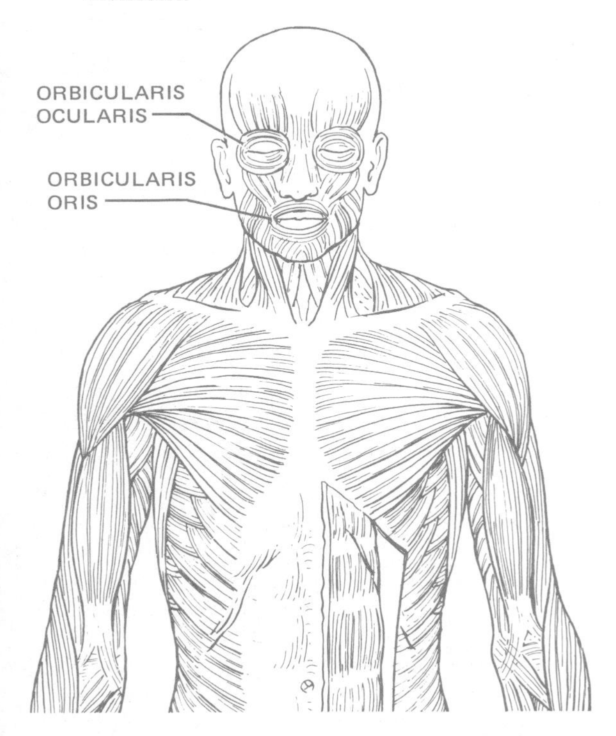

Figure 4-6 Muscles named for their location.

Muscles Named for Their Location

Many muscles are named for their location on the body or the organ they are near.

For example, **orbicularis oris** (or-**bick**-you-**LAY**-riss **OR**-iss) is the circular muscle that surrounds the mouth. (**Oris** means mouth or oral. **Orbicularis** means circular.)

Muscles Named for Their Shape

Some muscles are named because they are shaped like a familiar object. For example, the **deltoid muscle,** which forms the shoulder cap, is shaped like an inverted triangle or the Greek letter D (delta).

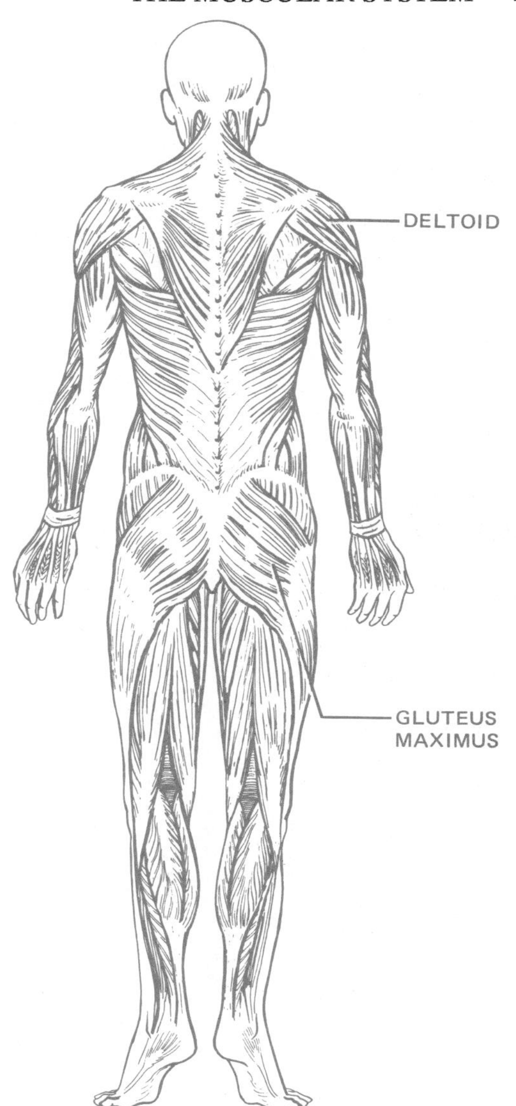

Figure 4-7 Muscles named for their size and shape.

Muscles Named for Their Size

Some muscles are named because they are broad or narrow, large or small. For example, **gluteus maximus** (**GLOO**-tee-us) is the largest muscle of the buttock. **Gluteus minimus** is the smallest muscle of the buttock.

DIAGNOSTIC PROCEDURES RELATED TO THE MUSCULAR SYSTEM

- **Electromyography,** (ee-**leck**-troh-my-**OG**-rah-fee), also known as EMG, records the strength of muscle contraction as a result of electrical stimulation. The resulting record is called an **electromyogram.**
- **Electroneuromyography** (ee-**leck**-troh-**new**-roh-my-**OG**-rah-fee) is a procedure for testing and recording neuromuscular activity by the electric stimulation of nerves.

PATHOLOGY OF THE MUSCULAR SYSTEM

Pathology of Fibers, Fascia and Tendons

- **Fibrositis** (**figh**-broh-**SIGH**-tis) is an inflammation of fibrous connective tissues that is usually characterized by a poorly defined set of symptoms.
- **Fasciitis** (**fas**-ee-**EYE**-tis) is inflammation of a fascia. (Be careful of the spelling on this one. There really are two letter *i*'s next to each other.)
- **Tendinitis** (**ten**-dih-**NIGH**-tis) is an inflammation of a tendon. (This may also be spelled tendonitis.)

Pathology of Muscle Action

- **Atonic** (ah-**TON**-ick) means lacking normal muscle tone.
- **Dystonia** (dis-**TOH**-nee-ah) is a condition of impaired muscle tone.
- **Myasthenia** (**my**-as-**THEE**-nee-ah) means muscle weakness.
- **Muscle atrophy** (**AT**-roh-fee) is muscle weakness and wasting caused by disuse of the muscle over a long period.
- **Ataxia** (ah-**TACK**-see-ah) is a lack of muscular coordination. (The combining form *TAX/O* means coordination.)
- **Myoparesis** (**my**-oh-**PAR**-eh-sis) is a weakness or slight paralysis of a muscle. (The suffix *-PARESIS* means slight paralysis.)
- **Paralysis** is the of loss sensation and voluntary muscle movements. It may be either temporary or permanent.
- **Tremors** are rhythmic, purposeless quivering movements.

Pathology of Muscles

- **Myalgia** (my-**AL**-jee-ah) is muscle tenderness or pain. (The suffix *-ALGIA* means pain.)
- **Myositis** (**my**-oh-**SIGH**-tis) means inflammation of a muscle or muscles. (May also be spelled myitis.)
- **Polymyositis** (**pol**-ee-**my**-oh-**SIGH**-tis) is the inflammation of several muscles at once.
- An **adhesion** is a band of fibers that holds structures together abnormally. Adhesions may form as the result of an injury or surgery. (The combining form *ADHES/O* means to stick to.)
- **Contracture** is an abnormal shortening of muscle tissues making the muscle resistant to stretching.
- **Myocele** (**MY**-oh-seel) is a protrusion of a muscle through its ruptured sheath or fascia. (The suffix *-CELE* means a tumor, cyst or hernia.)
- A **hernia** (**HER**-nee-ah) is the rupture and abnormal protrusion of an organ through its containing muscular wall.
- **Torticollis** (**tor**-tih-**KOL**-is), also known as **wryneck,** is a stiff neck due to spasmodic contraction of the sternocleidomastoid muscle, causing the head to be pulled to the af-

fected side. (The combining form *TORT/I* means twisted.)

- **Myomalacia** (**my**-oh-mah-**LAY**-she-ah) is abnormal softening of muscle tissue.
- **Myosclerosis** (**my**-oh-skle-**ROH**-sis) is abnormal hardening of muscle tissue.
- **Myosarcoma** (**my**-oh-sahr-**KOH**-mah) is a malignant tumor derived from muscle tissue.
- **Myasthenia gravis** (**my**-as-**THEE**-nee-ah **GRAH**-vis) is a chronic neuromuscular disease characterized by great muscular weakness and a progressive paralysis of the muscular system.
- **Muscular dystrophy** (**DIS**-troh-fee) is a group of inherited diseases characterized by progressive weakness and degeneration of muscle fibers without involvement of the nervous system.

PROCEDURES RELATED TO THE MUSCULAR SYSTEM

- **Fasciectomy** (**fas**-ee-**ECK**-toh-me) is the surgical removal of fascia.
- **Fascioplasty** (**fash**-ee-oh-**PLAS**-tee) is the surgical repair of a fascia.
- **Tenodesis** (ten-**ODD**-eh-sis) means to suture the end of a tendon to bone. (The suffix *-DESIS* means to bind or tie together.)
- **Tenolysis** (ten-**OL**-ih-sis) means to free a tendon from adhesions. (The suffix *-LYSIS* means to set free. It also means breaking down or detachment.)
- **Tenoplasty** (**TEN**-oh-**plas**-tee) is the surgical repair of a tendon.
- **Myoplasty** (**MY**-oh-**plas**-tee) is the surgical repair of a muscle.
- **Myotomy** (my-**OT**-oh-me) is an incision into a muscle. A **myotome** is an instrument used to cut muscle.
- **Myorrhaphy** (my-**OR**-ah-fee) is the suture of a muscle wound.
- **Herniorrhaphy** (**her**-nee-**OR**-ah-fee) is the surgical suturing of a defect in a muscular wall such as the repair of a hernia.
- **Lysis of adhesions** is surgery performed to free tissues from adhesions.

IMPORTANT TERMS: THE MUSCULAR SYSTEM

This list will help you identify and review the major terms from this chapter.

When you work with the audio tape for this chapter, listen to the word, repeat it and then place a ✓ next to it on the list below.

- ☐ **Aponeurosis** (**ap**-oh-new-**ROH**-sis)
- ☐ **Ataxia** (ah-**TACK**-see-ah)
- ☐ **Atonic** (ah-**TON**-ick)
- ☐ **Atrophy** (**AT**-roh-fee)
- ☐ **Brachii** (**BRAY**-kee-eye)
- ☐ **Dystonia** (dis-**TOH**-nee-ah)
- ☐ **Dystrophy** (**DIS**-troh-fee)
- ☐ **Electromyography** (ee-**leck**-troh-my-**OG**-rah-fee)
- ☐ **Electroneuromyography** (ee-**leck**-troh-**new**-roh-my-**OG**-rah-fee)
- ☐ **Fascia** (**FASH**-ee-ah)
- ☐ **Fasciectomy** (**fas**-ee-**ECK**-toh-me)
- ☐ **Fasciitis** (**fas**-ee-**EYE**-tis)
- ☐ **Fascioplasty** (**fash**-ee-oh-**PLAS**-tee)
- ☐ **Femoris** (**FEM**-or-iss)
- ☐ **Fibrositis** (**figh**-broh-**SIGH**-tis)
- ☐ **Flexion** (**FLECK**-shun)

- ☐ **Gluteus** (**GLOO**-tee-us)
- ☐ **Hernia** (**HER**-nee-ah)
- ☐ **Herniorrhaphy** (**her**-nee-**OR**-ah-fee)
- ☐ **Kinesiology** (kih-**nee**-see-**OL**-oh-jee)
- ☐ **Levatores costarum** (**lev**-ah-**TOH**-reez kahs-**TAH**-rum)
- ☐ **Myalgia** (my-**AL**-jee-ah)
- ☐ **Myasthenia** (**my**-as-**THEE**-nee-ah)
- ☐ **Myasthenia gravis** (**my**-as-**THEE**-nee-ah **GRAH**-vis)
- ☐ **Myocardium** (**my**-oh-**KAR**-dee-um)
- ☐ **Myocele** (**MY**-oh-seel)
- ☐ **Myomalacia** (**my**-oh-mah-**LAY**-she-ah)
- ☐ **Myoneural** (**my**-oh-**NEW**-ral)
- ☐ **Myoparesis** (**my**-oh-**PAR**-eh-sis)
- ☐ **Myoplasty** (**MY**-oh-**plas**-tee)
- ☐ **Myorrhaphy** (my-**OR**-ah-fee)
- ☐ **Myosarcoma** (**my**-oh-sahr-**KOH**-mah)
- ☐ **Myosclerosis** (**my**-oh-skle-**ROH**-sis)
- ☐ **Myositis** (**my**-oh-**SIGH**-tis)
- ☐ **Myotomy** (my-**OT**-oh-me)
- ☐ **Oblique** (oh-**BLEEK**)
- ☐ **Orbicularis oris** (or-**bick**-you-**LAY**-riss **OR**-iss)
- ☐ **Polymyositis** (**pol**-ee-**my**-oh-**SIGH**-tis)
- ☐ **Pronation** (proh-**NAY**-shun)
- ☐ **Rectus** (**RECK**-tus)
- ☐ **Sphincter** (**SFINK**-ter)
- ☐ **Sternocleidomastoid** (**ster**-no-**kly**-doh-**MASS**-toid)
- ☐ **Striated** (**STRY**-ayt-ed)
- ☐ **Supination** (**soo**-pih-**NAY**-shun)
- ☐ **Tendinitis** (**ten**-dih-**NIGH**-tis)
- ☐ **Tenodesis** (ten-**ODD**-eh-sis)
- ☐ **Tenolysis** (ten-**OL**-ih-sis)
- ☐ **Tenoplasty** (**TEN**-oh-**plas**-tee)
- ☐ **Tonus** (**TOH**-nus)
- ☐ **Torticollis** (**tor**-tih-**KOL**-is)

EXERCISES

DEFINING WORD PARTS

Write the definition for each of these word parts.

1. *AB-* ____________
2. *AD-* ____________
3. *-CELE* ____________
4. *-DESIS* ____________
5. *DUCT/O* ____________
6. *EX-* ____________
7. *FASCI/O* ____________
8. *FIBROS/O* ____________
9. *FLEX/O* ____________
10. *KINESI/O, -KINESIS* ____________
11. *LEV/O, LEVAT/O* ____________
12. *-LYSIS* ____________
13. *MY/O* ____________
14. *-PARESIS* ____________
15. *PRESS/O* ____________

16. *TAX/O* ______________________________

17. *TEN/O, TEND/O, TENDIN/O* ______________________________

18. *TENS/O* ______________________________

19. *TON/O* ______________________________

20. *TORT/I* ______________________________

DEFINITIONS

Circle the letter next to the correct answer.

1. ______________ muscles are so named because they are under the control of the autonomic nervous system.
   a) Involuntary
   b) Striated
   c) Visceral
   d) Voluntary

2. Muscle origin is ______________
   a) the more fixed attachment.
   b) the place where the muscle begins.
   c) toward the midline.
   d) a, b and c.

3. Rectus means ______________
   a) depressor.
   b) levator.
   c) slanted at an angle.
   d) straight.

4. The orbicularis oris ______________
   a) closes the eye.
   b) is a circular muscle.
   c) surrounds the mouth.
   d) b and c.

5. The point(s) of insertion for the sternocleidomastoid muscle is/are the ______________
   a) clavicle.
   b) mastoid.
   c) sternum.
   d) a and c.

6. The quadriceps femoris ______________
   a) assists in extending the leg.
   b) is formed from four divisions.
   c) is the large muscle of the anterior thigh.
   d) a, b and c.

7. A ______________ is a narrow band of fibrous tissue that attaches a muscle to bone.
   a) fascia
   b) ligament
   c) muscle fiber
   d) tendon

8. An aponeurosis is ______________
   a) a specialized form of voluntary muscle.
   b) a specialized tendon to attach muscles to bone.
   c) specialized fascia to bind muscles together.
   d) b and c.

9. The hamstrings are examples of ______________
   a) cartilage.
   b) fascia.
   c) ligaments.
   d) tendons.

10. Contraction ______________
    a) causes the muscle to become shorter and thicker.
    b) is a specialized function of muscle.
    c) is the tightening of a muscle.
    d) a, b and c.

MISSING WORDS

Write the missing word on the line.

1. ______________________ is the fibrous sheet of connective tissue that covers, supports, and separates muscles.

2. ______________________ is a circular movement of a limb at the far end such as the movement of the head of the femur within the hip joint.

3. A/an ______________________ is a muscle that raises a body part.

4. Each muscle consists of a group of fibers held together by connective tissue and enclosed in a ______________________ sheath.

5. A/an ______________________ is a ring-like muscle that tightly constricts the opening of a passageway.

6. A/an ______________________ is a muscle that moves a body part toward the midline.

7. The ______________________ muscle forms the shoulder cap.

8. ______________________ is a condition of a lack of muscle coordination.

9. ______________________ is the study of muscular activity and the movement of body parts.

10. The ______________________ brachii is the muscle of the posterior upper arm.

11. Muscle tone, also known as ______________________, is the normal state of balanced tension that is present in the body when one is awake.

12. The gluteus ______________________ is the largest muscle of the buttock.

13. ______________________ is the surgical repair of a tendon.

14. ______________________ is the abnormal softening of a muscle.

15. Cardiac muscle is also known as ______________________.

SPELLCHECK

Select the correct spelling and write it on the line.

1. ______________________ is also known as a wryneck.
   Tortacollis
   Tortecollis
   Torticollis

2. ______________________ is a malignant tumor derived from muscle tissue.
   Miosarcoma
   Myelosarcoma
   Myosarcoma

3. An ______________________ is a record of the strength of muscle contraction as a result of electrical stimulation.
   electromyelogram
   electriomyogram
   electromyogram

4. Muscular ______________________ is a group of inherited diseases characterized by progressive weakness and degeneration of muscle fibers without the involvement of the nervous system.
   destrophy
   distrophy
   dystrophy

5. ______________________ is the inflammation of several muscles at once.
   Polimyositis
   Polymyitis
   Polymyositis

6. The anal ______________________ closes the rectum.
   sfincter
   sphinctar
   sphincter

7. ______________________ is the circular motion of a limb at the far end.
   Circumduction
   Cirkumduction
   Sercumduction

8. ______________________ is an inflammation of a fascia.
   Fasciitis
   Fascitis
   Fasitis

9. An ______________________ is a band of fiber that holds structure together abnormally.
   adhesion
   adhesive
   Adhision

10. ______________________ is the loss of sensation and voluntary muscle movements.
    Paralysis
    Parelysis
    Parilysis

11. A ______________________ is the rupture and abnormal protrusion of an organ through its containing muscular wall.
    herinea
    hernea
    hernia

12. ______________________ are rhythmic, purposeless, quivery movements.
    Tremers
    Tremors
    Tremours

13. ______________________ means muscle weakness.
    Myasthenia
    Myesthenia
    Myoesthenia

14. The ______________________ muscle helps to flex the neck and rotate the head.
    sternalcleidomastoid
    sternocleidomastoid
    sternocliedomastoid

15. ______________________ means slanted outward, at an angle, from the midline.
    Obleque
    Oblike
    Oblique

CASE STUDIES

Write the correct answer on the line.

1. Immediately after his stroke Warren Hilgartner suffered temporary ______________________ and lost all sensation and voluntary control of the muscles on the right side of his body.
2. Nina Burleson suffers from the chronic neuromuscular disease ______________________ gravis.
3. A/an ______________________ was performed to repair Douglas Ryan's inguinal hernia.
4. Due to the lack of exercise while he was confined to bed, Gerald Hasting's experienced muscle ______________________.
5. Jill Franklin has an abnormal hardening of muscle tissue, which is called ______________________.
6. Ruth Vaugh was diagnosed as suffering from ______________________ which is an inflammation of a muscle or muscles.
7. Juan Romeriez suffers from the rupture of a muscle through its sheath or fascia. This is called a/an ______________________.
8. Hugo Edwards underwent ______________________ for the surgical removal of fascia.
9. After her the abdominal surgery, Wilma Huggins suffered from ______________________ which abnormally held the structures together.

10. After he was stabbed, ______________________ was required to suture Roscoe Baxter's muscle wounds.

11. Jamie Vaughn suffers from ______________________ which is a lack of muscle coordination.

12. George Quinton suffered from ______________________ which is commonly known as wryneck.

13. Several months after the accident, Margo Brooks underwent ______________________ to free the tendons in her arm from the adhesions caused by her injury.

14. ______________________, by the electrical stimulation of nerves, was used to test and record the neuromuscular activity of Gregory Harris's injured leg.

15. Mr. Hoski's ______________________, an inflammation of the fibrous connective tissues, is characterized by a poorly defined set of symptoms.

WORD BUILDING

Write the correct word or word part on the line.

1. Muscle of the heart
   a) The combining form ______________________ means muscle.
   b) The combining form ______________________ means heart.
   c) The term ______________________ means heart muscle.

2. Muscle pain
   a) The combining form ______________________ means muscle.
   b) The suffix ______________________ means pain.
   c) The term ______________________ means muscle tenderness or pain.

3. Inflammation of the fascia
   a) The combining form ______________________ means fascia.
   b) The suffix ______________________ means inflammation.
   c) The term ______________________ means inflammation of a fascia.

4. Freeing a tendon from adhesions (Be careful on this one!)
   a) The combining form ______________________ means tendon.
   b) The suffix ______________________ means to set free.
   c) The term ______________________ means to free a tendon from adhesions.

5. The study of movements
   a) The combining form ______________________ means movement or motion.
   b) The suffix ______________________ means the study of.
   c) The term ______________________ means the study of the movement of body parts.

LABELING EXERCISES

Identify the muscle movements that are numbered on this diagram.

1. ______________________________
2. ______________________________
3. ______________________________
4. ______________________________
5. ______________________________

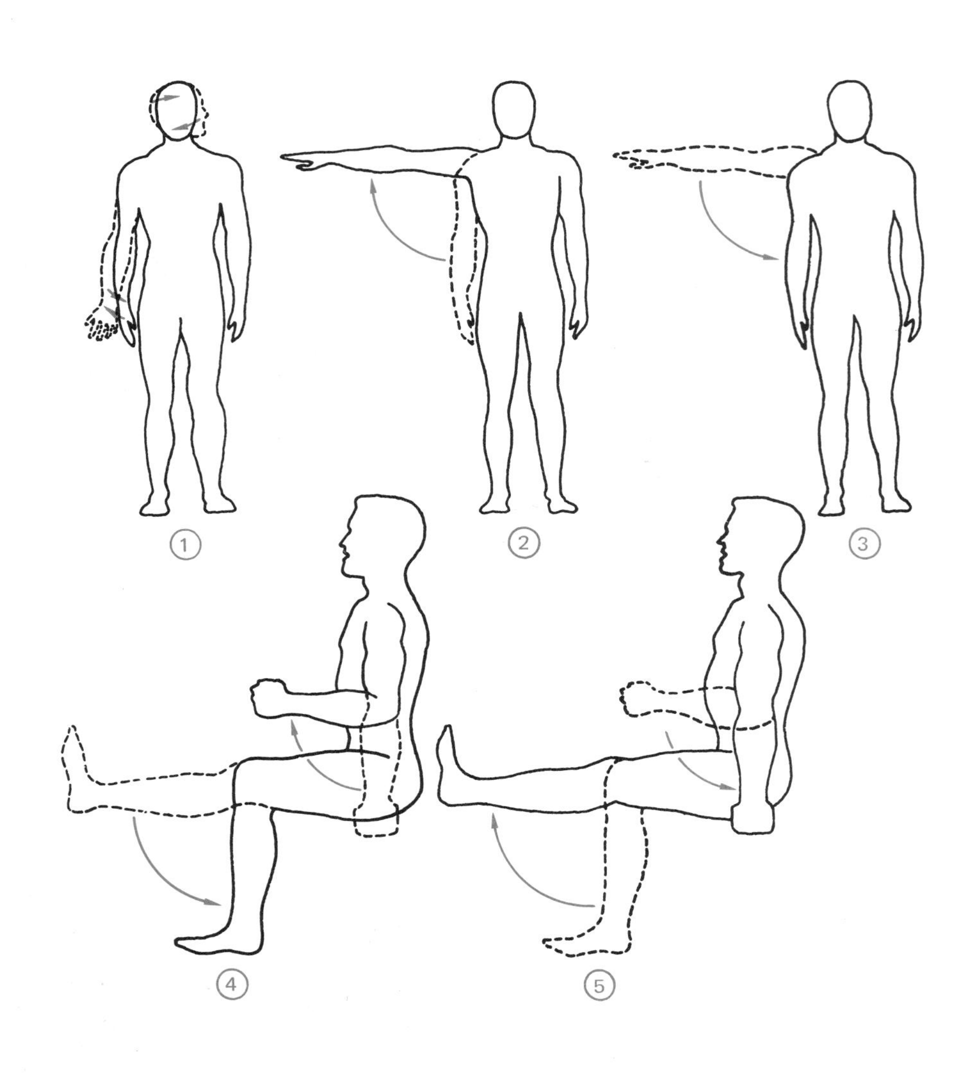

5

THE CARDIOVASCULAR SYSTEM

LEARNING GOALS

In this chapter you will learn to:

- describe the heart in terms of: chambers, valves, the heartbeat and heart sounds.
- differentiate between the three different types of blood vessels and describe the major function of each.
- identify the major components of blood and the major functions of each.
- state the difference between pulmonary and systemic circulation.
- recognize and define the terms related to the diagnosis, pathology and treatment of disorders of the cardiovascular system.

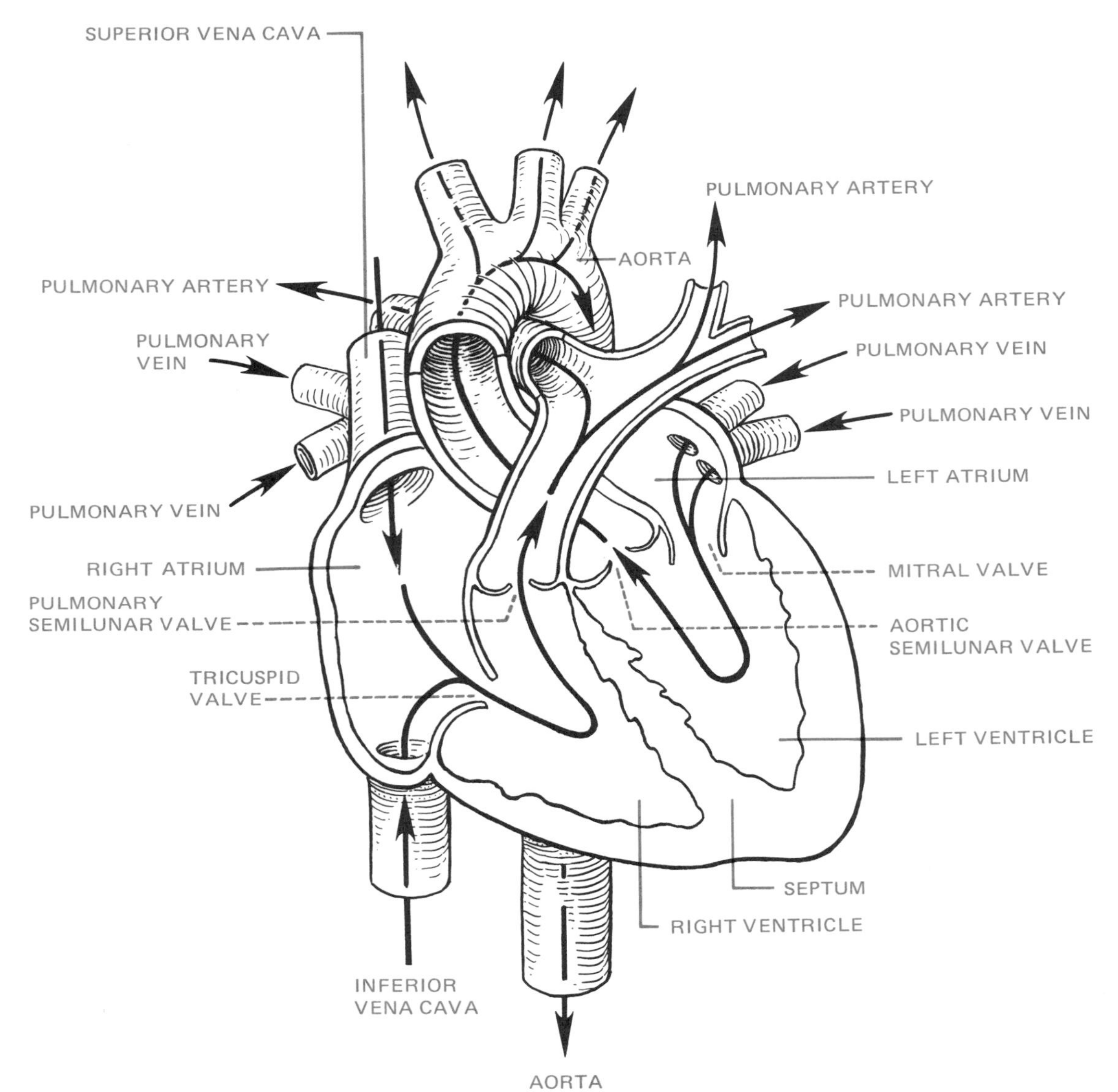

Figure 5-1 The structures and blood flow of the heart.

STRUCTURES OF THE CARDIOVASCULAR SYSTEM

The term cardiovascular means pertaining to the heart and the blood vessels.

The work of this system is carried out by three major parts. These are the heart, the blood vessels and the blood.

THE HEART

The heart is a hollow muscular organ that furnishes the power to maintain the circulation of the blood. It acts as a compound pump placed between, and connecting, pulmonary circulation and systemic circulation.

The heart, which is protected by the thoracic cavity, is located between the lungs and above the diaphragm. (The combining form *CARDI/O* means heart.)

The Pericardium

The heart is enclosed in a double-walled membranous sac known as the pericardium. **Pericardial fluid** between the layers prevents friction when the heart beats.

The Walls of the Heart

The **epicardium (ep**-ih-**KAR**-dee-um) is the external layer of the heart and is also part of the inner layer of the pericardial sac. (The prefix *EPI-* means upper.)

The **myocardium (migh**-oh-**KAR**-dee-um), the muscular middle layer, is the thickest of the three layers. (The combining form *MY/O* means muscle.)

The **endocardium (en**-doh-**KAR**-dee-um), is the inner layer that is lined with endothelium and forms the inner surface of the heart. (The combining form *END/O* means within.)

The Chambers of the Heart

The heart is divided into left and right sides. Each side is subdivided thus forming a total of four chambers.

The **atria (AY**-tree-ah), which are the upper chambers of the heart, are separated by the **interatrial septum.** The atria are the receiving chambers, and all the vessels coming into the heart enter here. (The combining form *ATRI/O* means atrium.) (Singular, **atrium**)

The **ventricles (VEN**-trih-kuhls), which are the lower chambers of the heart, are separated by the **interventricular septum.**

The ventricles are the pumping chambers and all vessels leaving the heart emerge from them. (The combining form *VENTRICUL/O* means ventricle and refers to both the ventricles of the heart and of the brain.)

The narrow tip of the heart is called the **cardiac apex.**

The Valves of the Heart

The valves heart control the flow of blood through the heart. (The combining forms *VALV/O* and *VALVUL/O* both mean valve.)

The **tricuspid valve** controls the opening between the right atrium and the right ventricle. (**Tricuspid** means having three points.)

The **pulmonary semilunar valve** is located between the right ventricle and the pulmonary artery. (**Semilunar** means resembling a half moon.)

The **mitral valve,** also known as the **bicuspid valve,** is located between the left atrium and left ventricle. (**Bicuspid** means having two points.)

The **aortic semilunar valve** is located between the left ventricle and the aorta.

BLOOD FLOW THROUGH THE HEART
The **RIGHT ATRIUM** receives blood from all tissues except the lungs through the **superior** and **inferior venae cavae.** Blood flows from the right atrium ,through the **tricuspid valve,** and into the right ventricle.
The **RIGHT VENTRICLE** receives blood from the right atrium and pumps it through the **pulmonary semilunar valve** and into the **pulmonary artery** which carries it to the lungs.
The **LEFT ATRIUM** receives oxygenated blood from the lungs through the four **pulmonary veins.** Blood flows through the **mitral valve,** into the left ventricle.
The **LEFT VENTRICLE** receives blood from the left atrium. From here blood goes out through the **aortic semilunar valve** and into the **aorta** and is pumped to all parts of the body, except the lungs.

The Heartbeat

The neuromuscular tissue of the heart comprises the sinoatrial (S-A) node, the atrioventricular (A-V) node, and the bundle of His.

The **sinoatrial node (sigh**-no-**AY**-tree-ahl) which is often called the **pacemaker** of the heart, is located in the upper wall of the right atrium.

The electrical impulses from the S-A node start each wave of muscle contraction in the heart. The impulse in the right atrium spreads over the muscles of both atria, causing them to contract simultaneously, sending blood into the ventricles.

These impulses also travel to the **atrioventricular node, (ay**-tree-oh-ven-**TRICK**-you-lahr) which is located beneath the endocardium of the right atrium. The A-V node then transmits the electric impulses on to the bundle of His.

The **bundle of His (HISS)** is located within the interventricular septum. Branches of this bundle carry the impulse to the right and left ventricles, causing them to contract.

Heart Sounds

When a stethoscope is used to listen to the heartbeat, two distinct sounds may be heard. They are referred to as the lubb dupp sounds.

The **lubb sound,** which is heard first, is caused by the valves slamming shut between the atria and the ventricles.

The **dupp sound,** heard second, is shorter and higher pitched. It is caused by the semilunar valves closing in the aorta and the pulmonary arteries.

A **heart murmur** is an extra sound, heard between normal heart sounds.

PULMONARY AND SYSTEMIC CIRCULATION

Pulmonary circulation includes the flow of blood through the right ventricle, pulmonary arterial system, lungs, pulmonary venous system and left atrium of the heart.

Systemic circulation includes blood flow to all parts of the body except the lungs. It consists of all the arteries, veins and capillaries of the body except those of the lungs.

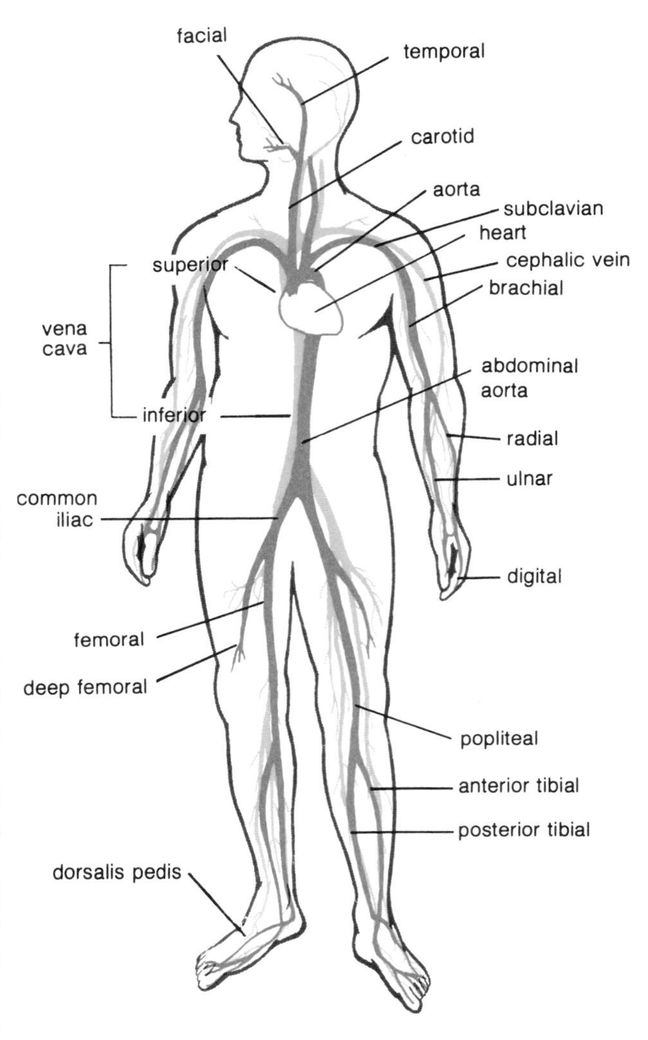

Figure 5-2 Systemic circulation.

BLOOD VESSELS

There are three major types of blood vessels in the body. They are the arteries, veins and capillaries. The combining forms *ANGI/O* and *VAS/O* both mean relating to the blood or lymph vessels.

The **lumen (LOO**-men) is the channel within the vessel that the blood flows through.

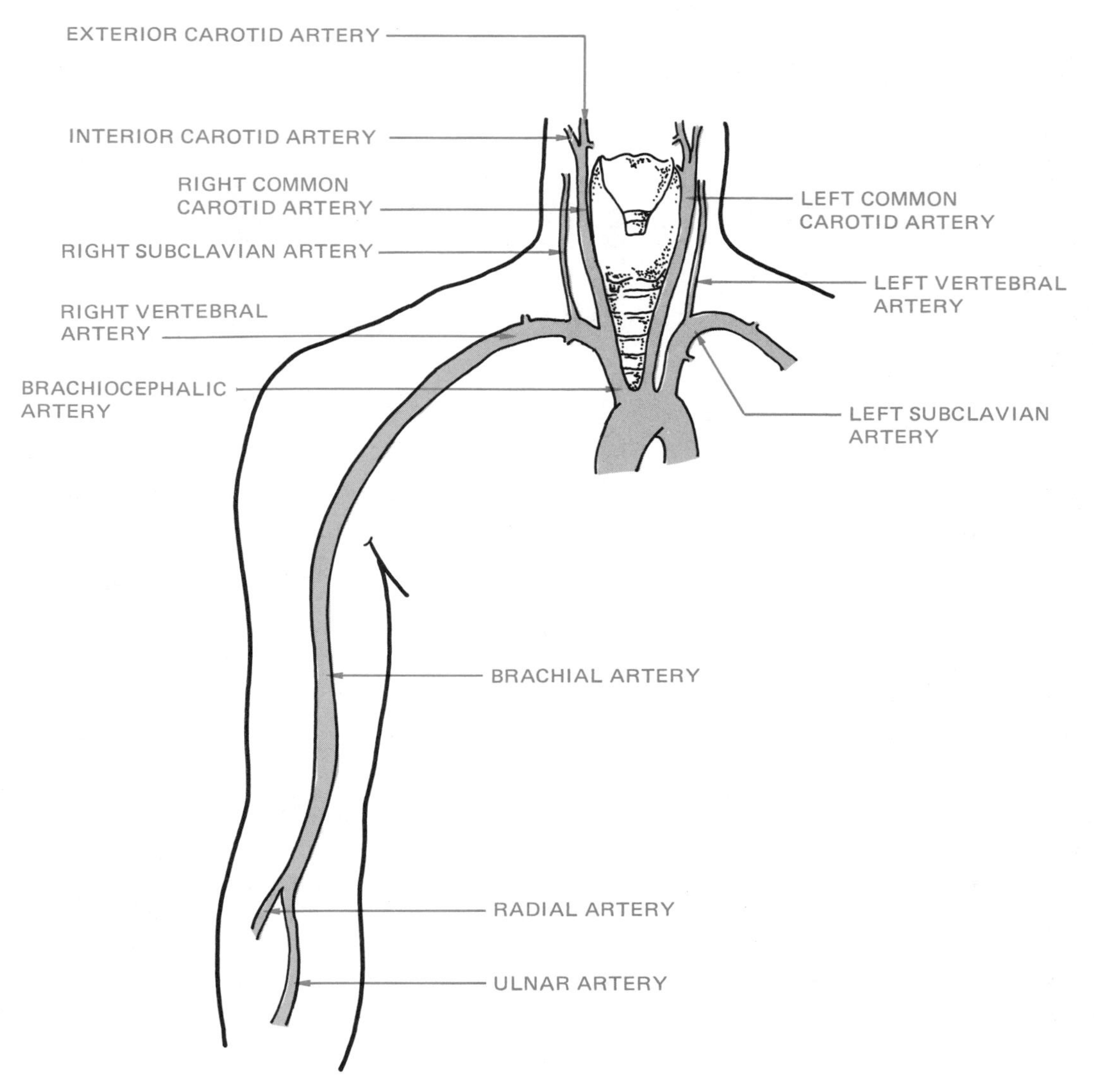

Figure 5-3 Major arteries of the upper chest, neck and arm.

Arteries

The arteries are the large blood vessels that carry blood away from the heart to all regions of the body. The term **endarterial** (**end**-ar-**TEE**-ree-al) means pertaining to the interior of an artery. (The combining form *ARTERI/O* means artery.)

The walls of the arteries are composed of three layers, and this structure makes them both muscular and elastic so they can expand and contract with the pumping beat of the heart.

The **aorta** (ay-**OR**-tah) is the largest of the arteries and it begins from the left ventricle of the heart. (The combining form *AORT/O* means aorta.)

The **coronary artery** branches from the aorta and supplies blood to the heart muscle.

The **arterioles** (are-**TEE**-ree-ohlz) are the smaller branches of arteries. Arterioles are thinner than arteries and carry the blood to the capillaries.

Capillaries

The capillaries are a system of microscopic vessels, only one epithelial cell in thickness. The capillaries serve as anatomic units connecting the arterial and venous system.

Blood flows rapidly along the arteries and veins; however, this flow is much slower through the expanded vascular bed provided by the capillaries.

This slower flow allows time for the exchange of oxygen, nutrients and waste materials between the tissue fluids and the surrounding cells.

Veins

The veins form a low-pressure collecting system to return the waste-filled blood to the heart. (The combining forms *VEN/O* and *PHLEB/O* mean vein.)

Small veins called **venules** (**VEN**-youls) join together to form the larger vessels called veins.

Veins have thinner walls and are less elastic then the arteries. They also have valves which allow blood to flow toward the heart, but prevent it from flowing away from the heart.

The two **venae cavae** (**VEE**-nee **KAY**-vee) are the large veins that enter the heart. The **superior vena cava** (**VEE**-nah **KAY**-vah) carries blood from the upper portion of the body. The **inferior vena cava** carries blood from the lower portion of the body.

The Pulse and Blood Pressure

The pulse is the rhythmic expansion and contraction of an artery produced by the pressure of the blood moving through the artery.

Blood pressure is a measurement of the amount of pressure exerted against the walls of the vessels.

Systolic pressure (sis-**TOL**-ick) is the highest pressure when the ventricles contract.

Diastolic pressure (dye-ah-**STOL**-ick) is the lowest pressure when the ventricles are relaxed.

THE BLOOD

Most of the blood is composed of the liquid plasma. Less than half of the blood's composition is made up of formed elements. (The combining forms *HEM/O* and *HEMAT/O* both mean blood or relating to the blood.)

The **formed elements,** also known as **blood corpuscles,** include the red blood cells, white blood cells and platelets.

Plasma

Plasma is a straw-colored fluid that transports nutrients, hormones, and waste products.

Plasma is 91 percent water. The remaining nine percent consists mainly of the plasma proteins including **albumin** (al-**BYOU**-min) and **globulin** (**GLOB**-you-lin).

Blood Clotting

Fibrinogen (fye-**BRIN**-oh-jen) and **prothrombin** (pro-**THROM**-bin) are clotting proteins found in plasma.

Fibrin is the protein formed by fibrinogen during the normal clotting of blood. **Coagulation** is the process of blood clot formation.

Serum (**SEE**-rum) is plasma with the clotting proteins removed.

Erythrocytes

Erythrocytes (eh-**RITH**-roh-sites) are also known as red blood cells or red corpuscles. (The combining form *ERYTHR/O* means red and the suffix *-CYTE* means cell.)

Erythrocytes contain the blood protein **hemoglobin** (**he**-moh-**GLOW**-bin), which plays an essential role in oxygen transport. (The suffix *-GLOBIN* means protein.)

A **reticulocyte** (reh-**TICK**-you-loh-**site**) is an immature erythrocyte that is characterized by a mesh-like pattern of threads. (The combining form *RETICUL/O* means network.)

A mature red blood cell has a shape resembling a doughnut, with a thin central portion instead of a hole. Erythrocytes are produced by the red bone marrow.

When erythrocytes are no longer useful they are destroyed by **macrophages** in the spleen, liver and bone marrow. (The suffix *-PHAGE* means a cell that destroys.)

Leukocytes

Leukocytes (**LOO**-koh-sites), also known as white blood cells or white corpuscles, have the primary function of fighting disease in the body. (The combining form *LEUK/O* means white.)

Leukocytes are classified as being granular and agranular. **Granulocytes** have granules in the cytoplasm of the cell. **Agranulocytes** do not have granules in the cytoplasm of the cell.

MAJOR GROUPS OF LEUKOCYTES
Basophils (**BAY**-soh-fills) are granular leukocytes whose exact function is unknown.
Eosinophils (ee-oh-**SIN**-oh-fills) are granular leukocytes that are increased in allergic conditions.
Lymphocytes (**LIM**-foh-sites) are agranular leukocytes that are important in the process of producing immunity to protect the body.
Monocytes (**MON**-oh-sites) are agranular leukocytes that act as macrophages that dispose of dead and dying cells and other debris.
Neutrophils (**NEW**-troh-fills) are granular leukocytes that fight disease by engulfing and swallowing up germs. (This process is called **phagocytosis.**)

Thrombocytes

Thrombocytes (**THROM**-boh-sites), also known as **platelets,** are the smallest formed elements of the blood.

Thrombocytes are manufactured in the bone marrow and play an important role in the clotting of blood. (The combining form *THROMB/O* means clot.)

Hemostasis (**he**-moh-**STAY**-sis) is the mechanism the body uses to control bleeding. (The suffix *-STASIS* means stopping or controlling.)

Blood Groups

The blood groups are A, AB, B, and O. In addition to matching these groups, the Rh factor must also be matched according to whether it is positive or negative.

The safe administration of blood from donor to recipient requires typing and cross-matching. A patient receiving blood incompatible with his own can experience a serious and possibly fatal reaction.

The Rh Factor

The Rh factor is an antigenic substance present in the erythrocytes of most people. A person having the factor is Rh positive. A person lacking the factor is Rh negative.

The Rh factor is an important consideration in blood typing and cross-matching and causes difficulties when an Rh positive infant is born to an Rh negative mother.

Blood Gases

A blood gas is a gas that is dissolved in the liquid part of the blood. Blood gases include **oxygen, carbon dioxide** and **nitrogen.**

DIAGNOSTIC PROCEDURES RELATED TO THE CIRCULATORY SYSTEM

- **Electrocardiography** (ee-**leck**-troh-kar-dee-**OG**-rah-fee), which is often identified by the initials EKG and ECG, is the process of recording the electrical activity of the myocardium. The resulting record is called a **cardiogram** or **electrocardiogram.**

- **Angiography (an-jee-OG-rah-fee)** is radiographic study of the blood vessels after the introduction of a contrast medium. The resulting film is called an **angiogram.**

- **Angiocardiography (an-jee-oh-kar-dee-OG-rah-fee)** is a diagnostic procedure involving the use of radiopaque dye and chest x-rays to show the dimensions of the heart and large blood vessels. The resulting film is called an **angiocardiogram.**

- **Digital subtraction angiography** (DSA) is an imaging technique that uses computer enhancement to produce clearer views of blood vessels injected with a contrast medium.

- **Arteriography (are-tee-ree-OG-rah-fee)** is a diagnostic procedure that involves the use of radiopaque dye and x-rays to study an artery or arteries. The resulting film is called an **arteriogram.**

- **Cardiac catheterization** is a radiographic study in which a radiopaque dye is introduced through a catheter into a vein or artery and is guided into the heart for purposes of detecting pressures and patterns of blood flow.

- **Echocardiography (eck-oh-kar-dee-OG-rah-fee)** is a diagnostic procedure that uses ultrasound for evaluating the structures of the heart.

- **Pericardiocentesis (per-ih-kar-dee-oh-sen-TEE-sis)**, which is also called **pericardicentesis,** is the drawing of fluid from the pericardial sac.

- **Phlebography (fleh-BOG-rah-fee)** is the technique of preparing an x-ray image of veins injected with a contrast medium material. The resulting film is a **phlebogram.**

- **Phonocardiography (foh-no-kar-dee-OG-rah-fee)** is a graphic representation of the heart sounds and murmurs produced by an electroacoustic device called a phonocardiograph. The resulting record is a **phonocardiogram.** (The combining form *PHON/O* means sound.)

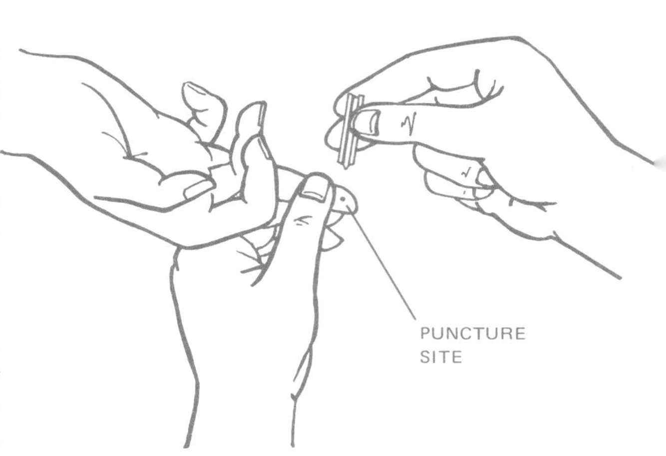

Figure 5-4 Capillary puncture.

Blood Tests

- A **capillary puncture,** also known as a finger stick, is the technique used when only a small amount of blood is needed as a specimen. A **lancet** is a sterile, sharp-pointed blade used to perform a capillary puncture.

- **Venipuncture (VEN-ih-punk-tyour)** is the use of a needle to puncture a vein to remove blood for diagnostic study or to administer drugs for intravenous therapy.

- **Serology (see-ROL-oh-jee)** is the laboratory study of serum and the reactions between antigens and antibodies. (The combining form *SER/O* means serum.)

  An **antigen** (AN-tih-jen) is a substance that causes the formation of antibodies. An **antibody** is an immunoglobulin molecule that interacts only with a specific antigen.

- **Agglutination** (ah-**gloo**-tih-**NAY**-shun) is the clumping together of cells or particles when mixed with incompatible blood.

- **Blood urea nitrogen** (BUN) is the amount of nitrogenous substance present in the blood as urea. It is a rough indicator of kidney function.

  Urea is a nitrogenous waste compound found in urine, blood and lymph.

- **Differential blood counts** are tests to determine the number of blood cells per cubic millimeter of blood.

  A **complete blood count** (CBC) is a determination of the number of red and white blood cells per cubic millimeter of blood.

  A **red blood count** (RBC) is a determination of the number of red blood cells per cubic millimeter of blood.

  A **white blood count** (WBC) is a determination of the number of white blood cells per cubic millimeter of blood.

  A **white blood cell differential** determines what percentage of the total white blood cell count is composed by each of the five types of white blood cells.

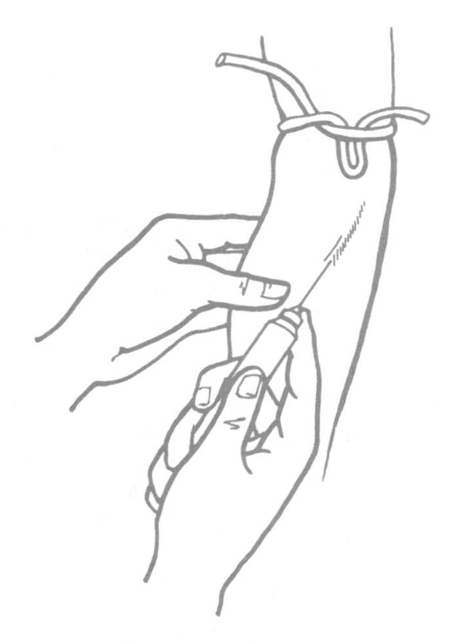

Figure 5-5 Venipuncture.

- **Erythrocyte Sedimentation Rate (ESR),** also known as **sedimentation rate,** is a test used to indicate the presence of inflammation in the body. It is based on the rate at which the erythrocytes (red blood cells) separate from the plasma and settle to the bottom of the container.

- **Fasting blood sugar** (FBS) level refers to the amount of sugar in the blood after the patient has fasted for several hours.

  A **glucose tolerance test** (GTT) measures the way sugars are handled by the body. A glucose tolerance test consists of a fasting blood sugar followed by oral or intravenous administration of a measured amount of glucose. Several times thereafter, blood sugar levels are determined.

- **Hematocrit** (he-**MAT**-oh-krit) means the volume percentage of erythrocytes in whole blood. (The suffix *-CRIT* means to separate.)

  A **centrifuge** (**SEN**-trih-fewj) is a machine which spins the specimen very rapidly to separate the elements from the plasma.

- **Lipid tests** measure the amounts of cholesterol and triglycerides in a blood sample. (**Cholesterol** (koh-**LES**-ter-ol) and **triglycerides** (try-**GLIS**-er-eyeds) are fatty substances that circulate in the blood stream.)

- **Prothrombin time** (pro-**THROM**-bin) is the number of seconds required for thromboplastin to coagulate plasma.

- **Serum enzyme tests** are used to measure the blood enzymes. These tests are useful as evidence of a myocardial infarction.

Specialized Blood Test Results

- **Acidosis** (ass-ih-**DOH**-sis) is an abnormal accumulation of acid in the blood and body tissues.

- **Hyperalbuminemia** (**high**-per-al-**byou**-mih-**NEE**-me-ah) is an abnormally high level of albumin in the blood.

- **Hyperbilirubinemia** (**high**-per-**bil**-ih-**roo**-bih-**NEE**-me-ah) is an excessive concentration of bilirubin in the blood.

- **Hyperlipidemia** (**high**-per-**lip**-ih-**DEE**-me-ah) is a general term for elevated concentrations of any or all of the lipids (fats) in the plasma. (The combining form *LIP/O* means fat.)

- **Hyperlipemia** (**high**-per-lye-**PEE**-me-ah) is an elevated concentration of triglycerides in the plasma.

- **Hyperuricemia** (**high**-per-**you**-rih-**SEE**-me-ah) is excessive uric acid in the bloodstream. (**Uric acid** is an end product of the metabolism of purine.)

PATHOLOGY OF THE CARDIOVASCULAR SYSTEM

Pathology of the Heart

- **Congenital heart diseases** are abnormalities in the heart that are present at birth. (The term **congenital** refers to conditions that are present at birth.)

- **Cardiac arrest** is the sudden cessation (stopping) of all cardiac output and effective circulation.

- **Congestive heart failure** (CHF) is a condition in which there is abnormal fluid retention so that the heart is unable to adequately maintain circulation.

- **Carditis** (kar-**DYE**-tis) is an inflammation of the heart.

  Pericarditis (**per**-ih-kar-**DYE**-tis) is an inflammation of the pericardium.

  Myocarditis (**my**-oh-kar-**DYE**-tis) is an inflammation of the myocardium.

  Endocarditis (**en**-doh-kar-**DYE**-tis) is an inflammation of the inner layer of the heart.

  Bacterial endocarditis is an inflammation of the inner lining of the heart caused by bacteria.

- **Cardiomegaly** (**kar**-dee-oh-**MEG**-ah-lee) is an enlargement of the heart. (The suffix *-MEGALY* means enlargement.)

- **Cardioplegia** (**kar**-dee-oh-**PLEE**-jee-ah) is paralysis of the heart. (The suffix *-PLEGIA* means paralysis.)

- **Cardiorrhexis** (**kar**-dee-oh-**RECK**-sis) is the rupture of the heart. (The suffix *-RRHEXIS* means rupture.)

Pathology of the Heart Valves

- **Valvulitis** (**val**-view-**LYE**-tis) is an inflammatory condition of a heart valve.

- **Mitral-valve prolapse** is a condition caused by an abnormal protrusion of the mitral value. This results in the incomplete closure of the valve. (**Prolapse** means falling down.)

- **Mitral stenosis** is an obstructive lesion in the mitral valve of the heart. (**Stenosis** (steh-**NO**-sis) is an abnormal narrowing or closing.)

- **Rheumatic heart disease** is heart disease caused by rheumatic fever. Damage may be done particularly to the heart valves.

Arrhythmias

- **Cardiac arrhythmia** (ah-**RITH**-me-ah), also called **dysrhythmia** (dis-**RITH**-me-ah), is any abnormal heart rhythm.

- **Palpitation** (**pal**-pih-**TAY**-shun) is a pounding or racing heart. This may be a normal response or associated with certain heart disorders.

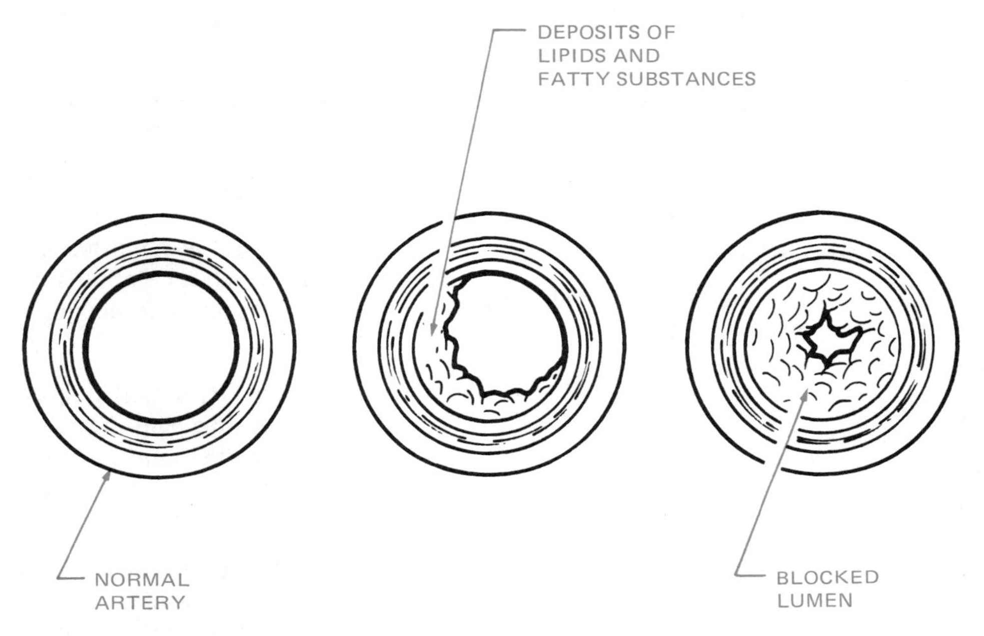

Figure 5-6 Atherosclerosis of an artery.

- **Fibrillation (fih-brih-LAY-shun)** is rapid, random and ineffective contractions of the heart.

- A **flutter** is a cardiac arrhythmia in which the atrial contractions are rapid but regular.

- **Bradycardia (brad-ee-KAR-dee-ah)** is an abnormally slow heartbeat. (The prefix *BRADY-* means slow.)

- **Tachycardia (tack-ee-KAR-dee-ah)** is an abnormally fast heartbeat. (The prefix *TACHY-* means fast, rapid.)

  Paroxysmal tachycardia is a fast heartbeat of sudden onset. **(Paroxysm (PAR-ock-sizm)** means convulsion or spasm.)

Pathology of the Blood Vessels

- **Coronary artery disease** is any one of the abnormal conditions that may affect the arteries of the heart.

- **Peripheral vascular disease** is any abnormal condition that affects the blood vessels outside the heart and lymphatic vessels.

- **Arteritis (ar-teh-RYE-tis)** is an inflammation of an artery.

- **Polyarteritis (pol-ee-ar-teh-RYE-tis)** is an inflammation involving several arteries. (The suffix *POLY-* means many.)

- An **infarct (IN-farkt)** is a localized area of necrosis in a tissue or organ caused by an interruption of the blood supply.

  A **myocardial infarction,** also known as a **heart attack** or **acute myocardial infarction,** is an occlusion of a coronary artery resulting in a necrotic area of the myocardium.

- **Arteriosclerosis (ar-tee-ree-oh-skleh-ROH-sis)** is hardening of the arteries, which reduces the flow of blood through these vessels.

- **Atherosclerosis (ath**-er-**oh**-sklee-**ROH**-sis) is hardening and narrowing of the arteries due to a buildup of cholesterol plaques.

  A **plaque (PLAK)** is a patch or flat area. (The combining form *ATHER/O* means plaque or fatty substance.)

- An **aneurysm** (AN-you-rizm) is a localized balloon-like enlargement of an artery.

- A **hemangioma** (heh-**man**-jee-**OH**-mah) is a benign tumor made up of newly formed blood vessels.

- **Angionecrosis (an**-jee-oh-neh-**KROH**-sis) is the necrosis of the walls of blood vessels. (**Necrosis** (neh-**KROH**-sis) means localized tissue death.)

- An **angiospasm (AN**-jee-oh-**spazm)** is a spasmodic contraction of the blood vessels.

- **Angiostenosis** (**AN**-jee-oh-stee-**NO**-sis) is the narrowing of a blood vessel.

- **Varicose veins** are abnormally swollen veins, usually occurring in the legs.

  A **varicosity (var**-ih-**KOS**-ih-tee) is one area of swelling. (Plural, **varices.)**

- **Hemorrhoids (HEM**-oh-roids), also known as piles, are varicose veins near the anus.

- A **thrombus (THROM**-bus) is a blood clot attached to the interior wall of a vein or artery.

  A **thrombosis** (throm-**BOH**-sis) is an abnormal condition in which a thrombus develops within a blood vessel.

  A **thrombotic occlusion** (throm-**BOT**-ick ah-**KLOO**-zhun) is the blocking of an artery by a clot. (In this context **occlusion** means a blockage in a canal, vessel or passageway in the body).

  A **coronary thrombosis** is blockage, and damage, in the heart caused by a blood clot.

- **Phlebitis** (fleh-**BYE**-tis), also known as **thrombophlebitis** (**throm**-boh-fleh-**BYE**-tis), is the inflammation of a vein that is often accompanied by the formation of a clot.

- An **embolus** (**EM**-boh-lus) is a foreign object, such as a quantity of air or gas, a bit of tissue or tumor or a piece of a thrombus. (Plural, **emboli.)**

- An **embolism** is an abnormal circulatory condition in which an embolus travels through the bloodstream and becomes lodged in a blood vessel.

- **Angina** (an-**JIGH**-nah) is spasmodic, choking or suffocating pain. The term is generally used to describe **angina pectoris,** which is usually due to interference with the supply of oxygen to the heart muscle.

- **Ischemic heart disease** is a pathologic condition of the myocardium caused by a lack of oxygen reaching the tissue cells.

  Ischemia (is-**KEY**-me-ah) is a deficiency in blood supply due to either the constriction or the obstruction of a blood vessel. (The combining form *ISCH/O* means to hold back.)

  A **transient ischemic attack** (TIA) is the temporary interruption in the blood supply to the brain.

  Raynaud's syndrome (ray-**NOHZ**), also known as **acrocyanosis** (**ak**-roh-**sigh**-ah-**NO**-sis), consists of intermittent attacks of ischemia of the extremities of the body. (The combining form *CYAN/O* means blue.)

- **Hypoperfusion (high**-poh-per-**FYOU**-zhun) is a deficiency of blood passing through an organ or body part.

  Perfusion means the flow of blood through the vessels of an organ.

- **Claudication (klaw**-dih-**KAY**-shun) is a weakness, limping and cramp-like pain of the leg muscles caused by poor circulation to the leg muscles.

Pathology of the Blood

- **Dyscrasia** (dis-**KRAY**-zee-ah) of the blood is any abnormal or pathological condition of the blood.
- **Hemorrhage** (**HEM**-or-idj) means the loss of a large amount of blood in a short time. (The suffix *-RRHAGE* means bursting forth.)
- **Hematoma** (**hem**-ah-**TOH**-mah) is a collection of blood trapped in the tissues of the skin or in an organ.
- **Epistaxis** (**ep**-ih-**STACK**-sis), also known as a **nosebleed,** is usually caused by an injury to the nose.
- **Hematemesis** (**hem**-ah-**TEM**-eh-sis) means vomiting blood. (The suffix *-EMESIS* means vomiting.)
- **Hemophilia** (**hee**-moh-**FILL**-ee-ah) is a group of hereditary bleeding disorders in which there is a lack of one of the factors needed to clot the blood.
- **Purpura** (**PUR**-pew-rah) is a disorder with bleeding beneath the skin that causes spontaneous bruising.
- **Hemarthrosis** (**hem**-ar-**THROH**-sis) is the condition of blood leaking into a joint. (The combining form *ARTHR/O* means joint.)
- **Erythrocytosis** (eh-**rith**-roh-sigh-**TOH**-sis) is an increase in the number of erythrocytes in proportion to the number of other blood cells.
- **Thrombocytopenia** (**throm**-boh-**sigh**-toh-**PEE**-nee-ah) is an abnormal hematological condition characterized by a decrease in the number of blood platelets.
- **Leukopenia** (**loo**-koh-**PEE**-nee-ah) is an abnormal decrease in the number of white blood cells. It may affect one or all kinds of white blood cells.
- **Leukemia** (loo-**KEY**-me-ah) is a malignant neoplasm of the blood-forming organs.
- **Anemia** (ah-**NEE**-me-ah) is a disorder characterized by lower than normal levels of red blood cells in the blood.

  Aplastic anemia is a form of anemia that is resistant to therapy and is marked by absence of regeneration of all formed blood elements.

  Hemolytic anemia (**he**-moh-**LIT**-ick) is due to the shortened survival of mature erythrocytes.

  Iron deficiency anemia is an anemia caused by an inadequate supply of iron within the body.

  Pernicious anemia (per-**NISH**-us) is a form of anemia that results from a failure of the body to absorb vitamin B_{12}.

  Sickle-cell anemia is a genetically determined defect of hemoglobin synthesis.

  Thalassemia (thal-ah-**SEE**-me-ah), also known as **Cooley's anemia,** is a hemolytic anemia characterized by short-lived red blood cells.

Hypertension

- **Essential hypertension,** also known as **primary hypertension** or **idiopathic hypertension** is consistently elevated blood pressure of unknown origin.
- **Secondary hypertension** is caused by some other problem such as a kidney problem or a tumor on the adrenal glands. When the other problem is cured, the secondary hypertension should be resolved.
- **Malignant hypertension** is an abnormal condition characterized by the sudden onset of severely elevated blood pressure. It commonly damages small vessels in the brain, retina, heart and kidneys.

PROCEDURES RELATED TO THE CARDIOVASCULAR SYSTEM

- **Percutaneous transluminal coronary angioplasty,** which is also called **balloon catheter dilation,** is a procedure in which a small balloon on the end of a catheter is used in an effort to improve the passage of blood.
- **Coronary bypass surgery** is a surgical procedure used to improve the blood supply to the heart muscle when narrowed coronary arteries reduce the flow of blood.
- **Anastomosis** (ah-**nas**-toh-**MOH**-sis) is the surgical joining of two ducts or blood vessels to allow flow from one to the other. (Plural, **anastomoses.**)
- **Angioplasty** (**AN**-jee-oh-**plas**-tee) is the surgical reconstruction of blood vessels.
- An **arteriectomy** (**ar**-teh-ree-**ECK**-toh-me), also spelled **arterectomy,** is the surgical removal of part of an artery.
- **Pericardiectomy** (per-ih-**kar**-dee-**ECK**- toh-me) is the surgical removal of a portion of the pericardium.
- **Valvuloplasty** (**VAL**-view-loh-**plas**-tee) is the surgical repair of a heart valve.
- **Cardiocentesis** (**kar**-dee-oh-sen-**TEE**-sis) is the surgical puncture or incision of the heart.
- **Hemorrhoidectomy** (**hem**-oh-roid-**ECK**-toh-me) is the surgical removal of hemorrhoids.
- **Cardiopulmonary resuscitation** (CPR) is an emergency procedure for life support consisting of artificial respiration and manual external cardiac massage that may be used in the event of cardiac arrest.
- **Defibrillation** is a treatment to stop cardiac arrhythmia and restore a more normal rhythm.
- A **tourniquet** (**TOOR**-nih-ket) is the use of a constricting band applied to a limb to control bleeding. A tourniquet is also used when drawing blood from a vein.
- A **transfusion** is the introduction into the bloodstream of the recipient of whole blood or blood components taken from a donor.
- **Plasmapheresis** (**plaz**-mah-feh-**REE**-sis) is the process of separating the plasma and formed elements from blood which has been withdrawn from the body. The formed elements are placed in an isotonic solution and reinfused into the donor.

IMPORTANT TERMS: THE CARDIOVASCULAR SYSTEM

This list will help you identify and review the major terms from this chapter.

When you work with the audio tape for this chapter, listen to the word, repeat it and then place a ✓ next to it on the list below.

- ☐ **Acidosis** (**ass**-ih-**DOH**-sis)
- ☐ **Acrocyanosis** (**ak**-roh- **sigh**-ah-**NO**-sis)
- ☐ **Agglutination** (ah-**gloo**-tih-**NAY**-shun)
- ☐ **Albumin** (al-**BYOU**-min)
- ☐ **Anastomosis** (ah-**nas**-toh-**MOH**-sis)
- ☐ **Anemia** (ah-**NEE**-me-ah)
- ☐ **Aneurysm** (**AN**-you-rizm)
- ☐ **Angina** (an-**JIGH**-nah)
- ☐ **Angiocardiography** (**an**-jee-oh-**kar**-dee-**OG**-rah-fee)
- ☐ **Angiography** (**an**-jee-**OG**-rah-fee)
- ☐ **Angionecrosis** (**an**-jee-oh-neh-**KROH**-sis)
- ☐ **Angioplasty** (**AN**-jee-oh-**plas**-tee)
- ☐ **Angiospasm** (**AN**-jee-oh-**spazm**)

- □ **Angiostenosis** (AN-jee-oh-stee-NO-sis)
- □ **Antigen** (AN-tih-jen)
- □ **Aorta** (ay-**OR**-tah)
- □ **Arrhythmia** (ah-**RITH**-me-ah)
- □ **Arteriectomy** (**ar**-teh-ree-**ECK**-toh-me)
- □ **Arteriography** (**are**-tee-ree-**OG**-rah-fee)
- □ **Arteriosclerosis** (ar-**tee**-ree-oh-skleh-**ROH**-sis)
- □ **Arterioles** (are-**TEE**-ree-ohlz)
- □ **Arteritis** (**ar**-teh-**RYE**-tis)
- □ **Atherosclerosis** (**ath**-er-**oh**-sklee-**ROH**-sis)
- □ **Atria** (**AY**-tree-ah)
- □ **Atrioventricular** (**ay**-tree-oh-ven-**TRICK**-you-lahr)
- □ **Basophils** (**BAY**-soh-fills)
- □ **Bradycardia** (**brad**-ee-**KAR**-dee-ah)
- □ **Cardiocentesis** (**kar**-dee-oh-sen-**TEE**-sis)
- □ **Cardiomegaly** (**kar**-dee-oh-**MEG**-ah-lee)
- □ **Cardioplegia** (**kar**-dee-oh-**PLEE**-jee-ah)
- □ **Cardiorrhexis** (**kar**-dee-oh-**RECK**-sis)
- □ **Carditis** (kar-**DYE**-tis)
- □ **Cholesterol** (koh-**LES**-ter-ol)
- □ **Claudication** (**klaw**-dih-**KAY**-shun)
- □ **Diastolic** (dye-ah-**STOL**-ick)
- □ **Dyscrasia** (dis-**KRAY**-zee-ah)
- □ **Echocardiography** (**eck**-oh-**kar**-dee-**OG**-rah-fee)
- □ **Electrocardiography** (ee-**leck**-troh-kar-dee-**OG**-rah-fee)
- □ **Embolus** (**EM**-boh-lus)
- □ **Endarterial** (**end**- ar-**TEE**-ree-al)
- □ **Endocarditis** (**en**-doh-kar-**DYE**-tis)
- □ **Endocardium** (**en**-doh-**KAR**-dee-um)
- □ **Eosinophils** (**ee**-oh-**SIN**-oh-fills)
- □ **Epicardium** (**ep**-ih-**KAR**-dee-um)
- □ **Epistaxis** (**ep**-ih-**STACK**-sis)
- □ **Erythrocytosis** (eh-**rith**-roh-sigh-**TOH**-sis)
- □ **Erythrocytes** (eh-**RITH**-roh-sites)
- □ **Fibrillation** (**fih**-brih-**LAY**-shun)
- □ **Fibrinogen** (fye-**BRIN**-oh-jen)
- □ **Globulin** (**GLOB**-you-lin)
- □ **Hemangioma** (heh-**man**-jee-**OH**-mah)
- □ **Hemarthrosis** (**hem**-ar-**THROH**-sis)
- □ **Hematemesis** (**hem**-ah-**TEM**-eh-sis)
- □ **Hematocrit** (he-**MAT**-oh-krit)
- □ **Hematoma** (**hem**-ah-**TOH**-mah)
- □ **Hemoglobin** (**he**-moh-**GLOW**-bin)
- □ **Hemolytic** (**he**-moh-**LIT**-ick)
- □ **Hemophilia** (**hee**-moh-**FILL**-ee-ah)
- □ **Hemorrhage** (**HEM**-or-idj)
- □ **Hemorrhoidectomy** (**hem**-oh-roid-**ECK**-toh-me)
- □ **Hemorrhoids** (**HEM**-oh-roids)
- □ **Hemostasis** (**he**-moh-**STAY**-sis)
- □ **Hyperalbuminemia** (**high**-per-al-**byou**-mih-**NEE**-me-ah)
- □ **Hyperbilirubinemia** (**high**-per-**bil**-ih-**roo**-bih-**NEE**-me-ah)
- □ **Hyperlipidemia** (**high**-per-**lip**-ih-**DEE**-me-ah)

- ☐ **Hyperlipemia** (**high**-per-lye-**PEE**-me-ah)
- ☐ **Hyperuricemia** (**high**-per-**you**-rih-**SEE**-me-ah)
- ☐ **Hypoperfusion** (**high**-poh-per-**FYOU**-zhun)
- ☐ **Ischemia** (is-**KEY**-me-ah)
- ☐ **Leukemia** (loo-**KEY**-me-ah)
- ☐ **Leukocytes** (**LOO**-koh-sites)
- ☐ **Leukopenia** (**loo**-koh-**PEE**-nee-ah)
- ☐ **Lumen** (**LOO**-men)
- ☐ **Lymphocytes** (**LIM**-foh-sites)
- ☐ **Monocytes** (**MON**-oh-sites)
- ☐ **Myocarditis** (**my**-oh-kar-**DYE**-tis)
- ☐ **Myocardium** (**migh**-oh-**KAR**-dee-um)
- ☐ **Necrosis** (neh-**KROH**-sis)
- ☐ **Neutrophils** (**NEW**-troh-fills)
- ☐ **Palpitation** (**pal**-pih-**TAY**-shun)
- ☐ **Pericardiectomy** (per-ih-**kar**-dee-**ECK**-toh-me)
- ☐ **Pericarditis** (**per**-ih-kar-**DYE**-tis)
- ☐ **Pericardiocentesis** (**per**-ih-**kar**-dee-oh-sen-**TEE**-sis)
- ☐ **Pernicious** (per-**NISH**-us)
- ☐ **Phlebitis** (fleh-**BYE**-tis)
- ☐ **Phlebography** (fleh-**BOG**-rah-fee)
- ☐ **Phonocardiography** (**foh**-no-**kar**-dee-**OG**-rah-fee)
- ☐ **Plasmapheresis** (**plaz**-mah-feh-**REE**-sis)
- ☐ **Polyarteritis** (**pol**-ee-**ar**-teh-**RYE**-tis)
- ☐ **Prothrombin** (pro-**THROM**-bin)
- ☐ **Purpura** (**PUR**-pew-rah)
- ☐ **Raynaud's** (ray-**NOHZ**)
- ☐ **Reticulocyte** (reh-**TICK**-you-loh-**site**)
- ☐ **Serology** (see-**ROL**-oh-jee)
- ☐ **Serum** (**SEE**-rum)
- ☐ **Sinoatrial** (**sigh**-no-**AY**-tree-ahl)
- ☐ **Stenosis** (steh-**NO**-sis)
- ☐ **Systolic** (sis-**TOL**-ick)
- ☐ **Tachycardia** (**tack**-ee-**KAR**-dee-ah)
- ☐ **Thalassemia** (thal-ah-**SEE**-me-ah)
- ☐ **Thrombocytes** (**THROM**-boh-sites)
- ☐ **Thrombocytopenia** (**throm**-boh-**sigh**-toh-**PEE**-nee-ah)
- ☐ **Thrombophlebitis** (**throm**-boh-fleh-**BYE**-tis)
- ☐ **Thrombotic occlusion** (throm-**BOT**-ick ah-**KLOO**-zhun)
- ☐ **Thrombosis** (throm-**BOH**-sis)
- ☐ **Thrombus** (**THROM**-bus)
- ☐ **Tourniquet** (**TOOR**-nih-ket)
- ☐ **Triglycerides** (try-**GLIS**-er-eyeds)
- ☐ **Valvulitis** (**val**-view-**LYE**-tis)
- ☐ **Valvuloplasty** (**VAL**-view-loh-**plas**-tee)
- ☐ **Varicosity** (**var**-ih-**KOS**-ih-tee)
- ☐ **Vena cava** (**VEE**-nah **KAY**-vah)
- ☐ **Venae cavae** (**VEE**-nee **KAY**-vee)
- ☐ **Venipuncture** (**VEN**-ih-**punk**-tyour)
- ☐ **Ventricles** (**VEN**-trih-kuhls)

5

EXERCISES

DEFINING WORD PARTS

Write the definition for each of these word parts.

1. *ANGI/O* ____________________
2. *AORT/O* ____________________
3. *ARTERI/O* ____________________
4. *ATHER/O* ____________________
5. *ATRI/O* ____________________
6. *BRADY-* ____________________
7. *CARDI/O* ____________________
8. *-CRIT* ____________________
9. *CYAN/O* ____________________
10. *-CYTE* ____________________
11. *-EMESIS* ____________________
12. *EPI-* ____________________
13. *ERYTHR/O* ____________________
14. *-GLOBIN* ____________________
15. *HEMAT/O, HEM/O* ____________________
16. *ISCH/O* ____________________

17. *LEUK/O* ______________________________

18. *-MEGALY* ______________________________

19. *-PHAGE* ______________________________

20. *PHLEB/O* ______________________________

21. *-PLEGIA* ______________________________

22. *-RRHAGE* ______________________________

23. *-RRHEXIS* ______________________________

24. *SER/O* ______________________________

25. *-STASIS* ______________________________

26. *TACHY-* ______________________________

27. *THROMB/O* ______________________________

28. *VALV/O, VALVUL/O* ______________________________

29. *VAS/O* ______________________________

30. *VEN/O* ______________________________

DEFINITIONS

Circle the letter next to the correct answer.

1. Leukocytes are ______________
   a) commonly known as white blood cells.
   b) destroyed in the spleen.
   c) important in fighting disease in the body.
   d) a and c.

2. The myocardium is the ______________
   a) external layer of the heart.
   b) innermost layer of the heart.
   c) muscular middle layer of the heart.
   d) sac surrounding the heart.

3. The ______________ is also called the pacemaker of the heart.
   a) atrioventricular node
   b) bundle of His
   c) sinoatrial node
   d) sinoventricular node

4. The ______________ valve is also known as the bicuspid valve.
   a) aortic semilunar
   b) mitral
   c) pulmonary semilunar
   d) sinomitral

5. The right ventricle ______________
   a) pumps blood to all parts of the body except the lungs.
   b) pumps blood to the lungs.
   c) receives blood from all tissues except the lungs.
   d) receives oxygenated blood from the lungs.

6. ______________ is the rapid, random and ineffective contractions of the heart.
   a) Bradycardia
   b) Fibrillation
   c) Flutter
   d) Tachycardia

7. Blood gases include ______________
   a) carbon dioxide.
   b) nitrogen.
   c) oxygen.
   d) a, b and c.

8. The term hemostasis means the ______________
   a) mechanism used by the body to control bleeding.
   b) percentage of formed elements in the blood.
   c) process of destroying worn-out red blood cells.
   d) process of forming new red blood cells.

9. Lipid tests ______________
   a) measure the amount of cholesterol in a blood sample.
   b) measure the amount of triglycerides in a blood sample.
   c) provide important evidence of a myocardial infarction.
   d) a and b.

10. ______________ is a surgical procedure used to improve the blood supply to the heart muscle when narrowed coronary arteries reduce the flow of blood.
    a) Anastomosis
    b) Balloon catheter
    c) Coronary bypass
    d) Vasodilation

MISSING WORDS

Write the missing word on the line.

1. ______________________ pressure is the highest blood pressure when the ventricles contract.
2. ______________________ is plasma with the clotting proteins removed.
3. ______________________ are commonly known as platelets.
4. The term ______________________ means the volume percentage of erythrocytes in whole blood.
5. ______________________ pressure is the lowest blood pressure when the ventricles are relaxed.
6. The blood protein ______________________ plays an essential role in oxygen transport.
7. ______________________ are a major group of leukocytes that fight disease by engulfing and swallowing up germs.
8. A/an ______________________ is a foreign object found in the circulatory system, such as a quantity of air or gas, a bit of tissue or tumor or a piece of a thrombus.
9. A/an ______________________ is a localized balloon-like enlargement of an artery.
10. The ______________________ ______________________ are the two large veins that enter the heart.

SPELLCHECK

Select the correct spelling and write it on the line.

1. ______________________ veins are abnormally swollen veins, usually occurring in the legs.
   Varicose
   Vericose
   Very course
2. ______________________ are commonly known as piles.
   Hemarroids
   Hemoroids
   Hemorrhoids
3. A coronary ______________________ is blockage, and damage, in the heart caused by a blood clot.
   thrombiosis
   thrombosis
   trombosis

4. ______________________ is the inflammation of a vein that is often accompanied by the formation of a clot.
   Fleabitis
   Pflebitis
   Phlebitis

5. ______________________ is an abnormally fast heartbeat.
   Tachicardia
   Tachycardia
   Tackycardia

6. ______________________ is a group of hereditary bleeding disorders in which there is a lack of one more or of the factors needed to clot blood.
   Hemaphilia
   Hemofilia
   Hemophilia

7. ______________________ is commonly known as a nosebleed.
   Epataxis
   Epitaxsis
   Epistaxis

8. ______________________ is an inflammatory condition of a heart valve.
   Valvolitis
   Valvitis
   Valvulitis

9. Cardiac ______________________ are any abnormal heart rhythms.
   arhythemias
   arrhythmias
   arrhythemias

10. ______________________ is a hemolytic anemia characterized by short-lived red blood cells.
    Thallassemia
    Thalasemia
    Thalassemia

11. ______________________ is a diagnostic procedure which uses ultrasound for evaluating the structures of the heart.
    Echocardigraphy
    Echocardiography
    Echocardiology

12. ______________________ heart disease is a pathological condition of the myocardium caused by a lack of oxygen reaching the tissue cells.
    Ischamic
    Ischemic
    Ishemic

13. ______________________ is the surgical reconstruction of blood vessels.
    Angiplasty
    Anginoplasty
    Angioplasty

14. ______________________ pectoris is usually due to interference with the supply of oxygen to the heart muscle.
    Angena
    Angina
    Anjena

15. ______________________ anemia is due to the shortened survival of mature erythrocytes.
    Hemalytic
    Hematolytic
    Hemolytic

CASE STUDIES

Write the correct answer on the line.

1. Ramon Martinez has ______________________ which is an abnormally fast heartbeat.
2. During her pregnancy, Polly Olson suffered from ______________________ veins (abnormally swollen veins) in her legs.
3. Roscoe Jackson has ______________________ which is hardening of the arteries due to a buildup of yellowish plaques of cholesterol.
4. Thomas Willis suffers from ______________________ which is spasmodic, choking or suffocating pain.
5. Herb Michaels died due to a ruptured ______________________ (balloon-like enlargement) of an artery in his brain.
6. Helen Grovenor was admitted to the hospital for ______________________ which means that she was vomiting blood.
7. Darlene Nolan has mitral ______________________ which is an obstructive lesion in the mitral valve of the heart.
8. ______________________ was used to stop cardiac arrhythmia and restore a more normal rhythm to Harry Young's heart.

9. Dave Orton has a/an ______________________ which is an extra sound heard between normal heart sounds.

10. Michael Lawson underwent ______________________ which is the surgical repair of a heart valve.

11. Jason Turner suffered from cardiac arrest and the paramedics used ______________________ ______________________ (CPR) as an emergency life support procedure.

12. Allen Franklin was rushed to the hospital when he suffered a/an ______________________ ______________________ which is commonly known as a heart attack.

13. Jenny Edwards was hospitalized after she suffered a transient ______________________ attack.

14. The process of ______________________ was used to produce a record of the electrical activity of the myocardium of Sam Harris's heart.

15. Gary Klein suffers from ______________________ which is a malignant neoplasm of the blood-forming organs.

WORD BUILDING

Write the correct word or word part on the line.

1. Paralysis of the heart
   a) The combining form ______________________ means heart.
   b) The suffix ______________________ means paralysis.
   c) The term ______________________ means paralysis of the heart.

2. The veins
   a) The combining form ______________________ means vein.
   b) The suffix ______________________ means inflammation.
   c) The term ______________________ means an inflammation of a vein.

3. Blood vessels
   a) The combining form ______________________ means blood vessels.
   b) The suffix ______________________ means surgical reconstruction or repair.
   c) The term ______________________ means the surgical reconstruction or repair of a blood vessel.

4. The arteries
   a) The combining form ______________________ means artery.
   b) The prefix ______________________ means many.
   c) The suffix ______________________ means inflammation.
   d) The term ______________________ means the inflammation of several arteries.

5. Enlargement of the heart
   a) The combining form ______________________ means heart.
   b) The suffix ______________________ means enlarged.
   c) The term ______________________ means an enlargement of the heart.

LABELING EXERCISES

Identify the numbered items on this diagram.

1. ______________________
2. ______________________
3. ______________________
4. ______________________
5. ______________________

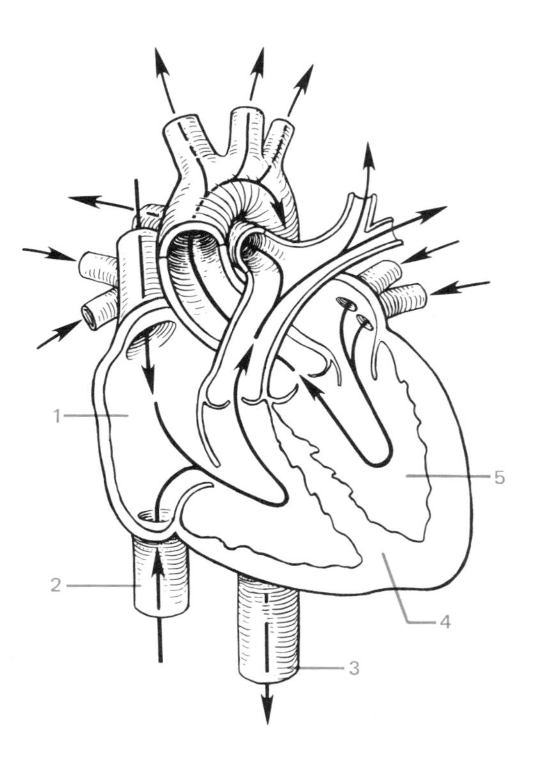

6

THE LYMPHATIC AND IMMUNE SYSTEMS

LEARNING GOALS

In this chapter you will learn to:

- describe the major functions and structures of the lymphatic system.
- recognize and identify the major terms related to the diagnosis, pathology and treatment of the lymphatic system.
- describe the major functions and structures of the immune system.
- identify the major types of immunity and describe how each is acquired.
- recognize and identify the major terms related to the diagnosis, pathology and treatment of disorders of the immune system.
- describe at least three types of pathogenic organisms and list six types of diseases.

THE LYMPHATIC SYSTEM

The major structures of the lymphatic system include the lymph vessels, lymph nodes and lymph fluid plus the tonsils and adenoids. (The combining form *LYMPH/O* means lymph.)

The spleen and thymus are also composed of lymphatic tissue and have important roles in the immune response. They are discussed later in this chapter under the immune system.

Lymph Vessels

Lymph capillaries, are thin-walled tubes that carry lymph from the tissue spaces to the larger **lymphatic vessels.** Like veins, lymphatic vessels have valves to prevent the backward flow of fluid.

Lymph fluid always flows toward the thoracic cavity. Here the **right lymphatic duct** and the **thoracic duct** empty lymph into veins in the upper thoracic region.

Specialized lymph vessels, called **lacteals** (LACK-tee-ahls), are located in the small intestine. The lacteals aid in the absorption of fats from the small intestine into the bloodstream.

Lymph passing through the lacteals is called **chyle (KYL)** and is milky in appearance because of the fats it has absorbed.

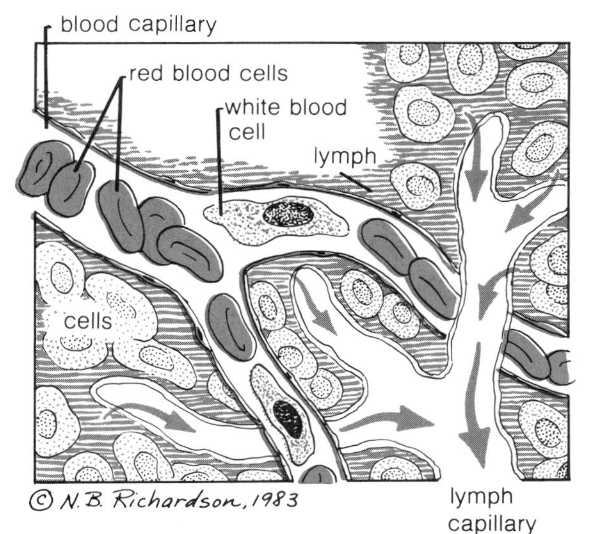

Figure 6-1 Lymph circulation.

Lymph Nodes

Lymph nodes are small round or oval structures located in lymph vessels.

Lymph nodes fight disease by producing antibodies, which are part of the immune reaction. The lymphocytes also purify the lymph by removing harmful substances such as bacteria or malignant cells.

In acute infections, the lymph nodes become swollen and tender due to the collection of lymphocytes gathered to destroy the invading substances.

Tumor cells may metastasize from the lymph nodes and spread to other sites in the body.

MAJOR LYMPH NODE SITES
CERVICAL LYMPH NODES (SER-vih-kal) are located in the neck. (The combining form *CERVIC/O* means neck.)
AXILLARY LYMPH NODES (AK-sih-**lar**-ee) are located under the arms. (The combining form *AXILL/O* means armpit.)
INGUINAL LYMPH NODES (ING-gwih-nal) are located in the inguinal (groin) area of the lower abdomen. (The combining form *INGUIN/O* means groin.)

Lymph Fluid

Lymph is a clear and colorless tissue fluid that is also known as **intercellular** or **interstitial fluid.** (The prefix *INTER-* means between and among.)

Lymph flows in the spaces between the cells and tissues so that it can carry the substances from these tissues back into the bloodstream.

Lymph fluid is composed of water, lymphocytes, digested nutrients, hormones, salts, carbon dioxide, oxygen and urea.

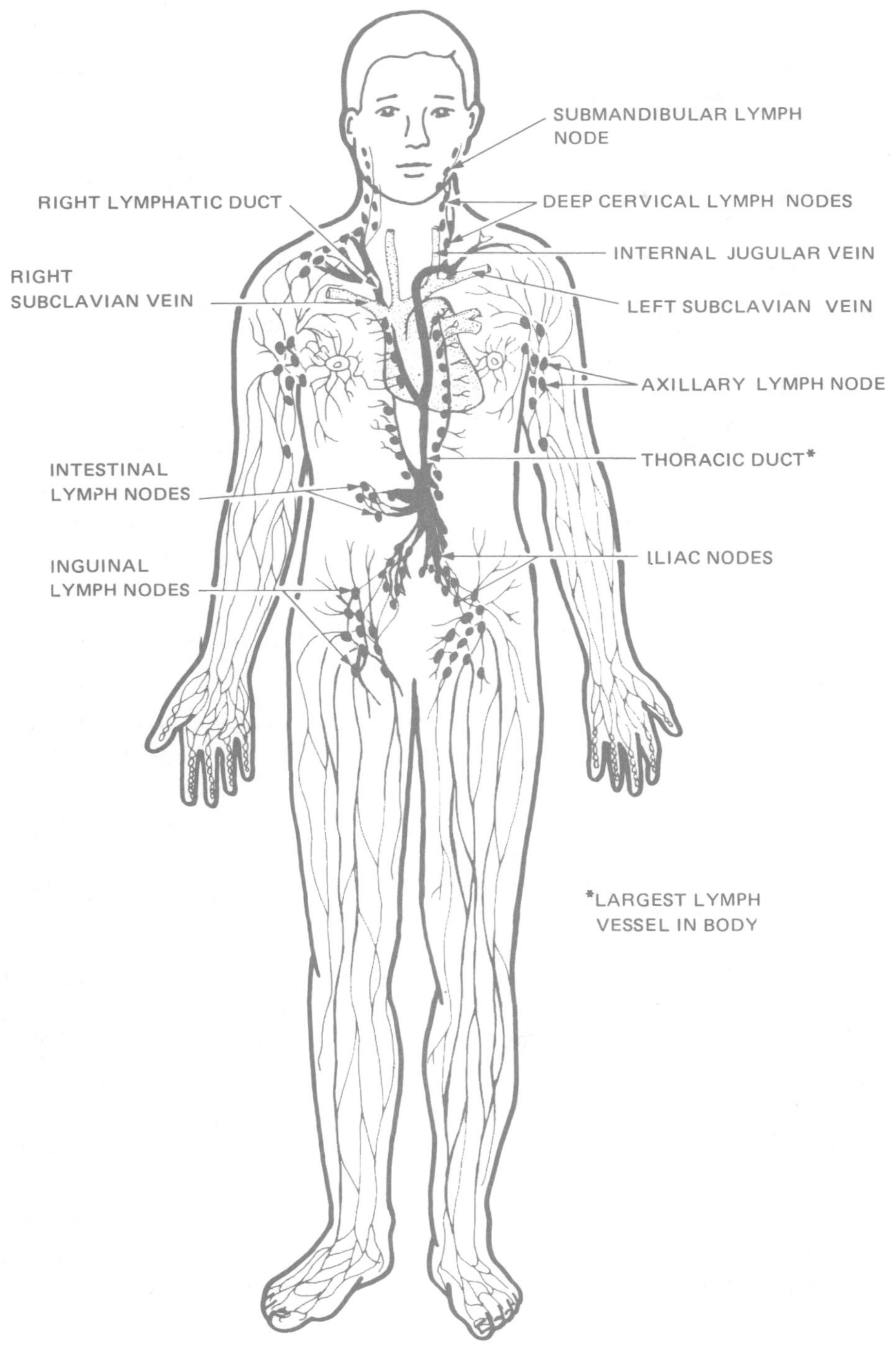

Figure 6-2 Lymphatic drainage. (From *Human Anatomy and Physiology* by Joan G. Creager. © 1983 by Wadsworth, Inc. Reprinted by permission of the publisher.)

Lymph Cells

Although the lymphatic system has its own vessels and fluid, it does not have cells or formed elements of its own. Instead, the cellular composition of lymph includes lymphocytes, monocytes and a few platelets and erythrocytes which are all blood cells. (See Chapter 5.)

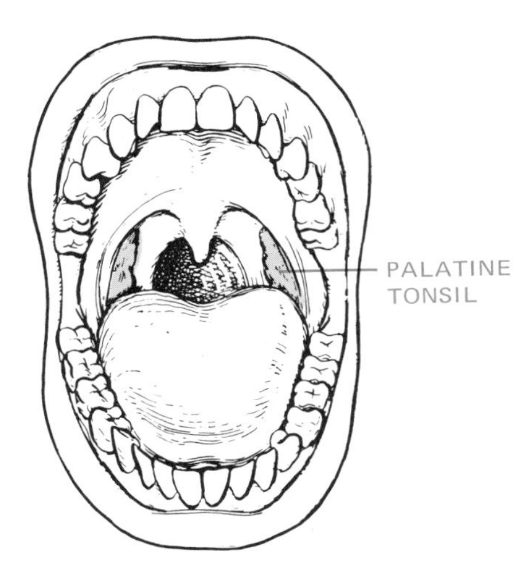

Figure 6-3 The palatine tonsils.

The Tonsils and Adenoids

The **tonsils** (**TON**-sils) and **adenoids** (**AD**-eh-noids) are masses of lymphatic tissue located in the upper portions of the nose and throat. (The combining form *TONSILL/O* means tonsil and *ADENOID/O* means adenoid.)

The adenoids, also known as the **nasopharyngeal tonsils** (**nay**-zoh-fah-**RIN**-jee-al), are found in the nasopharynx. (The combining form *NAS/O* means nose.)

The **palatine tonsils** are located in the oropharynx and are visible through the mouth. (The combining form *PALAT/O* means palate or roof of the mouth.)

The **lingual tonsils** are located on the back of the tongue. (The combining form *LINGU/O* means tongue.)

DIAGNOSTIC PROCEDURES RELATED TO THE LYMPHATIC SYSTEM

- **Lymphangiography** (lim-**fan**-jee-**OG**-rah-fee) is the radiographic examination of the lymphatic channels after introduction of a contrast medium. (The combining form *LYMPHANGI/O* means lymph vessel.)

PATHOLOGY OF THE LYMPHATIC SYSTEM

- **Lymphadenitis** (lim-**fad**-eh-**NIGH**-tis), also known as swollen glands, is an inflammation of the lymph nodes.
- **Adenoiditis** (**ad**-eh-noid-**EYE**-tis) is an inflammation of the adenoidal tissue of the nasopharynx.
- **Tonsillitis** (**ton**-sih-**LYE**-tis) is an inflammation of the tonsils.
- **Lymphoma** (lim-**FOH**-mah) is a general term that is applied to any tumor made up of lymphatic tissue.
- An **angioma** (**an**-jee-**OH**-mah), also known as a **lymphangioma** (lim-**fan**-jee-**OH**-mah), is a tumor composed of newly formed lymph spaces and channels.
- **Lymphosarcoma** (**lim**-foh-sar-**KOH**-mah) is a general term applied to malignant neoplastic disorders of lymphoid tissue, but not including Hodgkin's disease.
- **Hodgkin's disease** is a malignant condition characterized by progressive enlargement of the lymph nodes, spleen and lymphoid tissue.
- **Mononucleosis** (**mon**-oh-**new**-klee-**OH**-sis) is marked by the presence of an abnormally large number of atypical lymphocytes. It is caused by the Epstein-Barr virus.

THE IMMUNE SYSTEM

The immune system works to protect the entire body from a variety of harmful substances such as pathogenic microorganisms, allergens, toxins and malignant cells.

Immunity is the state of being resistant or not susceptible to a disease. (The combing form *IMMUN/O* means immune, protected and safe.)

Antigen-Antibody Reactions

An **antigen** is a substance such as a virus, bacterium or toxin that stimulates the production of antibodies. (A **toxin** is a poison.)

Antibodies are substances developed by the body in response to the presence of a specific antigen.

The **antigen-antibody reaction,** also known as the **immune reaction,** involves the binding of antigens to antibodies to form antigen-antibody complexes that may render the toxic antigen harmless.

STRUCTURES OF THE IMMUNE SYSTEM

Unlike other body systems, the immune system is not contained within a set of organs or vessels. Instead it involves many systems, organs and tissues including the skin, respiratory system, spleen, thymus and lymphocytes.

The Skin

The skin is the body's first line of defense against invading organisms because it acts as a physical barrier to prevent their entry into the body. It also triggers a response from the immune system to counteract any invaders that do penetrate the skin.

The Respiratory System

Foreign matter that is breathed in is trapped by nostril hairs and by the moist mucous membrane that lines the respiratory system. The mucus secreted by these membranes continually flushes away this trapped debris.

The Spleen

The spleen is a sac-like mass of lymphatic tissue that is located in the left upper quadrant of the abdomen, just below the diaphragm and behind the stomach. (The combining form *SPLEN/O* means spleen.)

The spleen is an important part of the immune system because it produces lymphocytes and monocytes. It also filters microorganisms and other foreign material from the blood.

Other functions include storing red blood cells and maintaining the appropriate balance between cells and plasma in the blood.

The spleen is **hemolytic (he-**moh-**LIT**-ick). This means that it removes and destroys worn-out red blood cells. (The suffix *-LYTIC* means to reduce or destroy.)

This hemolytic activity in the spleen causes bilirubin to be formed. (**Bilirubin** (bill-ih-**ROO**-bin) is the orange-yellow pigment of bile.)

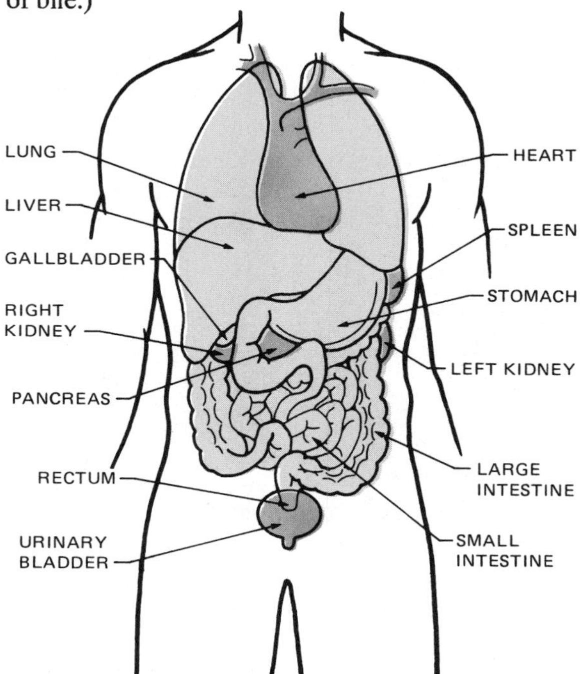

Figure 6-4 The spleen is located posterior to the stomach.

Figure 6-5 The thymus is located above the heart.

The Thymus

The thymus gland is composed largely of lymphatic tissue and is located in the upper anterior portion of the thorax above the heart.

The thymus produces lymphocytes and plays an important role in the body's immunologic system, especially in fetal life and the early years of growth. (The thymus also functions as an endocrine gland. This is discussed in chapter 13.)

Lymphocytes

Lymphocytes (**LIM**-foh-sights) are agranular leukocytes (white blood cells) that play an important part in the lymphatic system.

Macrophages

Monocytes are agranular lymphocytes that are formed in the bone marrow and transported to other parts of the body where they become macrophages. (The combining form *PHAG/O* means eating or swallowing.)

Macrophages are phagocytic cells that protect the body by ingesting (eating) invading bacteria and by interacting with the other cells of the immune system.

Histiocytes (HIS-tee-oh-**sights)** are the large macrophages found in loose connective tissue.

T-LYMPHOCYTES

T-lymphocytes, also known as **T-cells,** are small circulating lymphocytes that are produced in the bone marrow. They mature in the thymus or as a result of exposure to thymosin which is secreted by the thymus.

T-cells live for years and their primary function is to indirectly aid cellular immune responses such as graft rejection, delayed hypersensitivity, the destruction of virus-infected cells and the destruction of cancer cells.

Helper T-cells are a type of T-cell that stimulates the production of antibodies by B-cells.

Suppressor T-cells are a type of T-cell that suppresses B-cell activity. (See B-Lymphocytes below.)

Lymphokines

Lymphokines (**LIM**-foh-keens), which are produced by the T-cells, are molecules, other than antibodies, that are involved in signalling between the cells of the immune system.

Lymphokines attract macrophages to the site of infection or inflammation and then prepare them for attack.

Interferon

Interferon (**in**-ter-**FEAR**-on), which is also produced by the T-cells, is a protein substance released by cells that have been invaded by a virus.

Interferon induces noninfected cells to form an antiviral protein that inhibits viral multiplication. It also enhances antiviral immunity and is capable of modifying immune responses.

B-LYMPHOCYTES

B-lymphocytes, also known as **B-cells,** are also produced in the bone marrow. When confronted with a specific type of antigen, they are transformed into plasma cells.

Plasma Cells

Plasma cells produce and secrete antibodies. Each antibody is specifically coded to match one antigen. They are effective against most free-floating agents such as viruses, bacteria and many types of bacterial toxins.

Immunoglobulins

The antibodies made by plasma cells are called immunoglobulins (Ig). An immunoglobulin (**im**-you-no-**GLOB**-you-lin) is any of five distinct antibodies present in the serum and external secretions of the body. There are five types of immunoglobulins.

- **Immunoglobulin A** (IgA) is the major antibody in the mucous membrane lining of the intestines. It is also found in the bronchi, saliva, and tears.
- **Immunoglobulin D** (IgD) is found in small amounts in serum tissue. Its precise function is not known.
- **Immunoglobulin E** (IgE) is concentrated in the lungs, the skin and the cells of mucous membranes. It provides the primary defense against environmental antigens.
- **Immunoglobulin G** (IgG) is a specialized protein synthesized in response to invasions by bacteria, fungi and viruses.
- **Immunoglobulin M** (IgM) is the first immunoglobulin the body produces when challenged by antigens and is found in circulating fluids.

Complement

Complement is a series of complex, enzymatic proteins occurring in normal serum. In an antigen-antibody reaction, complement causes **lysis.** This is the destruction of a cell by penetrating the cell wall, allowing fluid to fill the cell and causing the cell to rupture.

Complement also aids phagocytes in the phagocytic destruction of antigens.

THE IMMUNE SYSTEM IN ACTION

STAGE ONE
• Viruses invade the body. Their goal is to invade cells where they can replicate.
• Macrophages consume some of the invading viruses.
• Helper T-cells are activated.

STAGE TWO
• Helper T-cells begin to multiply.
• They attract complement to the area.
• They also stimulate the multiplication of B-cells sensitive to the virus.
• B-cells start producing antibodies.

STAGE THREE
• Complement proteins break open cells invaded by the virus and spill the viral contents.
• Antibodies produced by the B-cells inactivate the viruses by binding with them.

STAGE FOUR
• As the infection is contained, suppressor T-cells halt the immune response.
• B-cells remain ready in case the same virus invades again.

ACQUIRED IMMUNITY

Acquired immunity is any form of immunity that is not innate and is obtained during life. (**Innate** means present at birth.)

Naturally acquired immunity is obtained by the development of antibodies resulting from an attack of infectious disease or by the transmission of the antibodies from the mother to the infant.

Artificially acquired immunity is obtained by vaccination or by the injection of antiserum.

PATHOLOGY OF THE IMMUNE SYSTEM

- **Immunodeficiency** (**im**-you-no-deh-**FISH**-en-see) is an abnormal condition of the immune system in which immunity is inadequate and resistance to infection is decreased.
- **Allergy** is a hypersensitive state acquired through exposure to a particular allergen.

  An **allergen** is a substance capable of inducing allergy or specific hypersensitivity.

  Anaphylactic shock (**an**-ah-fih-**LACK**-tick) is an unusual, severe and sometimes fatal allergic reaction to a foreign protein or other substance such as a drug, food, insect venom or chemical.
- An **autoimmune disorder** is what happens when the body forms antibodies against proteins that are not foreign, but are already part of the body. Autoimmune disorders are marked by inflammation and injury to body cells.
- **Acquired immune deficiency syndrome** (AIDS) is a disease caused by the **human immunodeficiency virus** (HIV). The disease destroys part of the body's immune system and leaves victims unable to defend themselves against opportunistic infections and certain cancers.
- An **opportunistic infection** is an infection caused by normally nonpathogenic organisms in a host whose resistance has been decreased by a different disorder.
- **AIDS-related complex** (ARC) consists of the indications of immune deficiency but which do not meet the criteria for AIDS.

Opportunistic Infections Related to AIDS and ARC

- **Kaposi's sarcoma** (**KAP**-oh-seez) is a malignant, multifocal neoplasm that begins as soft papules on the feet and slowly spreads in the skin, metastasizing to the lymph nodes and viscera.
- **Persistent generalized lymphadenopathy** is the continued presence of diffuse enlargement of lymph nodes.

  Lymphadenopathy (lim-**fad**-eh-**NOP**-ah-thee) means disease of the lymph nodes.
- **Pneumocystosis** (**new**-moh-sis-**TOH**-sis) is a form of pneumonia caused by an infection with the parasite *Pneumocystis carinii.*
- **Aspergillosis** (**as**-per-jil-**OH**-sis) is an infection caused by a fungus of the genus *Aspergillus.* It may cause inflammation and lesions on, or in, any organ.
- **Candidiasis** (**kan**-dih-**DYE**-ah-sis) is an infection caused by a species of *Candida,* a fungus.
- **Cryptococcal meningitis** (**krip**-toh-**KOCK**-al **men**-in-**JIGH**-tis) is a form of meningitis (an inflammation of the meninges of the brain) caused by the fungus *Cryptococcus neoformans.*
- **Cytomegalovirus** (**sigh**-toh-**meg**-ah-loh-**VYE**-rus) is an infection caused by a group of large herpes-type viruses with a wide variety of disease effects.
- **Nocardiosis** (no-kar-dee-**OH**-sis) is an infection with the bacterium *Nocardia asteroides* which is characterized by pneumonia and chronic abscesses of the brain and subcutaneous tissue.
- **Toxoplasmosis** (**tock**-soh-plaz-**MOH**-sis) is an infection with the protozoan parasite *Toxoplasma gondii,* which is characterized by lesions of the central nervous system.

Procedures Related to the Immune System

- **Immunosuppression** (**im**-you-no-sup-**PRESH**-un) is the administration of agents that significantly interfere with the ability of the immune system to respond to antigenic stimulation.

  This may be done with drugs or radiation as treatment for cancer or to prevent the rejection of donor tissue.

- **Immunotherapy** (ih-**myou**-no-**THER**-ah-pee) is a special treatment of allergic responses that administers increasingly large doses of the offending allergens to gradually develop immunity.

- **Vaccination,** also know as **inoculation,** is the administration of a weakened or dead microorganism to induce immunity or to reduce the effects of associated infectious diseases (for example, vaccination against smallpox or poliomyelitis).

DISEASES AND DISEASE TRANSMISSION

Types of Diseases

- An **infectious disease** is an illness caused by a pathogenic organism. The term **virulence** (**VIR**-you-lens) is used to describe the degree of pathogenicity of an organism.

- A **communicable disease,** also known as a **contagious disease,** is any disease transmitted from one person to another either by direct contact or indirectly by contact with contaminated objects.

- An **acute** disease or symptom has a sudden onset or short duration.

  A **chronic** disease or symptom lasts for a long time.

- An **organic disease** involves actual pathological changes in one or more organs.

  In a **functional disease,** the patient is sick despite the fact that there are no observable pathological changes in any organ.

- An **iatrogenic illness** (eye-**at**-roh-**JEN**-ick) is one that results from treatment during the process of medical care.

- An **idiopathic disorder** (**id**-ee-oh-**PATH**-ick) is an illness without known cause. (The combining form *IDI/O* means peculiar to the individual or organ.)

- A **hereditary disease** is one transmitted genetically by a parent or parents to their child.

- A **congenital disease** is present at birth but is not due to genetic factors.

- **Deficiency diseases** are disorders of nutrition that result from a deficiency of one or more nutrients in the diet.

- **Metabolic diseases** are disorders caused by a disturbance of one or more endocrine glands.

Pathogenic Organisms

- A **microorganism** is a living organism that is so small it can only be seen with the aid of a microscope.

- A **pathogen** is a microorganism that causes a disease. (Not all microorganisms are pathogens. Some are very important to our well-being.)

- **Bacteria** (back-**TEE**-ree-ah) are a large group of microscopic, unicellular organisms that may cause disease in man. Most bacterial infections are treated with antibiotics. (Singular, **bacterium.**) (See next page for examples of bacterial infections.)

- A **fungus** (**FUNG**-gus) is a simple parasitic plant. Some fungi are pathogenic. (The combining forms *FUNG/I, MYC/E* and *MYC/O* all mean fungus.) (Plural, **fungi.**)

Most fungal infections are mild; however, in debilitated or immunosuppressed patients they may become systemic and life-threatening. (**Debilitated** means weakened.)

Tinea pedis, also known as athlete's foot, is an example of a fungus infection.

- A **yeast** is a type of fungus and some yeasts are pathogenic.

  Candidiasis albicans is an example of a yeast infection.

- A **parasite** (**PAR**-ah-sight) is a plant or animal that lives upon or within another living organism at the expense of that organism.

  Malaria (mah-**LAY**-ree-ah) is an example of a disease which is caused by a parasite.

- A **rickettsia** (rih-**KET**-see-ah) is a small bacterium that lives in lice, fleas, ticks and mites. They transmit the infection to humans. (Plural, **rickettsiae.**)

  Rocky Mountain spotted fever is an example of a disease transmitted by tick-bite.

- A **spirochete** (**SPY**-roh-keet) is a type of bacterium which may cause diseases in man.

  Syphilis (**SIF**-ih-lis) is an example of a disease caused by spirochetes.

- **Viruses** (**VYE**-rus-ez) are extremely small infectious agents that grow by invading living cells where they reproduce.

Examples of Bacterial Diseases

- **Gangrene** (**GANG**-green) is tissue death usually associated with a loss of circulation and followed by bacterial invasion and putrefaction. (The combining form *GANGREN/O* means gangrene or eating sore.)

  Putrefaction (pyou-treh-**FACK**-shun) is decay that produces foul-smelling compounds.

- **Septicemia** (sep-tih-**SEE**-me-ah), also known as **blood poisoning,** is the presence and persistence of pathogenic microorganisms or their toxins in the blood. (The combining form *SEPT/O* means infection.)

  Sepsis (**SEP**-sis) means infection or contamination. (The combining form *SEPS/O* also means infection.)

Examples of Viral Diseases

- **Mumps** is an acute viral disease characterized by swelling of the parotid glands.

- **Chickenpox,** also known as **varicella,** is an acute highly contagious viral disease characterized by fever and pustules. It is caused by the herpes virus Varicella zoster.

- **Measles** is an acute, highly contagious viral disease involving the respiratory tract and characterized by a spreading cutaneous rash and Koplik's spots which are present on the oral mucosa.

- **Rubella** (roo-**BELL**-ah), also known as **German measles** or **three-day measles,** is a viral infection characterized by fever and a diffuse, fine, red rash.

- **Rabies** (**RAY**-beez) is an acute viral infection that is transmitted to people by the blood, tissue or saliva of an infected animal.

RELATED TERMINOLOGY

Symptoms and Signs

- A **symptom** (**SIMP**-tum) is any subjective evidence of a disease, such as pain or a headache, that is observed by the patient.

- A **sign** is objective evidence of disease, such as fever, that can be observed by someone other than the patient.

Manifestations and Syndromes

- **Manifestations** are the set of signs or symptoms through which a condition makes itself known. For example, the manifestations of a heart attack usually include chest pain.

- A **syndrome** (SIN-drome) refers to a set of symptoms that occur together. For example, irritable bowel syndrome consists of many symptoms that occur together.

Diagnosis and Prognosis

- **Diagnosis** (dye-ag-NO-sis) is the process of determining the cause of a disease.

  A **differential diagnosis** attempts to determine which one of several diseases may be producing the symptoms.

- **Prognosis** (pragh-NO-sis) is a forecast, or prediction, of the probable course and outcome of a disorder.

Endemic, Epidemic and Pandemic

- **Endemic** (en-DEM-ick) means a persistent (chronic) presence of a disease within a population, group or area. For example, the common cold is endemic because it is always present within the population.
- An **epidemic** (ep-ih-DEM-ick) is a sudden and wide spread outbreak of a disease within a population group or area. For example, a sudden and wide-spread outbreak of measles is an epidemic.
- **Pandemic** (pan-DEM-ick) means occurring over a large geographic area, possibly worldwide. For example, the spread of AIDS is pandemic.

IMPORTANT TERMS: THE LYMPHATIC AND IMMUNE SYSTEMS

This list will help you identify and review the major terms from this chapter.

When you work with the audio tape for this chapter, listen to the word, repeat it and then place a ✓ next to it on the list below.

- ☐ **Adenoiditis** (ad-eh-noid-EYE-tis)
- ☐ **Adenoids** (AD-eh-noids)
- ☐ **Anaphylactic** (an-ah-fih-LACK-tick)
- ☐ **Angioma** (an-jee-OH-mah)
- ☐ **Aspergillosis** (as-per-jil-OH-sis)
- ☐ **Axillary** (AK-sih-lar-ee)
- ☐ **Bacteria** (back-TEE-ree-ah)
- ☐ **Bilirubin** (bill-ih-ROO-bin)
- ☐ **Candidiasis** (kan-dih-DYE-ah-sis)
- ☐ **Cervical** (SER-vih-kal)
- ☐ **Chyle** (KYL)
- ☐ **Cryptococcal meningitis** (krip-toh-KOCK-al men-in-JIGH-tis)
- ☐ **Cytomegalovirus** (sigh-toh-meg-ah-loh-VYE-rus)
- ☐ **Diagnosis** (dye-ag-NO-sis)
- ☐ **Endemic** (en-DEM-ick)
- ☐ **Epidemic** (ep-ih-DEM-ick)
- ☐ **Fungus** (FUNG-gus)
- ☐ **Gangrene** (GANG-green)
- ☐ **Hemolytic** (he-moh-LIT-ick)
- ☐ **Histiocytes** (HIS-tee-oh-sights)
- ☐ **Iatrogenic** (eye-at-roh-JEN-ick)

- ☐ **Idiopathic (id**-ee-oh-**PATH**-ick)
- ☐ **Immunodeficiency (im**-you-no-deh-**FISH**-en-see)
- ☐ **Immunoglobulin (im**-you-no-**GLOB**-you-lin)
- ☐ **Immunosuppression (im**-you-no-sup-**PRESH**-un)
- ☐ **Immunotherapy** (ih-**myou**-no-**THER**-ah-pee)
- ☐ **Inguinal (ING**-gwih-nal)
- ☐ **Interferon (in**-ter-**FEAR**-on)
- ☐ **Kaposi's (KAP**-oh-seez)
- ☐ **Lacteals (LACK**-tee-ahls)
- ☐ **Lymphadenitis** (lim-**fad**-eh-**NIGH**-tis)
- ☐ **Lymphadenopathy** (lim-**fad**-eh-**NOP**-ah-thee)
- ☐ **Lymphangiography** (lim-**fan**-jee-**OG**-rah-fee)
- ☐ **Lymphangioma** (lim-**fan**-jee-**OH**-mah)
- ☐ **Lymphocytes (LIM**-foh-sights)
- ☐ **Lymphokines (LIM**-foh-keens)
- ☐ **Lymphoma** (lim-**FOH**-mah)
- ☐ **Lymphosarcoma (lim**-foh-sar-**KOH**-mah)
- ☐ **Malaria** (mah-**LAY**-ree-ah)
- ☐ **Mononucleosis (mon**-oh-**new**-klee-**OH**-sis)
- ☐ **Nasopharyngeal** (**nay**-zoh-fah-**RIN**-jee-al)
- ☐ **Nocardiosis** (no-kar-dee-**OH**-sis)
- ☐ **Pandemic** (pan-**DEM**-ick)
- ☐ **Parasite (PAR**-ah-sight)
- ☐ **Pneumocystosis** (**new**-moh-sis-**TOH**-sis)
- ☐ **Prognosis** (pragh-**NO**-sis)
- ☐ **Putrefaction** (**pyou**-treh-**FACK**-shun)
- ☐ **Rabies (RAY**-beez)
- ☐ **Rickettsia** (rih-**KET**-see-ah)
- ☐ **Rubella** (roo-**BELL**-ah)
- ☐ **Sepsis (SEP**-sis)
- ☐ **Septicemia (sep**-tih-**SEE**-me-ah)
- ☐ **Spirochete (SPY**-roh-keet)
- ☐ **Symptom (SIMP**-tum)
- ☐ **Syndrome (SIN**-drome)
- ☐ **Tonsillitis (ton**-sih-**LYE**-tis)
- ☐ **Tonsils (TON**-sils)
- ☐ **Toxoplasmosis (tock**-soh-plaz-**MOH**-sis)
- ☐ **Virulence (VIR**-you-lens)
- ☐ **Viruses (VYE**-rus-ez)

6

EXERCISES

DEFINING WORD PARTS

Write the definition for each of these word parts.

1. *ADENOID/O* ______
2. *AXILL/O* ______
3. *CERVIC/O* ______
4. *FUNG/I* ______
5. *GANGREN/O* ______
6. *IDI/O* ______
7. *IMMUN/O* ______
8. *INGUIN/O* ______
9. *LINGU/O* ______
10. *LYMPH/O* ______
11. *LYMPHANGI/O* ______
12. *-LYTIC* ______
13. *MYC/E* ______
14. *MYC/O* ______
15. *NAS/O* ______
16. *PALAT/O* ______

17. *PHAG/O* ______________________________

18. *SEPS/O* ______________________________

19. *SEPT/O* ______________________________

20. *SPLEN/O* ______________________________

DEFINITIONS

Circle the letter next to the correct answer.

1. The spleen ______________
   a) is hemolytic.
   b) produces lymphocytes.
   c) stores red blood cells.
   d) a, b and c.

2. ______________ is also known as swollen glands.
   a) Adenoiditis
   b) Lymphadenitis
   c) Lymphoma
   d) Mononucleosis

3. Immunosuppression is ______________
   a) a type of complex protein found in serum.
   b) formed by B-cells.
   c) formed by T-cells
   d) used to prevent the rejection of donor tissue.

4. A congenital disease is ______________
   a) hereditary.
   b) not due to genetic factors.
   c) present at birth.
   d) b and c.

5. Syphilis is caused by a ______________
   a) fungus.
   b) parasite.
   c) spirochete.
   d) virus.

6. A prognosis is _______________
   a) a prediction of the probable course and outcome of a disorder.
   b) a set of signs by which a disease makes itself known.
   c) a set of symptoms that occur together.
   d) the process of determining the cause of a disease.

7. Lymph is also known as _______________
   a) intercellular fluid.
   b) interstitial fluid.
   c) serum.
   d) a and b.

8. Lacteals are located in the _______________
   a) groin.
   b) small intestine.
   c) under the arms.
   d) a and c.

9. A/an _______________ is an antigen that stimulates the production of antibodies.
   a) B-cell
   b) immunoglobulin
   c) monocyte
   d) virus

10. Interferon _______________
    a) is a type of macrophage.
    b) is produced by T-cells.
    c) suppresses B-cell activity.
    d) b and c.

MISSING WORDS

Write the missing word on the line.

1. _______________________ is the state of being resistant or not susceptible to a disease.

2. The antigen-antibody reaction is also known as the _______________________ reaction.

3. A/an _______________________ disease is one that results from treatment during the process of medical care.

4. The nasopharyngeal tonsils are also known as the _______________________.

5. The _______________________ lymph nodes are located in the groin area.

6. _______________________ is the orange-yellow pigment of bile.

7. ________________________ are agranular leukocytes that play an important part in the lymphatic system.

8. The ________________________ is an endocrine gland that plays an important role in the body's immunological system especially in fetal life and the early years of growth.

9. ________________________ are molecules, other than antibodies, that are involved in signalling between the cells of the immune system.

10. ________________________ is a series of complex, enzymatic proteins occurring in normal serum.

SPELLCHECK

Select the correct spelling and write it on the line.

1. ________________________ are antibodies made by plasma cells.
   Immuneglobulins
   Immunoglobulins
   Imunoglobulins

2. ________________________ shock is an unusual, severe and sometimes fatal allergic reaction.
   Anaphylactic
   Annaphylactic
   Anopylactic

3. ________________________ is an infection caused by a species of fungus.
   Candiasis
   Candidiasis
   Candiliasis

4. ________________________ is a general term applied to malignant neoplastic disorders of lymphoid tissue.
   Lymphisarcoma
   Lymphosarcoma
   Lymphosarkoma

5. ________________________ is a form of pneumonia caused by an infection with a parasite.
   Pneumicystosis
   Pneumocystosis
   Pnumocytosis

6. A ________________________ is a small bacterium that lives in lice, fleas, ticks and mites.
   reckittsia
   rickettsia
   rickittsea

7. ______________________ means weakened.
   Debilitated
   Debillitated
   Dibillitated

8. ______________________ diseases are disorders caused by a disturbance of one or more endocrine glands.
   Metabolic
   Metebollic
   Metobolic

9. A ______________________ refers to a set of symptoms that occur together.
   sindrome
   syndrome
   synidrome

10. An ______________________ is a sudden and wide spread outbreak of a disease.
    epademic
    epedemic
    epidemic

11. ______________________, also known as German measles, is a viral infection.
    Robella
    Ruballa
    Rubella

12. ______________________ is also known as blood poisoning.
    Septacemia
    Septecemia
    Septicemia

13. The ______________________ lymph nodes are located under the arm.
    auxillary
    axillary
    axilliary

14. ______________________ is caused by a spirochete.
    Siffillis
    Syphilis
    Syphillis

15. ______________________ disorders are marked by inflammation and injury to body cells.
    Autoemmune
    Autoimmune
    Autoimune

CASE STUDIES

Write the correct answer on the line.

1. John Fogelman suffers from AIDS. He was recently hospitalized with pneumocystosis which is a/an ______________________ infection.

2. When Dr. Wei saw the Koplik's spots in Peggy Martin's mouth, he was certain that her rash was ______________________.

3. Jose Sanchez received a/an ______________________ to assure his immunity to polio.

4. Jessica Parsons is allergic to bee stings. Recently she was stung and required prompt treatment for ______________________ shock.

5. Frank Black has AIDS and recently developed ______________________ sarcoma, which is a malignant neoplasm that began as soft papules on his feet.

6. ______________________, using increasingly large doses of the offending allergens, was helpful in the treatment of Alice Clawson's allergies.

7. It was necessary to amputate Mr. Grossman's toe because of the ______________________ that resulted from impaired circulation in the area.

8. Dorothy Mullins has the ______________________. This viral infection is characterized by swelling of the parotid glands.

9. After a recent camping trip Roger Thompson developed Rocky Mountain ______________________ ______________________. Apparently during the trip he had been bitten by an infected tick.

10. Dr. Ricardo examined Ruth Nolan. Ruth's primary ______________________ was a severe headache of long duration.

11. Because her breast cancer was not detected before it had spread to other parts of her body, the ______________________ for Gertrude Vogel's recovery is poor.

12. Bobby Harris was bitten by an infected dog, and the doctors fear that Bobby may be infected with ______________________.

13. Mr. Lanning has ______________________ disease, which is a malignant condition characterized by progressive enlargement of the lymph nodes, spleen and lymphoid tissue.

14. Nancy Inglis complained that the glands in her neck were swollen. Dr. Neilson explained that these are the ______________________ lymph nodes.

15. Public health officials describe the rapid spread of AIDS as possibly being of ______________________ proportions.

WORD BUILDING

Write the correct word or word part on the line.

1. Without known cause
   a) The combining form ______________________ means peculiar to the individual or organ.
   b) The suffix ______________________ means pertaining to disease.
   c) The term ______________________ means an illness without known cause.

2. A lymphatic tumor
   a) The combining form ______________________ means lymph.
   b) The suffix ______________________ means tumor.
   c) The term ______________________ means a tumor made up of lymphatic tissue.

3. An inflammation of the adenoids
   a) The combining form ______________________ means adenoids.
   b) The suffix ______________________ means inflammation.
   c) The term ______________________ means an inflammation of the adenoids.

4. Destroying red blood cells
   a) The combining form ______________________ means pertaining to the blood.
   b) The suffix ______________________ means to reduce or destroy.
   c) The term ______________________ means to destroy worn-out red blood cells.

LABELING EXERCISES

Identify the numbered items on this diagram.

1. Deep ______________________ lymph nodes
2. ______________________ lymph nodes
3. ______________________ duct
4. ______________________ lymph nodes
5. ______________________ duct

SUBMANDIBULAR LYMPH NODE
1
5
INTERNAL JUGULAR VEIN
RIGHT SUBCLAVIAN VEIN
LEFT SUBCLAVIAN VEIN
4
3
INTESTINAL LYMPH NODES
ILIAC NODES
2

(From *Human Anatomy and Physiology* by Joan G. Creager.
© 1983 by Wadsworth, Inc.
Reprinted by permission of the publisher.)

7

THE RESPIRATORY SYSTEM

LEARNING GOALS

In this chapter you will learn to:

- describe the major structures and functions of the respiratory system.
- identify the two kinds of respiration and define the major terms associated with respiration.
- recognize and define the major terms related to the diagnosis, pathology and treatment of disorders of the respiratory system.

STRUCTURES OF THE RESPIRATORY SYSTEM

The Nose

Air enters the body through the nose and passes through the **nasal cavity.** The nose is divided by a wall of cartilage called the **nasal septum** (NAY-zal SEP-tum). (The combining form *NAS/O* means nose.)

The nose and respiratory system are lined with **mucous membrane** which is a specialized form of epithelial tissue. The incoming air is filtered by the **cilia** (SIL-ee-ah), which are thin hairs attached to the mucous membrane just inside the nostrils.

Mucus (MYOU-kus) secreted by the mucous membranes helps to moisten and warm the air as it enters the nose. (Notice the different spellings of mucous and mucus.)

The **olfactory receptors** (ol-FAK-toh-ree) are nerve endings located in the mucous membrane in the upper part of the nasal cavity. They are the receptors for the sense of smell. (The combining form *OLFACT/O* means smell or sense of smell.)

The Sinuses

The four pairs of sinuses are air-containing spaces within the skull that communicate with the nasal cavity. They are also known as the **paranasal sinuses**, (The combining form *SINUS/O* means sinus or cavity.)

The sinuses have a mucous membrane lining and their functions include providing mucus, making the bones of the skull lighter, and helping to produce sound. The sinuses are named for the bones in which they are located.

- The **maxillary sinuses** are the largest of the paranasal sinuses.
- The **frontal sinuses** are located just above the eyes.
- The **ethmoid sinuses** are irregularly shaped air cells, separated from the orbital (eye) cavity only by a very thin layer of bone.
- The **sphenoid sinuses** are located close to the optic nerves, and an infection here can damage vision.

The Pharynx

After passing through the nasal cavity, the air reaches the **pharynx** (FAR-inks), commonly known as the **throat.** (The combining form *PHARYNG/O* means pharynx or throat.) There are three divisions of the pharynx:

- The **nasopharynx** (nay-zoh-FAR-inks) is the division nearest to the nasal cavities.
- The **oropharynx** (oh-roh-FAR-inks) is the second division and is the part of the throat that is visible when looking into the mouth. (The combining form *OR/O* means mouth.)
- The **laryngopharynx** (lah-ring-goh-FAR-inks), also known as the **hypopharynx** (high-poh-FAR-inks), is the third division and is located near the larynx.

The Epiglottis

The oropharynx and laryngopharynx serve as a common passageway for both food from the mouth and air from the nose.

In the act of swallowing, the **epiglottis** (ep-ih-GLOT-is), acts as a lid and covers the larynx so that food does not enter the lungs.

The Larynx

The larynx (LAR-inks), also known as the **voice box,** contains the structures which make speech possible. (The combining form *LARYNG/O* means voice box or larynx.)

The **glottis** is the vocal apparatus. It consists of the **vocal bands,** also known as **vocal cords,** and the space between them.

The larynx is protected and held open by a series of nine separate cartilages. The **thyroid cartilage** is the largest and its prominent projection is commonly known as the **Adam's apple.**

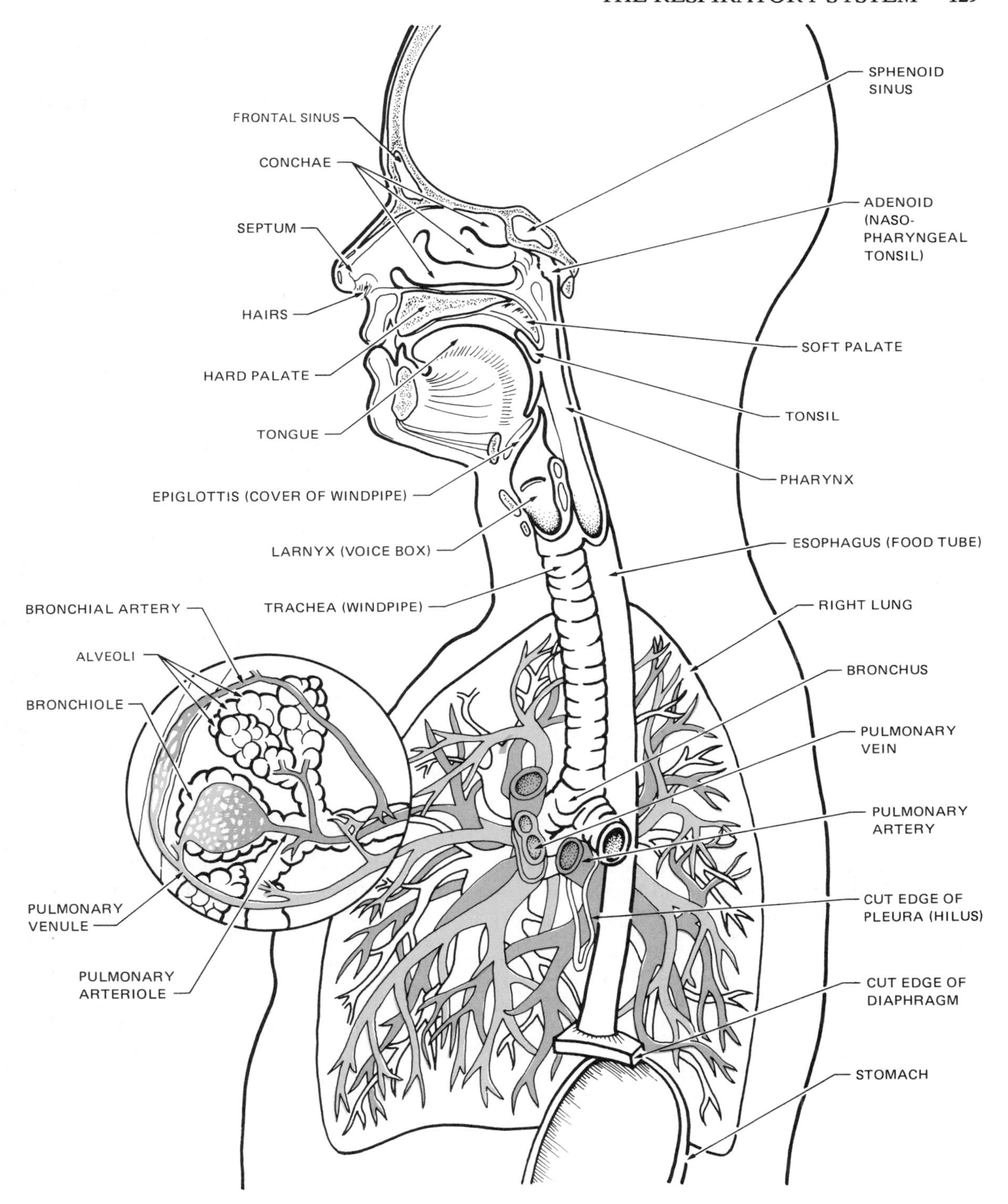

Figure 7-1 The structures of the respiratory system.

The Trachea

Air passes from the larynx to the **trachea (TRAY-kee-ah)**, commonly known as the **windpipe.** (The combining form *TRACHE/O* means trachea.)

The trachea extends from the neck into the chest, directly in front of the esophagus.

The trachea is held open by a series of C-shaped cartilage rings. The wall between these rings is elastic, enabling the trachea to adjust to different body positions.

The Bronchi

The region between the lungs is called the **mediastinum (me-dee-as-TYE-num)**. It contains the heart, aorta, esophagus, bronchial tubes and thymus.

In this region, the trachea divides into two branches called **bronchi (BRONG-kye)**. (The combining forms *BRONCH/O* and *BRONCHI/O* refer to the bronchial tubes.) (Singular, **bronchus.)**

Each bronchus leads to a separate lung and, like the branches of a tree, divides and subdivides into increasingly smaller bronchi.

Bronchioles (BRONG-kee-ohlz) are the smallest branches of the bronchi. (The combining form *BRONCHIOL/O* refers to the bronchioles.)

The Alveoli

Alveoli (al-VEE-oh-lye), also known as **air sacs,** are the very small grape-like clusters found at the end of each bronchiole. (The combining form *ALVEOL/O* means air sac.) (Singular, **alveolus.)**

The membrane walls of the alveoli are only one cell thick and are surrounded by a network of microscopic capillaries.

During respiration, it is here that the gas exchange takes place between the alveolar air and the pulmonary capillary blood.

The Lungs

Together the structures of the bronchial tree form the organs known as the lungs. A **lobe** is a division of the lungs. (The combining form *LOB/O* means lobe.)

The right lung has three lobes: the superior, middle, and inferior. The left lung has two lobes: the superior and inferior.

The combining forms *PNEUM/O* and *PNEUMON/O* both pertain to the lungs and air, and the prefix *PNEU-* has the same meaning. *PULM/O* and *PULMON/O* are additional combining forms that mean of, or pertaining to, the lungs.

The Pleura

Each lung, with its blood vessels and nerves, is enclosed in a many-layered membrane called the **pleura (PLOOR-ah)**. (The combining form *PLEUR/O* means pleura or side of body.) (Plural, **pleurae.)**

The **parietal pleura** is the outer layer that lines the thoracic cavity and forms the sac containing each of the lungs.

The **visceral pleura** is the inner layer of pleura that closely surrounds the lung tissue.

The **pleural space,** also known as the **pleural cavity,** is the airtight space between the folds of the pleural membranes. It contains a lubricating fluid to prevent friction when the membranes rub together during respiration.

The Diaphragm

The **diaphragm** is the muscle separating the chest and abdomen. Breathing action is caused primarily by the contraction of the diaphragm producing a vacuum within the thoracic cavity to draw in air. When the diaphragm returns to its relaxed state, air is forced out of the lungs.

The **phrenic nerve (FREN-ick)** innervates the diaphragm. (The combining form *PHREN/O* means diaphragm; however, it also means relating to the mind.)

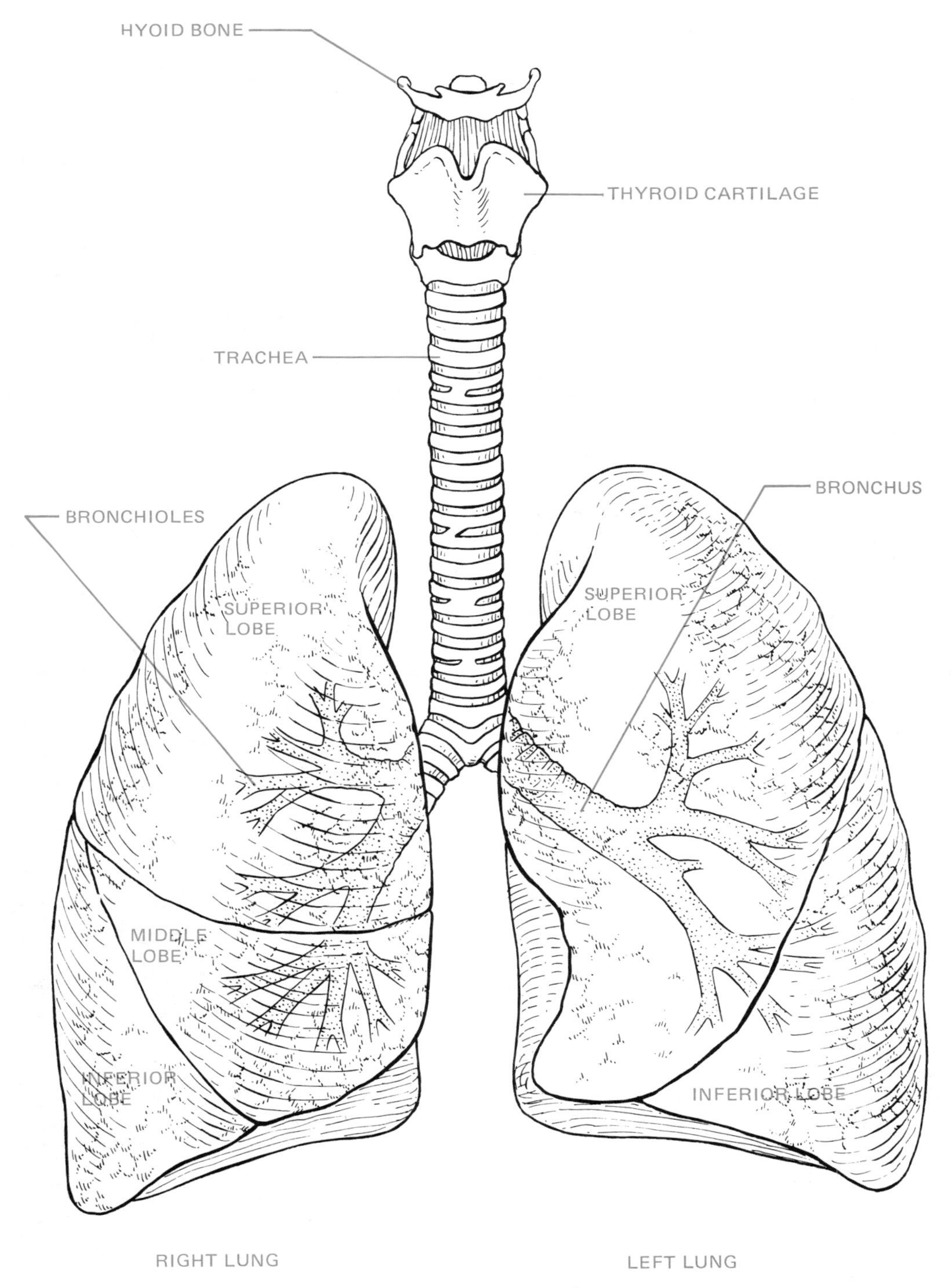

Figure 7-2 The lungs and surrounding tissues.

RESPIRATION

External Respiration

External respiration is the exchange of gases in the lungs. Here air is inhaled into the alveoli, and the oxygen immediately passes into tiny surrounding capillaries and is carried to all body cells.

At the same time, the waste product carbon dioxide passes from the capillaries into the airspaces of the lungs to be exhaled.

Internal Respiration

Internal respiration is the exchange of gases within the cells of all the body organs and tissues.

In this process, oxygen passes out of the bloodstream and into the tissue cells. At the same time, carbon dioxide passes from the tissue cells into the blood stream.

DIAGNOSTIC PROCEDURES RELATED TO THE RESPIRATORY SYSTEM

- **Phlegm (FLEM)** is the thick mucus secreted by the tissues that line the respiratory passages.

  When this matter is ejected through the mouth it is called **sputum (SPYOU**-tum). Sputum may be used for diagnostic purposes.

- **Bronchoscopy** (brong-**KOS**-koh-pee) is the visual examination of the bronchi using a **bronchoscope.**

- **Laryngoscopy (lar**-ing-**GOS**-koh-pee) is the visual examination of the larynx using a **laryngoscope.**

- **Pulmonary function tests** are a group of tests used to measure lung volume during a specified period of time. A **spirometer** is used to measure the air taken in and out of the lungs.

- **Thoracocentesis (thoh**-rah-koh-sen-**TEE**-sis), also called **thoracentesis,** is the puncture of the chest wall with a needle to obtain fluid from the pleural cavity for diagnostic studies.

- A **lung scan** is an examination using radioactive material, either through intravenous injection or inhalation, primarily to evaluate pulmonary emboli (clots) or to determine the capacity of the lung for ventilation.

PATHOLOGY OF THE RESPIRATORY SYSTEM

Inflammations of the Respiratory System

- **Sinusitis (sigh**-nuh-**SIGH**-tis) is an inflammation of the sinuses.

- **Acute nasopharyngitis (nay**-zoh-**far**-in-**JYE**-tis) is one of the terms used to describe the common cold.

- **Pharyngitis (far**-in-**JYE**-tis), also known as a sore throat, is an inflammation of the pharynx.

- **Laryngitis (lar**-in-**JYE**-tis) is an inflammation of the larynx.

- **Epiglottitis (ep**-ih-glot-**TYE**-tis) is an inflammation of the epiglottis.

- **Tracheitis (tray**-kee-**EYE**-tis) is an inflammation of the trachea.

- **Bronchitis** (brong-**KYE**-tis) is an inflammation of the bronchial walls.

General

- **Upper respiratory infection** is one of the terms used to describe the **common cold.**

- **Influenza (in**-flew-**EN**-zah), also known as **flu,** is an acute, highly contagious respiratory infection that usually occurs during the colder months.

- **Allergic rhinitis** (rye-NIGH-tis) is an allergic reaction to airborne allergens.
- **Peritonsillar abscess** (per-ih-TON-sih-lar), also known as **Quinsy sore throat,** is an infection of tissue between the tonsil and pharynx.
- **Laryngoplegia** (lar-ing-goh-PLEE-jee-ah) is the paralysis of the larynx. (The suffix *-PLEGIA* means paralysis.)
- **Dysphonia** (dis-FOH-nee-ah) is any voice impairment. (The prefix *DYS-* means difficult or painful. The combining form *PHON/O* means sound or voice.)
- **Aphonia** (ah-FOH-nee-ah) is the loss of the ability to produce normal speech sounds.
- **Diphtheria** (dif-THEE-ree-ah) is an acute infectious disease of the throat and upper respiratory tract caused by the presence of diphtheria bacteria.
- **Pertussis** (per-TUS-is), also known as **whooping cough,** is a contagious bacterial infection of the upper respiratory tract that is characterized by a paroxysmal cough.

  Paroxysmal (par-ock-SIZ-mal) means sudden or spasm-like.
- **Croup** (KROOP) is an acute respiratory syndrome in children and infants that is characterized by obstruction of the larynx, hoarseness and a barking cough.
- **Bronchiectasis** (brong-kee-ECK-tah-sis) is an abnormal condition of the bronchial tree, characterized by irreversible dilation and destruction of the bronchial walls. (The suffix *-ECTASIS* means stretching, dilation, enlargement.)
- **Dyspnea** (DISP-nee-ah) is difficult or labored breathing.
- **Rales** (RAHLZ) are abnormal respiratory sounds heard while listening to the chest during inspiration.
- **Rhonchus** (RONG-kus), also known as a **wheeze,** is an abnormal respiratory sound heard when the airway is obstructed by thick secretions, a muscular spasm, a neoplasm or external pressure. (Plural, **rhonchi.**)
- **Stridor** (STRYE-dor) is an abnormal, high-pitched, harsh sound heard during inspiration when the larynx is obstructed.
- **Singultus** (sing-GUL-tus), also known as **hiccups,** is a characteristic sound caused by the involuntary contraction of the diaphragm.

Lung Disorders

- **Asthma** (AZ-mah) is a chronic allergic disorder that is characterized by spasms, which narrow the bronchioles, and by increased mucus secretions, which block passageways of air.
- **Hypoxia** (high-POCK-see-ah) is the condition of having inadequate oxygen in the cells. (The combining forms *OX/I, OX/O* and *OX/Y* all mean oxygen.)
- **Asphyxia** (as-FICK-see-ah) is severe hypoxia that results in loss of consciousness and, if not corrected, in death.
- **Asphyxiation** (as-fick-see-AY-shun), also known as **suffocation,** is defined as any interruption of breathing that may result in the loss of consciousness and/or death.
- **Cyanosis** (sigh-ah-NO-sis) is a bluish discoloration of the skin caused by a lack of adequate oxygen. (The combining form *CYAN/O* means blue.)
- **Hypopnea** (high-poh-NEE-ah) is shallow or slow respiration. (The suffix *-PNEA* means breathing.)
- **Apnea** (ap-NEE-ah) is the absence of spontaneous respiration.

- **Emphysema** (**em**-fih-**SEE**-mah) is an irreversible enlargement of the air spaces in the lungs due to destruction of the alveoli walls.

- **Pneumonia** (new-**MOH**-nee-ah) is an acute inflammation and infection of the alveoli.

  Lobar pneumonia is a form of pneumonia which involves one or more lobes of a lung.

  Bronchopneumonia (**brong**-koh-new-**MOH**-nee-ah) is a form of pneumonia that begins in the bronchioles.

- **Pulmonary edema** (eh-**DEE**-mah) is an accumulation of fluid in lung tissues.

- **Tuberculosis** (too-**ber**-kew-**LOH**-sis) is an infectious disease caused by *Mycobacterium tuberculosis*. The lungs are the major seat of infection; however, the disease may also affect other parts of the body.

- **Pleurisy** (**PLOOR**-ih-see) is an inflammation of the visceral and parietal pleura in the thoracic cavity.

- **Pneumothorax** (**new**-moh-**THOR**-racks) is an accumulation of air or gas in the pleural space causing the lung to collapse. (The suffix *-THORAX* means pleural cavity or chest.)

- **Atelectasis** (**at**-ee-**LEK**-tah-sis) is the incomplete expansion of a lung. It may also mean the collapse of a lung.

- **Pleural effusion** (eh-**FEW**-zhun) is the abnormal escape of fluid into the pleural cavity.

  Effusion means the escape of fluid into a body cavity.

- **Empyema** (**em**-pye-**EE**-mah) is an accumulation of pus in the pleural cavity. (The prefix *EM-* means in and the combining form *PY/O* means pus.)

- **Hemothorax** (**he**-moh-**THOH**-racks) is an accumulation of blood in the pleural cavity. (The combining form *HEM/O* means blood.)

- **Pneumoconiosis** (**new**-moh-**koh**-nee-**OH**-sis) is an abnormal condition caused by dust in the lungs that usually develops after years of environmental or occupational contact. These disorders are named for the causative agents.

  Anthracosis (**an**-thrah-**KOH**-sis), also known as **black-lung disease,** is caused by coal dust in the lungs.

  Asbestosis (**as**-beh-**STOH**-sis), is caused by asbestos particles in the lungs and is found in workers from the shipbuilding and construction trades.

  Byssinosis (**biss**-ih-**NO**-sis), also known as **brown-lung disease,** is caused by cotton, flax, or hemp dust in the lungs.

  Silicosis (**sill**-ih-**KOH**-sis), also known as **grinder's disease,** is caused by silica dust or glass in the lungs.

PROCEDURES RELATED TO THE RESPIRATORY SYSTEM

- **Rhinoplasty** (**RYE**-no-**plas**-tee) is plastic surgery of the nose. (The combining form *RHIN/O* means nose.)

- **Septoplasty** (**sep**-toh-**PLAS**-tee) is the surgical reconstruction of the nasal septum.

- **Laryngoplasty** (lah-**RING**-goh-**plas**-tee) is the surgical repair of the larynx.

- **Laryngectomy** (**lar**-in-**JECK**-toh-me) is the surgical removal of the larynx.

- **Pneumonectomy** (**new**-moh-**NECK**-toh-me) is the surgical removal of all or part of a lung.

- **Endotracheal intubation** (**en**-doh-**TRAY**-kee-al) is a form of treatment in which a tube is placed through the mouth, pharynx, and larynx into the trachea to establish an airway.

- **Tracheotomy** (**tray**-kee-**OT**-oh-me) is an emergency procedure in which an incision is made into the trachea to gain access to the airway below a blockage.

- A **tracheostomy** (**tray**-kee-**OS**-toh-me) is cutting an opening into the trachea and inserting a tube to facilitate the passage of air or the removal of secretions. Placement of this tube may be temporary or permanent. The resulting opening is called a stoma.

  A **stoma** (**STOH**-mah) is an opening on a body surface. A stoma may occur naturally, for example a pore in the skin, or it may be created surgically, for example as the result as a tracheostomy.
- A **lobectomy** (loh-**BECK**-toh-me) is the surgical removal of a lobe of the lung.
- **Thoracocentesis** (**thoh**-rah-koh-sen-**TEE**-sis) is the puncture of the chest wall with a needle to obtain fluid from the pleural cavity, to drain pleural effusions, or to re-expand a collapsed lung.
- **Respiratory therapy** includes a variety of treatments to support, assist or control the patient's breathing.

IMPORTANT TERMS: THE RESPIRATORY SYSTEM

This list will help you identify and review the major terms from this chapter.

When you work with the audio tape for this chapter, listen to the word, repeat it and then place a ✓ next to it on the list below.

- ☐ **Alveoli** (al-**VEE**-oh-lye)
- ☐ **Anthracosis** (**an**-thrah-**KOH**-sis)
- ☐ **Aphonia** (ah-**FOH**-nee-ah)
- ☐ **Apnea** (ap-**NEE**-ah)
- ☐ **Asbestosis** (**as**-beh-**STOH**-sis)
- ☐ **Asphyxiation** (as-**fick**-see-**AY**-shun)
- ☐ **Asphyxia** (as-**FICK**-see-ah)
- ☐ **Asthma** (**AZ**-mah)
- ☐ **Atelectasis** (**at**-ee-**LEK**-tah-sis)
- ☐ **Bronchitis** (brong-**KYE**-tis)
- ☐ **Bronchi** (**BRONG**-kye)
- ☐ **Bronchiectasis** (**brong**-kee-**ECK**-tah-sis)
- ☐ **Bronchioles** (**BRONG**-kee-ohlz)
- ☐ **Bronchoscopy** (brong-**KOS**-koh-pee)
- ☐ **Bronchopneumonia** (**brong**-koh-new-**MOH**-nee-ah)
- ☐ **Byssinosis** (**biss**-ih-**NO**-sis)
- ☐ **Croup** (**KROOP**)
- ☐ **Cyanosis** (**sigh**-ah-**NO**-sis)
- ☐ **Diphtheria** (dif-**THEE**-ree-ah)
- ☐ **Dysphonia** (dis-**FOH**-nee-ah)
- ☐ **Dyspnea** (**DISP**-nee-ah)
- ☐ **Effusion** (eh-**FEW**-zhun)
- ☐ **Emphysema** (**em**-fih-**SEE**-mah)
- ☐ **Empyema** (**em**-pye-**EE**-mah)
- ☐ **Endotracheal** (**en**-doh-**TRAY**-kee-al)
- ☐ **Epiglottis** (**ep**-ih-**GLOT**-is)
- ☐ **Epiglottitis** (**ep**-ih-glot-**TYE**-tis)
- ☐ **Hemothorax** (**he**-moh-**THOH**-racks)
- ☐ **Hypopharynx** (**high**-poh-**FAR**-inks)
- ☐ **Hypopnea** (**high**-poh-**NEE**-ah)
- ☐ **Hypoxia** (high-**POCK**-see-ah)
- ☐ **Influenza** (**in**-flew-**EN**-zah)
- ☐ **Laryngectomy** (**lar**-in-**JECK**-toh-me)
- ☐ **Laryngitis** (**lar**-in-**JYE**-tis)
- ☐ **Laryngopharynx** (lah-**ring**-goh-**FAR**-inks)
- ☐ **Laryngoscopy** (**lar**-ing-**GOS**-koh-pee)

- **Laryngoplasty** (lah-**RING**-goh-**plas**-tee)
- **Laryngoplegia** (**lar**-ing-goh-**PLEE**-jee-ah)
- **Larynx** (**LAR**-inks)
- **Lobectomy** (loh-**BECK**-toh-me)
- **Mediastinum** (**me**-dee-as-**TYE**-num)
- **Mucus** (**MYOU**-kus)
- **Nasal septum** (**NAY**-zal **SEP**-tum)
- **Nasopharyngitis** (**nay**-zoh-**far**-in-**JYE**-tis)
- **Nasopharynx** (**nay**-zoh-**FAR**-inks)
- **Olfactory** (ol-**FAK**-toh-ree)
- **Oropharynx** (**oh**-roh-**FAR**-inks)
- **Paroxysmal** (**par**-ock-**SIZ**-mal)
- **Peritonsillar** (**per**-ih-**TON**-sih-lar)
- **Pertussis** (per-**TUS**-is)
- **Pharyngitis** (**far**-in-**JYE**-tis)
- **Pharynx** (**FAR**-inks)
- **Phlegm** (**FLEM**)
- **Phrenic** (**FREN**-ick)
- **Pleura** (**PLOOR**-ah)
- **Pleurisy** (**PLOOR**-ih-see)
- **Pneumoconiosis** (**new**-moh-**koh**-nee-**OH**-sis)
- **Pneumonia** (new-**MOH**-nee-ah)
- **Pneumonectomy** (**new**-moh-**NECK**-toh-me)
- **Pneumothorax** (**new**-moh-**THOR**-racks)
- **Rales** (**RAHLZ**)
- **Rhinitis** (rye-**NIGH**-tis)
- **Rhinoplasty** (**RYE**-no-**plas**-tee)
- **Rhonchus** (**RONG**-kus)
- **Septoplasty** (**sep**-toh-**PLAS**-tee)
- **Silicosis** (**sill**-ih-**KOH**-sis)
- **Singultus** (sing-**GUL**-tus)
- **Sinusitis** (**sigh**-nuh-**SIGH**-tis)
- **Sputum** (**SPYOU**-tum)
- **Stoma** (**STOH**-mah)
- **Stridor** (**STRYE**-dor)
- **Thoracocentesis** (**thoh**-rah-koh-sen-**TEE**-sis)
- **Trachea** (**TRAY**-kee-ah)
- **Tracheitis** (tray-kee-**EYE**-tis)
- **Tracheostomy** (**tray**-kee-**OS**-toh-me)
- **Tracheotomy** (**tray**-kee-**OT**-oh-me)
- **Tuberculosis** (too-**ber**-kew-**LOH**-sis)

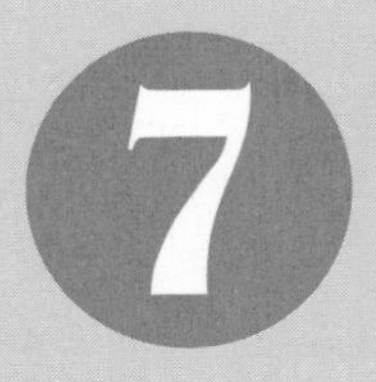

EXERCISES

DEFINING WORD PARTS

Write the definition for each of these word parts.

1. *ALVEOL/O* ______
2. *BRONCH/O, BRONCHI/O* ______
3. *CYAN/O* ______
4. *LOB/O* ______
5. *NAS/O* ______
6. *OLFACT/O* ______
7. *OR/O* ______
8. *OX/I, OX/O, OX/Y* ______
9. *PHARYNG/O* ______
10. *PHON/O* ______
11. *PHREN/O* ______
12. *PLEUR/O* ______
13. *PNEUM/O, PNEUMON/O, PNEU-* ______
14. *PULM/O, PULMON/O* ______
15. *TRACHE/O* ______

DEFINITIONS

Circle the letter next to the correct answer.

1. The mediastinum ______________
   a) contains the heart, aorta, esophagus, and bronchial tubes.
   b) is the division between the chest and abdominal cavities.
   c) is the region between the lungs in the chest cavity.
   d) a and c.

2. The epiglottis ______________
   a) is commonly known as the Adam's apple.
   b) is commonly known as the voice box.
   c) serves as a lid to prevent food from entering the lungs.
   d) a and c.

3. The pleura is ______________
   a) a many-layered membrane surrounding each lung.
   b) the nerve that innervates the diaphragm.
   c) the site of external respiration.
   d) a and c.

4. The oropharynx ______________
   a) is located just below the nasolarynx.
   b) is visible when looking in the mouth.
   c) protects the epiglottis.
   d) b and c.

5. The alveoli are ______________
   a) also known as air sacs.
   b) composed of lymphatic tissue.
   c) located at the end of each bronchiole.
   d) a and c.

6. The trachea divides into two branches called ______________
   a) alveoli.
   b) bronchi.
   c) bronchus.
   d) bronchioles.

7. Stridor is ______________
   a) an abnormal sound heard when the larynx is obstructed.
   b) a paroxysmal cough.
   c) characteristic of croup.
   d) b and c.

8. Pneumothorax means _______________
   a) an abnormal lung condition caused by dust.
   b) an accumulation of air or gas in the pleural space.
   c) inflammation of the thorax.
   d) inhalation of air into the thoracic cavity.

9. The _______________ is sometimes called the hypopharynx.
   a) epiglottis
   b) laryngopharynx
   c) nasopharynx
   d) oropharynx

10. Pulmonary edema is a collection of _______________ in lung tissue.
   a) air
   b) fluid
   c) gas
   d) pus

MISSING WORDS

Write the missing word on the line.

1. _______________________ is also known as suffocation.
2. The _______________________ are the thin hairs just inside the nose.
3. _______________________ is also known as hiccups.
4. The suffix _______________________ means breathing.
5. _______________________ means an absence of spontaneous respiration.
6. _______________________ is also known as whooping cough.
7. _______________________ is the material coughed up from the lungs and expectorated through the mouth.
8. The _______________________ is also known as the windpipe.
9. _______________________ is severe hypoxia that results in unconsciousness and possibly death.
10. _______________________ is an abnormal lung condition caused by dust in the lungs that usually develops after years of environmental or occupational contact.
11. _______________________ function tests are a group of tests used to measure lung volume.
12. The _______________________ are smallest branches of the bronchi.
13. The _______________________ is the muscle separating the chest and abdomen.

14. One function of the ______________________ is to make the bones of the skull lighter.

15. ______________________ is a collection of blood in the pleural cavity.

SPELLCHECK

Select the correct spelling and write it on the line.

1. ______________________, also known as black-lung disease, is caused by coal dust in the lungs.
   Anthracosis
   Anthracossis
   Anthrocossis

2. ______________________ is an accumulation of pus in the pleural cavity.
   Empyema
   Emphyema
   Imphysema

3. ______________________ is an acute infectious disease of the throat and upper respiratory tract.
   Diphtheria
   Diptheria
   Dyptheria

4. A ______________________ is cutting an opening into the trachea and inserting a tube to facilitate the passage of air or the removal of secretions.
   tracheotomy
   tracheostomy
   trachiostomy

5. ______________________ begins in the bronchioles.
   Bronchioneumonia
   Bronchipnumonia
   Bronchopneumonia

6. ______________________ is an irreversible enlargement of the air spaces in the lungs.
   Amphysema
   Emphysema
   Empysema

7. ______________________ is also known as brown-lung disease.
   Bissinosis
   Bysinosis
   Byssinosis

8. In ______________________, the chest wall is punctured with a needle to obtain fluid from the pleural cavity.
   thoraciocentesis
   thoracocentesis
   thoraxocentesis

9. ______________________ intubation is a form of treatment in which a tube is placed into the trachea to establish an airway.
   Endotracheal
   Endotrachial
   Endotrachioeal

10. ______________________ is an inflammation of the larynx.
    Laryingitis
    Laringoitis
    Laryngitis

11. ______________________ is the visual examination of the bronchi.
    Bronchiscopy
    Bronchioscopy
    Bronchoscopy

12. ______________________ is the thick mucus secreted by the tissues that line the respiratory passages.
    Fleam
    Phlegm
    Plegm

13. Acute ______________________ is one of the terms used to describe the common cold.
    nasiopharyngitis
    nasopharyngitis
    nasopharyngoitis

14. ______________________ is a bluish discoloration of the skin caused by a lack of adequate oxygen.
    Cianosis
    Cyanosis
    Cyenosis

15. The lungs are the major seat of infection for ______________________; however, it may also affect other parts of the body.
    tuberculiosis
    tuberculosis
    tuberoculosis

CASE STUDIES

Write the correct answer on the line.

1. Mrs. Jamison has a running nose caused by an allergy to airborne allergens. Her condition is diagnosed as allergic ______________________.
2. George Farrington has a ______________________ abscess, which is also known as Quinsy sore throat.
3. Dr. Timkins used a/an ______________________ to visually examine Helen Barron's larynx.
4. When Dr. Jamison listened to Mr. Leigh's chest he heard abnormal respiratory sounds during inspiration. These sounds are called ______________________.
5. Walter Lawson has smoked cigarettes for most of his life. Now he suffers from ______________________ which is an irreversible enlargement of the air spaces in the lungs due to destruction of the alveolar walls.
6. Marion Douglass had ______________________ performed to improve the appearance of her nose.
7. The doctor's examination showed that Jean Marshall has an accumulation of blood in the pleural cavity. This diagnosis is recorded on her chart as ______________________.
8. Harry Vaughn had a/an ______________________ performed to correct damage to the septum of his nose.
9. The Klein baby has been sick with ______________________. This is characterized by obstruction of the larynx, hoarseness, and a barking cough.
10. Ted Coleman required an emergency ______________________ because of an obstruction in his windpipe.
11. Mr. Parker received what is commonly known as a flu shot to prevent ______________________.
12. Donna Kirkman has ______________________ which is an inflammation of the pleura of the thoracic cavity.
13. Ronald Grossman has a sinus infection. This diagnosis is recorded on his chart as ______________________.
14. Susanne Holderman is suffering from an inflammation of the bronchial walls. Susanne's condition is ______________________.
15. Beverly Andrews has ______________________ which is a chronic allergic disorder characterized by spasms that narrow the bronchioles.

WORD BUILDING

Write the correct word or word part on the line.

1. The larynx
   a) The combining form ______________________ means voice box or larynx.
   b) The suffix ______________________ means paralysis.
   c) The term ______________________ means paralysis of the larynx.
2. The remove of a lobe
   a) The combining form ______________________ means lobe.
   b) The suffix ______________________ means the surgical removal.
   c) The term ______________________ means surgical removal of a lobe.
3. The voice
   a) The prefix ______________________ difficult or painful.
   b) The combining form ______________________ means voice.
   c) The term ______________________ means any voice impairment.
4. The pharynx
   a) The combining form ______________________ means pharynx.
   b) The suffix ______________________ means inflammation.
   c) The term ______________________ means an inflammation of the pharynx and is commonly known as a sore throat.
5. Air or gas in the pleural cavity
   a) The combining form ______________________ means lungs and air.
   b) The suffix ______________________ means thorax.
   c) The term ______________________ means an accumulation of air or gas in the pleural space causing the lung to collapse.

LABELING EXERCISES

Identify the parts of numbered items on this diagram.

1. ______________________________
2. ______________________________
3. ______________________________
4. ______________________________
5. ______________________________

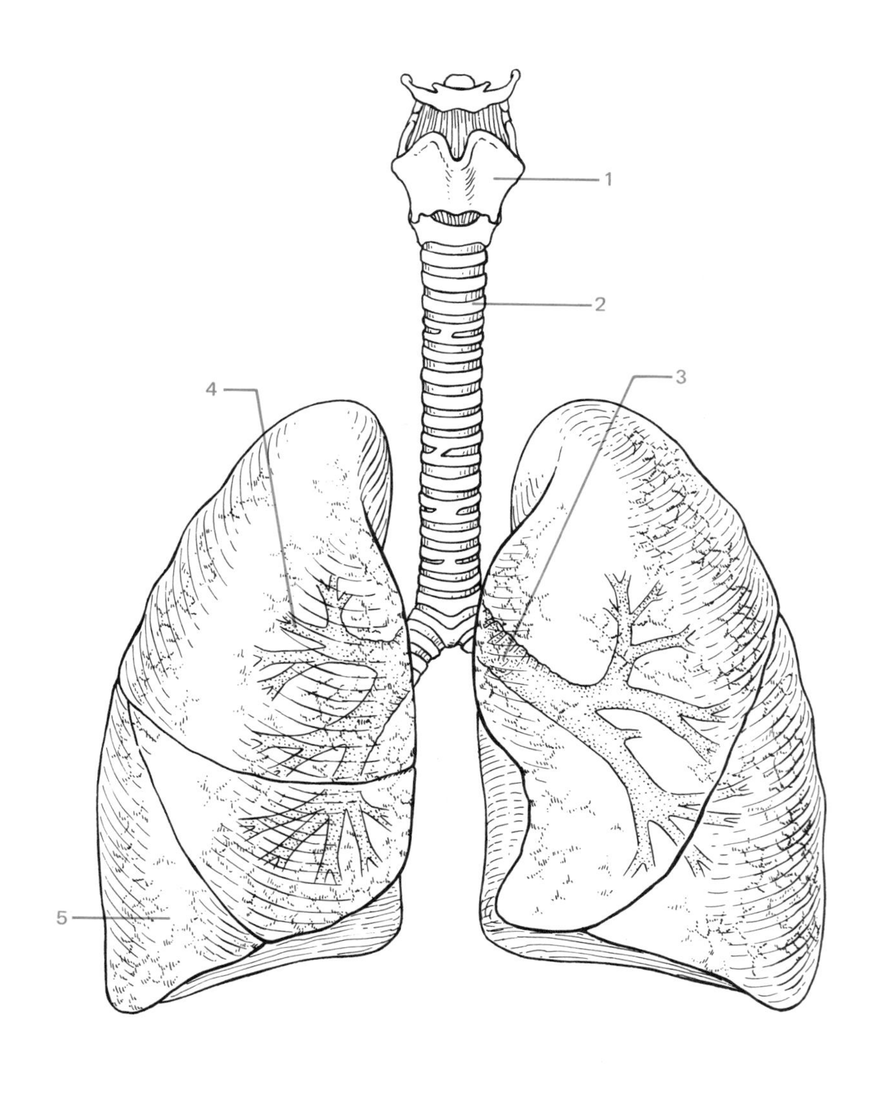

8

THE DIGESTIVE SYSTEM

LEARNING GOALS

In this chapter you will learn to:

- describe the structures and functions of the organs of the digestive system.
- describe the processes of digestion, absorption and metabolism.
- recognize and define terms relating to the diagnosis, pathology and treatment of disorders of the digestive system.

OVERVIEW OF THE DIGESTIVE SYSTEM

The digestive system is also known as the **alimentary canal. (al-**ih-**MEN-**tar-ee) (The combining form *ALIMENT/O* means to nourish.)

Another name for it is the **gastrointestinal tract.** (The combining form *GASTR/O* means stomach and *INTESTIN/O* means intestine.)

The primary functions of the digestive system are the digestion and absorption of food taken into the body, and the elimination of solid waste products.

The major parts of the digestive system are the oral cavity, pharynx, esophagus, stomach and small and large intestines. Related organs include the liver, gallbladder and pancreas.

The Peritoneum

The organs located in the abdominal cavity are protected and suspended in place by the layers of the **peritoneum (per-**ih-toh-**NEE-**um).

The **parietal peritoneum** (pah-**RYE-**eh-tal) is the outer layer and it lines the abdominal cavity. (The combining form *PARIET/O* means a wall.)

The **visceral peritoneum (VIS-**er-al) is the inner layer and it surrounds the organs. (The combining form *VISCER/O* means viscera or internal organs.)

THE ORAL CAVITY

The Lips and Cheeks

The oral cavity, also known as the mouth, is lined with mucous membrane. (The combining form *OR/O* means the mouth.)

The cheeks form the walls of the oral cavity. The term **buccal** means pertaining to or directed toward the cheek. (The combining form *BUCC/O* means cheek.)

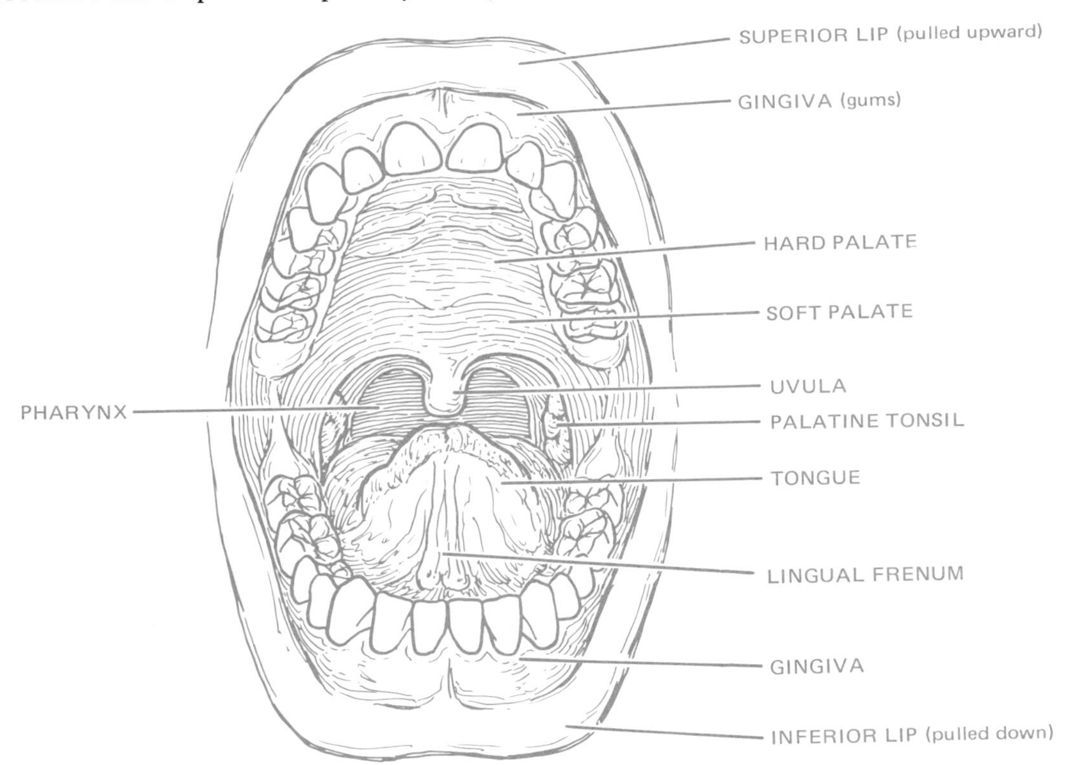

Figure 8-1 The mouth and its structures.

The **labia** (**LAY**-bee-ah), also known as the lips, form the opening to the oral cavity. (The combining forms *CHEIL/O* and *LABI/O* both mean lip.) (Singular, **labium.**)

A **frenum** (**FREE**-num) is a narrow band of tissue that connects two structures. For example, the **lingual frenum** connects the tongue to the floor of the mouth. (The combining form *FREN/O* means frenum or any device that limits motion.) (Plural, **frena.**)

The Palate

The palate (**PAL**-at), also known as the **roof of the mouth,** consists of two parts. (The combining form *PALAT/O* means palate.)

The **hard palate** forms the bony anterior portion of the palate. The **soft palate** forms the flexible posterior portion of the palate.

The **rugae** (**ROO**-gay) are irregular ridges or folds in the mucous membrane. In the mouth, rugae cover the anterior portion of the hard palate. (The combining form *RUG/O* means a wrinkle or fold.) (Singular, **ruga.**)

The **uvula** (**YOU**-view-lah), which hangs from the free edge of the soft palate, helps in producing sounds and speech. (The combining form *UVUL/O* means little grape, and the uvula does look like a grape.)

The Tongue

The tongue, which aids in speech and moves food during chewing and swallowing, consists of a very flexible group of muscles that are attached only at the posterior end. (The combining form *LINGU/O* means tongue.)

The tongue is covered by a series of small projections called papillae. Each **papilla** (pah-**PILL**-ah) contains cells which are the receptors for the sense of taste. (Plural, **papillae.**)

The Teeth

The teeth are arranged into the upper **maxillary arch** and lower **mandibular arch.** The term **dentition** refers to the natural teeth arranged in these arches. (The combining forms *DENT/I* and *DENT/O* mean teeth).

The **anterior teeth,** which are used for biting and tearing, include the central and lateral **incisors** and the **canines** (also known as **cuspids).**

The **posterior teeth,** which are used for chewing and grinding, include the **premolars** (also known as **bicuspids**), and **molars.**

The **primary dentition,** also known as the **deciduous dentition** (dee-**SID**-you-us) or baby teeth, consists of 20 teeth (eight incisors, four cuspids and eight molars).

The primary teeth are shed normally and are replaced by the permanent teeth. (The combining form *DECIDU/O* means falling off or shedding.)

The **permanent dentition** consists of 32 teeth (eight incisors, four cuspids, eight premolars and twelve molars) that are designed to last a lifetime.

The Structure of the Teeth

The crown of the tooth is the part that is visible in the mouth. It is covered by **enamel** which is the hardest substance in the body. The root of the tooth is covered by **cementum** (see-**MEN**-tum).

The bulk of the tooth consists of **dentin** (**DEN**-tin). These tissues all surround, and protect, the sensitive **pulp** which contains nerves and blood vessels.

The Periodontium

The periodontium (**per**-ee-oh-**DON**-she-um) consists of the hard and soft tissues that surround and support the teeth.

Each tooth has its own socket, within the bony **alveolar ridge** (al-**VEE**-oh-lar) that forms the dental arch.

Each tooth is surrounded by its own **periodontal ligament** (**per**-ee-oh-**DON**-tal) which cushions it and holds it in place.

The **gingiva (JIN-jih-vah)**, also known as the **gums,** is the specialized mucous membrane that surrounds the teeth, covers the alveolar bone and continues to form the lining of the mouth. (The combining form *GINGIV/O* means gum.)

Salivary Glands

Saliva, which is secreted by the salivary glands, helps to moisten food, start the digestive process and cleanse the mouth. (The combining forms *SIAL/O* and *SIALADEN/O* mean saliva and salivary glands.)

There are three pairs of salivary glands. The **parotid glands** (pah-**ROT**-id) are located on the face in front of, and slightly lower than, each ear.

The **sublingual glands** are located under the tongue, and the **submandibular glands** are located on the floor of the mouth.

THE PHARYNX

The pharynx, which is a common passageway for both respiration and digestion, is discussed in Chapter 7.

THE ESOPHAGUS

The esophagus (eh-**SOF**-ah-gus), also known as the **gullet,** is a collapsible tube that leads from the pharynx to the stomach. (The combining form *ESOPHAG/O* means esophagus.)

The **cardiac sphincter** is the muscle ring located around the opening from the esophagus into the stomach. This muscle controls the flow between the two structures.

THE STOMACH

The stomach is a sac-like organ which is composed of the **fundus** (upper, rounded part), **body** (main portion), and **antrum** (lower part).

Rugae are the folds in the mucosa lining the stomach. Glands located within these folds produce the gastric juices that aid in digestion and the mucus that forms the protective coating of the lining of the stomach.

The **pylorus** (pye-**LOR**-us) is the narrow passage connecting the stomach with the small intestine. (The combining form *PYLOR/O* means pylorus or gatekeeper.)

The **pyloric sphincter** controls the flow from the stomach to the duodenum.

THE SMALL INTESTINE

The small intestine, also known as the **small bowel,** extends from the pyloric sphincter to the first part of the large intestine. (The combining form *ENTER/O* means small intestine.)

The **villi (VILL-eye)** are the tiny hair-like projections that line the walls of the small intestine. (The combining form *VILL/I* means tuft of hair.) (Singular, **villus.)**

The **ileocecal valve (ill-ee-oh-SEE-**kull) is the valve between the ileum and the large intestine. This valve prevents the back flow of waste into the small intestine.

Parts of the Small Intestine

The small intestine consists of three parts:

- The **duodenum (dew-oh-DEE-**num) (The combining forms *DUODEN/I* and *DUODEN/O* mean duodenum.)
- The **jejunum** (jeh-**JOO**-num) (The combining form *JEJUN/O* means jejunum.)
- The **ileum (ILL-ee-um)** (The combining form *ILE/O* means ileum.)

THE LARGE INTESTINE

The large intestine extends from the end of the ileum of the small intestine to the anus. (The combining forms *COL/O* and *COLON/O* mean colon and large intestine.)

The large intestine is divided into four major parts: the **cecum,** the **colon,** the **sigmoid colon,** the **rectum** and **anus.**

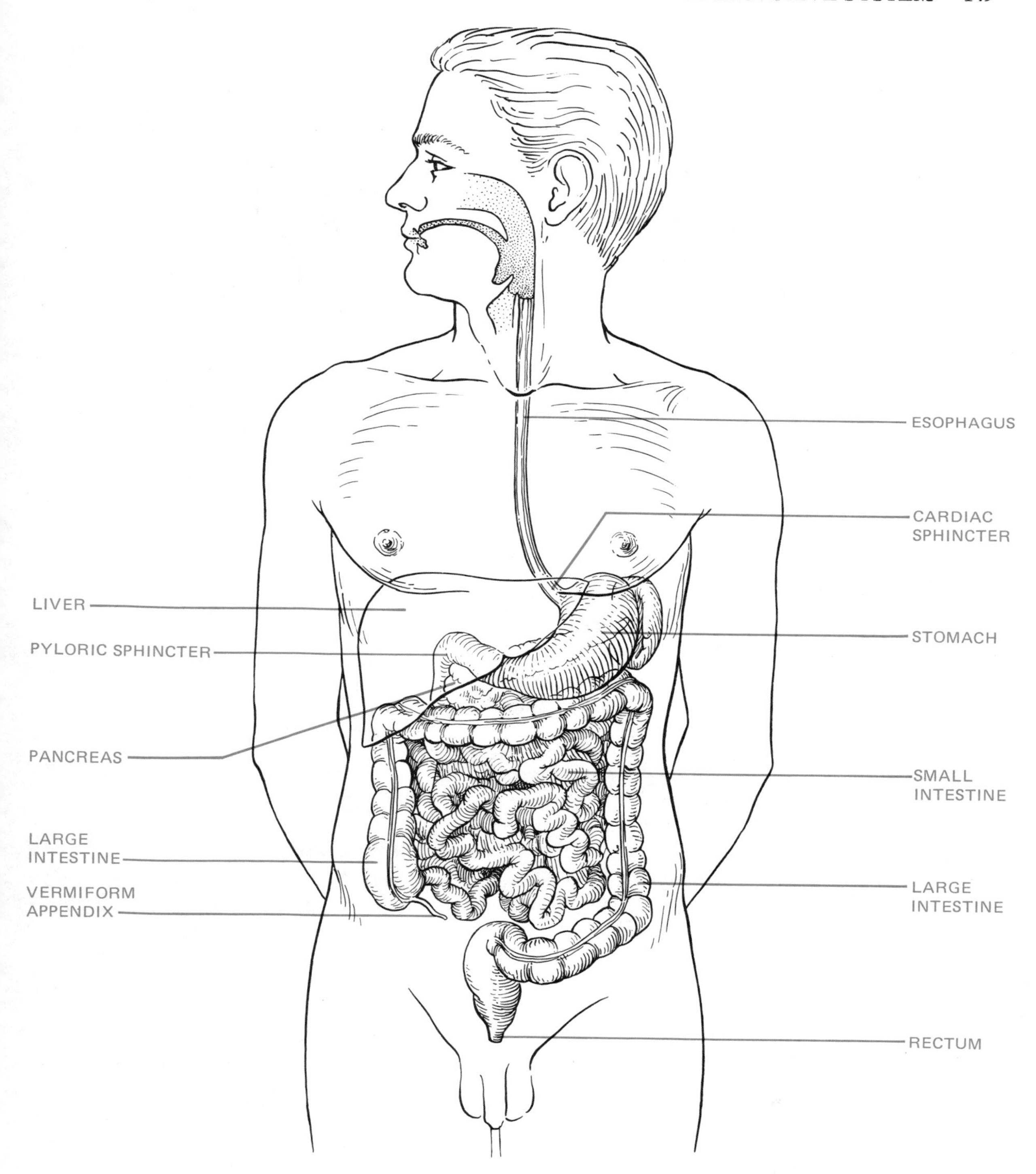

Figure 8-2 Structures of the digestive system.

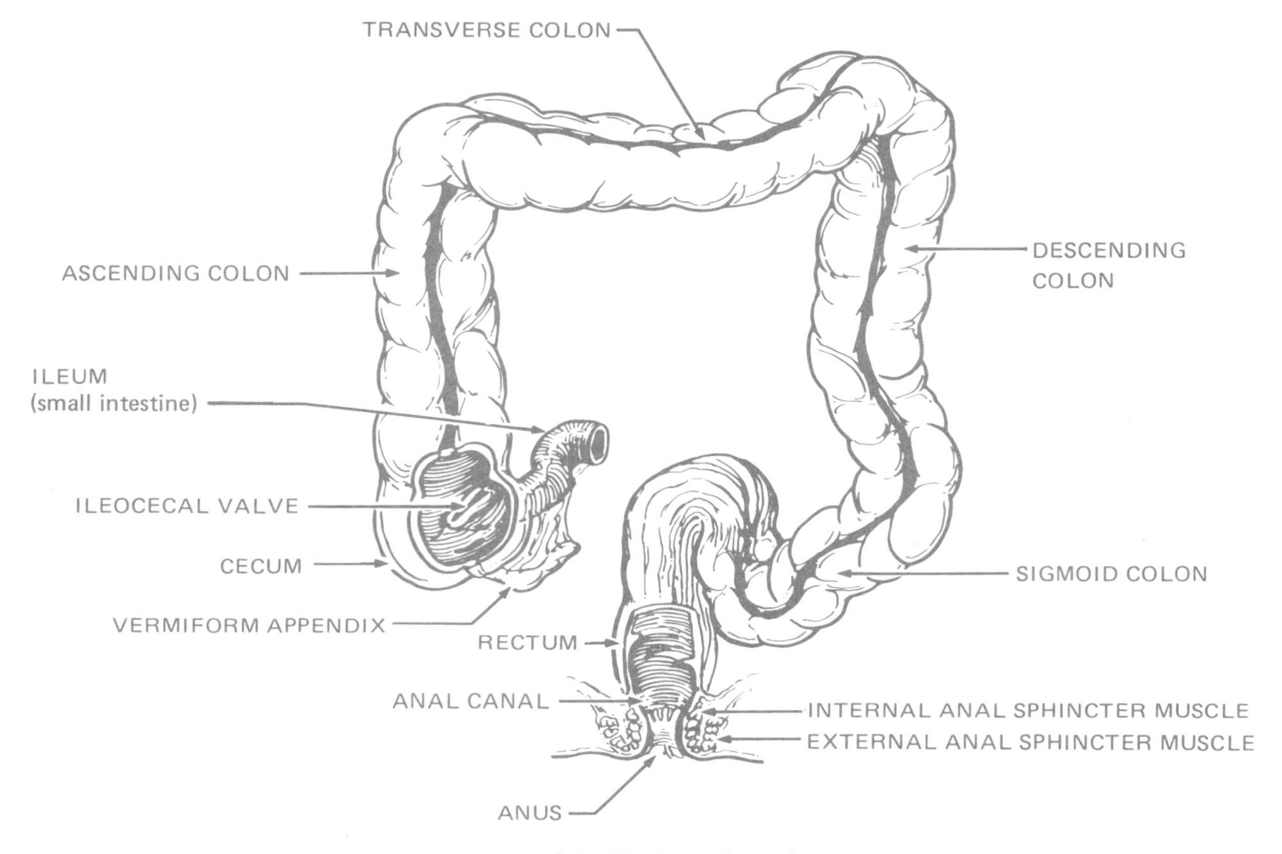

Figure 8-3 The large intestine.

The Cecum

The cecum (**SEE**-kum) is a pouch which lies on the right side of the abdomen. It is connected to the ileum by the **ileocecal sphincter.** (The combining form *CEC/O* means cecum or blind gut.)

The **vermiform appendix** hangs from the cecum. (The combining forms *APPEND/O* and *APPENDIC/O* both mean appendix.)

The Colon

The colon is subdivided into three divisions:

- the **ascending colon** extends from the cecum to the under surface of the liver;
- the **transverse colon** which passes horizontally to the left toward the spleen; and
- the **descending colon** travels down the left side of the abdominal cavity.

The Sigmoid Colon

The sigmoid colon (**SIG**-moid) is the third major part of the large intestine. It goes from the descending colon and leads into the rectum. (The combining form *SIGMOID/O* means sigmoid colon.)

The Rectum

The rectum, which is the last division of the large intestine, terminates in the lower opening of the gastrointestinal tract, the anus. (The combining form *RECT/O* means rectum or straight.)

The Anus

The anus is the lower opening of the digestive tract. It is controlled by two **anal sphincter** muscles. (The combining form *AN/O* means anus.)

The term **anorectal (ah-no-RECK-tal)** refers to the anus and rectum as a single unit.

THE LIVER

The liver is located in the right upper quadrant of the abdomen and has several important functions. (The combining form *HEPAT/O* means liver.)

The liver removes excess **glucose (GLOO-kohs)** (sugar) from the bloodstream and stores it as **glycogen (GLYE-koh-jen)** (starch). When the blood sugar level is low, the liver converts the glycogen back into glucose and releases it for use by the body.

The liver destroys old erythrocytes, removes poisons from the blood and manufactures some blood proteins. It also manufactures **bile,** which is a digestive juice.

Bile travels down the **hepatic duct** to the **cystic duct** which leads to the gallbladder where the bile is stored.

Bilirubin (bill-eh-**ROO**-bin), a pigment that is produced from the destruction of hemoglobin, is released by the liver in bile.

THE GALLBLADDER

The gallbladder is a pear-shaped sac located under the liver. It stores and concentrates the bile for later use. (The combining form *CHOL/E* means bile or gall and *CYST/O* means cyst or a sac filled with fluid.)

When bile is needed, the gallbladder contracts, forcing the bile out the **cystic duct** into the **common bile duct.**

THE PANCREAS

The pancreas **(PAN-**kree-as) produces pancreatic juices which are filled with the digestive enzymes. (The combining form *PANCREAT/O* means pancreas.)

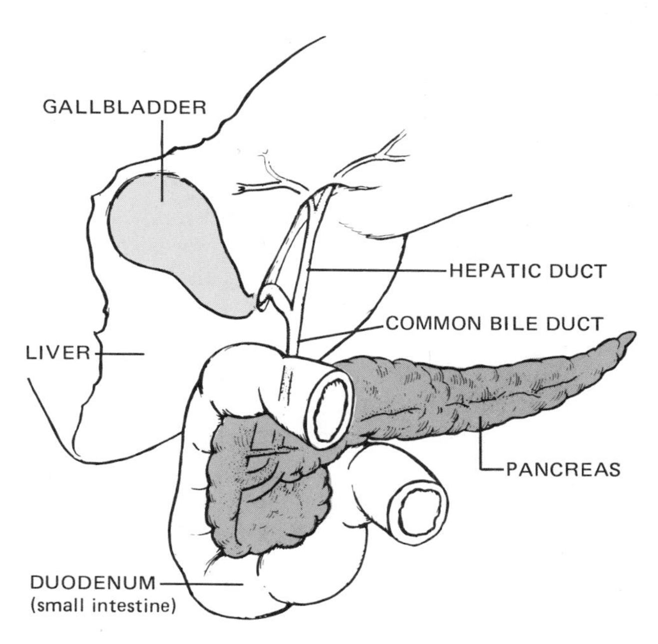

Figure 8-4 The gall bladder, liver and pancreas.

The pancreatic juices leave the pancreas through the **pancreatic duct** and join the common bile duct just before the entrance to the duodenum.

The pancreas also has a role in the endocrine system and this is discussed in Chapter 13.

DIGESTION

Digestion is the process by which complex foods are broken down into nutrients in a form that the body can utilize.

Enzymes (EN-zimes) are responsible for the chemical changes that break foods down into simpler forms which can be utilized by the body.

The term **metabolism** (meh-**TAB**-oh-lizm) includes all of the processes involved in the body's use of these nutrients. (The prefix *META-* means to change.)

Anabolism (an-**NAB**-oh-lizm) is the process of converting nutrients to build body cells and substances. **Catabolism** (kah-**TAB**-oh-lizm) is just the opposite. It is the process of breaking down body cells or substances.

The Role of the Mouth

Mastication (**mass**-tih-**KAY**-shun), also known as **chewing,** breaks food down into smaller pieces, and mixes it with saliva. Saliva contains the enzyme **salivary amylase** (**AM**-ih-lays) which begins the chemical breakdown of starches.

Deglutition (**dee**-gloo-**TISH**-un), also known as **swallowing,** is the action that moves the food bolus from the mouth into the pharynx and on into the esophagus. (A **bolus** is a soft round mass of chewed food.)

During swallowing the **epiglottis** closes off the entrance to the trachea and allows the bolus to move safely into the esophagus.

After it has been swallowed, food is moved through the digestive system by peristaltic action. (**Peristalsis** (**per**-ih-**STAL**-sis) is a series of wave-like contractions of smooth muscles. The suffix *-STALSIS* means contraction.)

The Role of the Stomach

The **gastric juices** of the stomach contain **hydrochloric acid** and the enzymes **protease** (**PROH**-tee-ays), **pepsin** (**PEP**-sin) and **lipase** (**LIP**-ays).

Very few nutrients enter the bloodstream through the walls of the stomach. Instead, the churning action of the stomach works with the gastric juices to convert the food to chyme which passes into the small intestine. (**Chyme** (**KYM**) is the semifluid mass of partly digested food.)

The Role of the Small Intestine

Digestion is completed in the duodenum after the chyme has been mixed with bile and pancreatic juice.

Bile breaks apart large fat globules so that enzymes from the pancreatic juice can digest the fats. Pancreatic juice contains the enzymes **trypsin** (**TRIP**-sin), **lipase** (**LIP**-ays) and **amylase** (**AM**-ih-lays).

This action is called **emulsification** and it must be completed before the nutrients can be absorbed into the body.

Absorption is the process by which completely digested nutrients are taken into the circulatory system by passing through the capillaries and lymph vessels in the villi of the small intestine.

The Role of the Large Intestine

The role of the entire large intestine is to receive the fluid waste products of digestion and store it until it is released from the body.

Water in the wastes is absorbed through the walls of the large intestine and solid feces are formed. (**Feces** (**FEE**-seez), also known as **stools,** are the solid body wastes that are expelled through the rectum.)

Defecation (**def**-eh-**KAY**-shun), also known as a **bowel movement,** is the evacuation or emptying of the bowels.

DIAGNOSTIC PROCEDURES RELATED TO THE DIGESTIVE SYSTEM

- **Abdominocentesis** (ab-**dom**-ih-no-sen-**TEE**-sis), also known as **paracentesis,** is the surgical puncture of the abdominal cavity which may be performed for diagnostic purposes or to remove excess fluids.
- **Anoscopy** (ah-**NOS**-koh-pee) is the visual examination of the anus and lower rectum using an **anoscope.**
- **Esophagoscopy** (eh-**sof**-ah-**GOS**-koh-pee) is the visual examination of the esophagus using an **esophagoscope.**
- **Gastroscopy** (gas-**TROS**-koh-pee) is the endoscopic examination of the interior of the stomach using a **gastroscope.**
- **Proctoscopy** (prock-**TOS**-koh-pee) is the direct visual examination of the interior of the anal canal and rectum using a **proctoscope.** (The combining form *PROCT/O* means rectum and anus.)

- **Sigmoidoscopy** (**sig**-moi-**DOS**-koh-pee) is the direct visual examination of the interior of the sigmoid colon using a **sigmoidoscope.**
- **Hemoccult** is a test for **occult blood** in the stools. (**Occult** means hidden or difficult to see.)

PATHOLOGY OF THE DIGESTIVE SYSTEM

Pathology of the Oral Cavity

- **Stomatitis** (stoh-mah-**TYE**-tis) is any inflammation of the mouth.
- **Aphthous stomatitis** (**AF**-thus), also known as **canker sores,** is an inflammation of the mouth associated with small ulcers.
- **Herpes labialis** (**HER**-peez **lay**-be-**AL**-iss), also known as **cold sores** or **fever blisters,** is caused by the herpes simplex virus.
- **Cheilitis** (kye-**LYE**-tis) is an inflammation of the lips.
- **Cheiloschisis** (kye-**LOHS**-kih-sis), also known as **harelip** or **cleft lip,** is a deep fissure of the lip that is present at birth. (A **fissure** is a deep groove.)
- **Cleft palate,** also known as **palatoschisis** (**pal**-ah-**TOS**-kih-sis), is a congenital fissure of the palate that may involve the soft palate, hard palate and upper lip.
- **Ankyloglossia** (**ang**-kih-loh-**GLAHS**-ee-ah), also known as **tongue-tied,** is an abnormal shortness of the lingual frenum.
- **Dentalgia** (den-**TAL**-jee-ah), also known as a **toothache,** is pain in a tooth.
- **Dental caries,** also known as **tooth decay,** is the progressive destruction of the structure of a tooth.
- **Bruxism** (**BRUCK**-sizm) is grinding of the teeth in other than chewing movements that usually occurs during sleep.
- **Edentulous** (ee-**DEN**-too-lus) means without teeth, after having lost the natural teeth.
- **Gingivitis** (**jin**-jih-**VYE**-tis) is an inflammation of the gums.
- **Periodontitis** (**per**-ee-oh-don-**TYE**-tis) is an inflammation of the gingiva and other tissues of the periodontium.
- **Sialadenitis** (**sigh**-al-**ad**-eh-**NIGH**-tis) is an inflammation of a salivary gland.

Pathology of the Esophagus

- **Dysphagia** (dis-**FAY**-jee-ah) is difficulty in swallowing.
- **Esophageal varices** (eh-**sof**-ah-**JEE**-al **VAYR**-ih-seez) are enlarged and swollen veins at the lower end of the esophagus.
- **Pyrosis** (pye-**ROH**-sis), also known as **heartburn,** is discomfort due to the regurgitation of stomach acid upward along the esophagus. (The combining form *PYR/O* means fever or fire.)
- A **hiatal hernia** (high-**AY**-tal **HER**-nee-ah) is a protrusion of part of the stomach through the esophageal opening in the diaphragm. (The combining form *HIAT/O* means opening.)

Pathology of the Stomach

- **Gastritis** (gas-**TRY**-tis) is an inflammation of the stomach.
- **Gastralgia** (gas-**TRAL**-jee-ah), also known as **gastrodynia** (**gas**-trow-**DIN**-ee-ah), means pain in the stomach.
- **Dyspepsia** (dis-**PEP**-see-ah), also known as **indigestion,** is an impairment of digestion.
- **Regurgitation** (ree-**gur**-jih-**TAY**-shun) is the return of swallowed food into the mouth.

- **Emesis (EM-**eh-sis), also known as **vomiting,** means to expel the contents of the stomach through the esophagus and out of the mouth.
- **Nausea** (**NAW**-see-ah) is the sensation that leads to the urge to vomit.
- **Hematemesis (hem-**ah-**TEM-**eh-sis) means the vomiting of blood. (The combining form *HEMAT/O* means blood.)
- **Anorexia (an-**oh-**RECK-**see-ah) is the lack or loss of the appetite for food.
- **Aerophagia (ay-**er-oh-**FAY-**jee-ah) is the spasmodic swallowing of air followed by eructations.

  Eructation (eh-ruk-**TAY-**shun) is the act of belching or raising gas orally from the stomach.
- **Flatus (FLAY-**tus) is gas in the stomach or intestines that is expelled through the anus.
- **Achlorhydria (ah-**klor-**HIGH-**dree-ah) is the absence of hydrochloric acid from gastric secretions.

Pathology of the Intestines

- **Gastroenteritis** (**gas-**troh-en-ter-**EYE-**tis) is an inflammation of the stomach and intestines, especially the small intestine.
- **Enteritis (en-**ter-**EYE-**tis) is an inflammation of the small intestine.
- **Ileitis (ill-**ee-**EYE-**tis) is an inflammation of the ileum.
- **Intussusception (in-**tus-sus-**SEP-**shun) is the telescoping of one part of the intestine into the opening of an immediately adjacent part.
- **Volvulus (VOL-**view-lus) is twisting of the intestine upon itself which causes an obstruction.
- **Crohn's disease** is a type of inflammatory bowel disease that usually affects the ileum and/or the colon.
- **Appendicitis** (ah-**pen-**dih-**SIGH-**tis) is an inflammation of the vermiform appendix.
- **Peritonitis (per-**ih-toh-**NIGH-**tis) is an inflammation of the peritoneum.
- **Diverticulitis (die-**ver-tick-you-**LYE-**tis) is an inflammation of a diverticulum.

  A **diverticulum** (**die-**ver-**TICK-**you-lum) is a pouch or sac occurring in the lining or wall of a tubular organ including the intestines. (Plural, **diverticula.**) (The combining form *DIVERT/I* means a turning aside or a bypath.)
- **Colitis** (koh-**LYE-**tis) is an inflammation of the colon.
- An **inguinal hernia** occurs when a small loop of bowel protrudes through a weak place in the lower abdominal wall or groin.
- **Colorectal polyps** are small growths that protrude from the mucous membrane lining of the colon and rectum.
- **Borborygmus** (**bor-**boh-**RIG-**mus) is the rumbling noise caused by the movement of gas in the intestine.
- An **anal fissure** is a crack-like lesion in the anus.
- An **anal fistula (FIS-**too-lah) is an abnormal opening in the skin surface near the anus.

  A **fistula** is an abnormal opening between two organs or from an organ through the skin.
- **Constipation** is a decrease in the frequency of bowel movements, usually accompanied by the difficult passage of stools.
- **Diarrhea** is loose or watery stools and an increase in bowel movements. Severe diarrhea can lead to dehydration.

Dehydration is a loss of the body's normal water content, which can affect both physical and mental functions.

- **Melena** (meh-**LEE**-nah) is the passage of black stools containing digested blood.

Infectious Diseases of the Intestines

- **Amebic dysentery** (ah-**ME**-bik) is an inflammation of the intestine caused by *Entamoeba histolytica* and is characterized by frequent, loose stools flecked with blood and mucus.
- **Botulism** (**BOCH**-oo-lizm), an often fatal form of food poisoning, is caused by eating food contaminated by *clostridium botulinum*.
- **Cholera** (**KOL**-er-ah) is an acute bacterial infection of the small intestine characterized by severe diarrhea and vomiting, muscular cramps and dehydration.
- **Salmonellosis** (**sal**-moh-nel-**LOH**-sis), also known as **salmonella**, is caused by eating food contaminated with a species of *Salmonella*. It is characterized by sudden abdominal pain, fever and bloody, watery diarrhea.
- **Shigellosis** (**shih**-gel-**LOH**-sis) is an acute infection of the bowel caused by a bacterium of the *Shigella* species. It is characterized by diarrhea, abdominal pain and fever.
- **Typhoid fever,** also known as **enteric fever,** is a bacterial infection usually caused by *Salmonella typhi*. It is characterized by headache, delirium, cough, watery diarrhea, rash and a high fever.

Pathology of the Liver, Gallbladder and Pancreas

- **Hepatitis** (**hep**-ah-**TYE**-tis) is an inflammation of the liver caused by a virus or by damage from toxic substances.
- **Hepatomegaly** (**hep**-ah-toh-**MEG**-ah-lee) is an enlargement of the liver.
- **Jaundice,** (**JAWN**-dis) also known as **icterus** (**ICK**-ter-us), is a yellow discoloration of the skin and other tissues caused by greater than normal amounts of bilirubin in the blood.
- **Cirrhosis** (sir-**ROH**-sis) is a chronic degenerative disease of the liver.
- **Cholelithiasis** (**koh**-lee-lih-**THIGH**-ah-sis) is the formation of gallstones.
- **Pancreatitis** (**pan**-kree-ah-**TYE**-tis) is an inflammation of the pancreas.

PROCEDURES RELATED TO THE DIGESTIVE SYSTEM

Procedures Related to the Oral Cavity and Esophagus

- **Cheiloplasty** (**KYE**-loh-**plas**-tee) is surgical repair of a defect of the lip.
- **Palatoplasty** (**PAL**-ah-toh-**plas**-tee) is surgical repair of the palate.
- A **frenectomy** (free-**NECK**-toh-me) is the surgical freeing of the frenum.
- An **odontectomy** (**oh**-don-**TECK**-toh-me), also known as an **extraction,** is the surgical removal of a tooth.
- **Gingivectomy** (**jin**-jih-**VECK**-toh-me) is the surgical removal of diseased gingival tissue.
- **Esophagoplasty** (eh-**SOF**-ah-go-**plas**-tee) is the surgical repair of the esophagus.

Procedures Related to the Stomach

- **Nasogastric intubation** is the placement of a tube through the nose and into the stomach.
- **Gastrectomy** (gas-**TRECK**-toh-me) is the surgical removal of all or a part of the stomach.

- A **gastrostomy** (gas-**TROS**-toh-me) is the surgical creation of an artificial opening into the stomach.
- **Pyloroplasty** (pye-**LOH**-roh-**plas**-tee) is the surgical repair of the pylorus.
- **Vagotomy** (vay-**GOT**-oh-me) is the surgical cutting of the vagus nerve, which stimulates acid secretion in the stomach.

Procedures Related to the Intestines

- An **appendectomy** (**ap**-en-**DECK**-toh-me) is the surgical removal of the vermiform appendix.
- A **colectomy** (koh-**LECK**-toh-me) is the surgical removal of all or part of the colon.
- A **colostomy** (koh-**LAHS**-toh-me) is the surgical creation of an opening between the colon and the body surface.
- **Diverticulectomy** (**die**-ver-**tick**-you-**LECK**-toh-me) is the surgical removal of a diverticulum.
- **Anastomosis** (ah-**nas**-toh-**MOH**-sis) is the surgical joining of two parts to allow flow from one to the other such as joining parts of the intestine. However, it may also be performed on blood vessels. (Plural, **anastomoses.**)
- **Enterocolostomy** (**en**-ter-oh-koh-**LAHS**-toh-me) is the surgical formation of a communication between the small intestine and the colon.
- An **ileostomy** (**ill**-ee-**OS**-toh-me) is the surgical creation of an opening into the wall of the ileum.
- **Proctectomy** (prock-**TECK**-toh-me) is the surgical removal of the rectum.
- **Proctoplasty** (**PROCK**-toh-**plas**-tee) is the surgical repair of the rectum.

Procedures Related to the Liver, Gallbladder and Pancreas

- **Hepatectomy** (**hep**-ah-**TECK**-toh-me) is the surgical removal of all or part of the liver.
- **Cholecystectomy** (**koh**-lee-sis-**TECK**-toh-me) is the surgical removal of the gallbladder.
- **Choledocholithotomy** (koh-**led**-uh-koh-lih-**THOT**-oh-me) is an incision in the common bile duct for the removal of gallstones.
- **Pancreatectomy** (**pan**-kree-ah-**TECK**-toh-me) is the surgical removal of the pancreas.

IMPORTANT TERMS: THE DIGESTIVE SYSTEM

This list will help you identify and review the major terms from this chapter.

When you work with the audio tape for this chapter, listen to the word, repeat it and then place a ✓ next to it on the list below.

- ☐ **Abdominocentesis** (ab-**dom**-ih-no-sen-**TEE**-sis)
- ☐ **Achlorhydria** (**ah**-klor-**HIGH**-dree-ah)
- ☐ **Aerophagia** (**ay**-er-oh-**FAY**-jee-ah)
- ☐ **Alimentary** (**al**-ih-**MEN**-tar-ee)
- ☐ **Alveolar** (al-**VEE**-oh-lar)
- ☐ **Amebic dysentery** (ah-**ME**-bik)
- ☐ **Amylase** (**AM**-ih-lays)
- ☐ **Anabolism** (an-**NAB**-oh-lizm)
- ☐ **Anastomosis** (ah-**nas**-toh-**MOH**-sis)
- ☐ **Ankyloglossia** (**ang**-kih-loh-**GLAHS**-ee-ah)
- ☐ **Anorectal** (**ah**-no-**RECK**-tal)
- ☐ **Anorexia** (**an**-oh-**RECK**-see-ah)
- ☐ **Anoscopy** (ah-**NOS**-koh-pee)
- ☐ **Aphthous** (**AF**-thus)

- ☐ **Appendectomy** (**ap**-en-**DECK**-toh-me)
- ☐ **Appendicitis** (ah-**pen**-dih-**SIGH**-tis)
- ☐ **Bilirubin** (bill-eh-**ROO**-bin)
- ☐ **Borborygmus** (**bor**-boh-**RIG**-mus)
- ☐ **Botulism** (**BOCH**-oo-lizm)
- ☐ **Bruxism** (**BRUCK**-sizm)
- ☐ **Catabolism** (kah-**TAB**-oh-lizm)
- ☐ **Cecum** (**SEE**-kum)
- ☐ **Cementum** (see-**MEN**-tum)
- ☐ **Cheilitis** (kye-**LYE**-tis)
- ☐ **Cheiloplasty** (**KYE**-loh-**plas**-tee)
- ☐ **Cheiloschisis** (kye-**LAHS**-kih-sis)
- ☐ **Cholecystectomy** (**koh**-lee-sis-**TECK**-toh-me)
- ☐ **Choledocholithotomy** (koh-**led**-uh-koh-lih-**THOT**-oh-me)
- ☐ **Cholelithiasis** (**koh**-lee-lih-**THIGH**-ah-sis)
- ☐ **Cholera** (**KOL**-er-ah)
- ☐ **Cirrhosis** (sir-**ROH**-sis)
- ☐ **Colectomy** (koh-**LECK**-toh-me)
- ☐ **Colitis** (koh-**LYE**-tis)
- ☐ **Colostomy** (koh-**LAHS**-toh-me)
- ☐ **Defecation** (**def**-eh-**KAY**-shun)
- ☐ **Deglutition** (**dee**-gloo-**TISH**-un)
- ☐ **Dentalgia** (den-**TAL**-jee-ah)
- ☐ **Diverticulectomy** (**die**-ver-**tick**-you-**LECK**-toh-me)
- ☐ **Diverticulitis** (**die**-ver-tick-you-**LYE**-tis)
- ☐ **Diverticulum** (**die**-ver-**TICK**-you-lum)
- ☐ **Duodenum** (**dew**-oh-**DEE**-num)
- ☐ **Dyspepsia** (dis-**PEP**-see-ah)
- ☐ **Dysphagia** (dis-**FAY**-jee-ah)
- ☐ **Edentulous** (ee-**DEN**-too-lus)
- ☐ **Emesis** (**EM**-eh-sis)
- ☐ **Enteritis** (**en**-ter-**EYE**-tis)
- ☐ **Enterocolostomy** (**en**-ter-oh-koh-**LAHS**-toh-me)
- ☐ **Eructation** (eh-ruk-**TAY**-shun)
- ☐ **Esophageal varices** (eh-**sof**-ah-**JEE**-al **VAYR**-ih-seez)
- ☐ **Esophagoscopy** (eh-**sof**-ah-**GOS**-koh-pee)
- ☐ **Esophagoplasty** (eh-**SOF**-ah-go-**plas**-tee)
- ☐ **Esophagus** (eh-**SOF**-ah-gus)
- ☐ **Feces** (**FEE**-seez)
- ☐ **Fistula** (**FIS**-too-lah)
- ☐ **Flatus** (**FLAY**-tus)
- ☐ **Frenectomy** (free-**NECK**-toh-me)
- ☐ **Frenum** (**FREE**-num)
- ☐ **Gastralgia** (gas-**TRAL**-jee-ah)
- ☐ **Gastrectomy** (gas-**TRECK**-toh-me)
- ☐ **Gastritis** (gas-**TRY**-tis)
- ☐ **Gastrodynia** (**gas**-trow-**DIN**-ee-ah)
- ☐ **Gastroenteritis** (**gas**-troh-en-ter-**EYE**-tis)
- ☐ **Gastroscopy** (gas-**TROS**-koh-pee)
- ☐ **Gastrostomy** (gas-**TROS**-toh-me)
- ☐ **Gingiva** (**JIN**-jih-vah)
- ☐ **Gingivectomy** (**jin**-jih-**VECK**-toh-me)
- ☐ **Gingivitis** (**jin**-jih-**VYE**-tis)
- ☐ **Glucose** (**GLOO**-kohs)

- ☐ **Glycogen** (**GLYE**-koh-jen)
- ☐ **Hematemesis** (**hem**-ah-**TEM**-eh-sis)
- ☐ **Hepatectomy** (**hep**-ah-**TECK**-toh-me)
- ☐ **Hepatitis** (**hep**-ah-**TYE**-tis)
- ☐ **Hepatomegaly** (**hep**-ah-toh-**MEG**-ah-lee)
- ☐ **Herpes labialis** (**HER**-peez lay-be-**AL**-iss)
- ☐ **Hiatal hernia** (high-**AY**-tal **HER**-nee-ah)
- ☐ **Ileitis** (**ill**-ee-**EYE**-tis)
- ☐ **Ileocecal** (**ill**-ee-oh-**SEE**-kull)
- ☐ **Ileostomy** (**ill**-ee-**OS**-toh-me)
- ☐ **Ileum** (**ILL**-ee-um)
- ☐ **Intussusception** (**in**-tus-sus-**SEP**-shun)
- ☐ **Jaundice** (**JAWN**-dis)
- ☐ **Jejunum** (jeh-**JOO**-num)
- ☐ **Labia** (**LAY**-bee-ah)
- ☐ **Lipase** (**LIP**-ays)
- ☐ **Mastication** (**mass**-tih-**KAY**-shun)
- ☐ **Melena** (meh-**LEE**-nah)
- ☐ **Metabolism** (meh-**TAB**-oh-lizm)
- ☐ **Odontectomy** (**oh**-don-**TECK**-toh-me)
- ☐ **Palatoplasty** (**PAL**-ah-toh-**plas**-tee)
- ☐ **Palatoschisis** (**pal**-ah-**TOS**-kih-sis)
- ☐ **Pancreatectomy** (**pan**-kree-ah-**TECK**-toh-me)
- ☐ **Pancreas** (**PAN**-kree-as)
- ☐ **Pancreatitis** (**pan**-kree-ah-**TYE**-tis)
- ☐ **Papilla** (pah-**PILL**-ah)
- ☐ **Parietal peritoneum** (pah-**RYE**-eh-tal **per**-ih-toh-**NEE**-um)
- ☐ **Parotid** (pah-**ROT**-id)
- ☐ **Pepsin** (**PEP**-sin)
- ☐ **Periodontitis** (**per**-ee-oh-don-**TYE**-tis)
- ☐ **Periodontal** (**per**-ee-oh-**DON**-tal)
- ☐ **Periodontium** (**per**-ee-oh-**DON**-she-um)
- ☐ **Peristalsis** (**per**-ih-**STAL**-sis)
- ☐ **Peritonitis** (**per**-ih-toh-**NIGH**-tis)
- ☐ **Proctectomy** (prock-**TECK**-toh-me)
- ☐ **Proctoplasty** (**PROCK**-toh-**plas**-tee)
- ☐ **Proctoscopy** (prock-**TOS**-koh-pee)
- ☐ **Protease** (**PROH**-tee-ays)
- ☐ **Pyloroplasty** (pye-**LOH**-roh-**plas**-tee)
- ☐ **Pylorus** (pye-**LOR**-us)
- ☐ **Pyrosis** (pye-**ROH**-sis)
- ☐ **Regurgitation** (ree-**gur**-jih-**TAY**-shun)
- ☐ **Rugae** (**ROO**-gay)
- ☐ **Salmonellosis** (**sal**-moh-nel-**LOH**-sis)
- ☐ **Shigellosis** (**shih**-gel-**LOH**-sis)
- ☐ **Sialadenitis** (**sigh**-al-**ad**-eh-**NIGH**-tis)
- ☐ **Sigmoid** (**SIG**-moid)
- ☐ **Sigmoidoscopy** (**sig**-moi-**DOS**-koh-pee)
- ☐ **Stomatitis** (stoh-mah-**TYE**-tis)
- ☐ **Trypsin** (**TRIP**-sin)
- ☐ **Uvula** (**YOU**-view-lah)
- ☐ **Vagotomy** (vay-**GOT**-oh-me)
- ☐ **Villi** (**VILL**-eye)
- ☐ **Visceral** (**VIS**-er-al)
- ☐ **Volvulus** (**VOL**-view-lus)

8

EXERCISES

DEFINING WORD PARTS

Write the definition for each of these word parts.

1. *ALIMENT/O* __________
2. *AN/O* __________
3. *BUCC/O* __________
4. *CEC/O* __________
5. *CHEIL/O* __________
6. *CHOL/E* __________
7. *COLON/O* __________
8. *CYST/O* __________
9. *DECIDU/O* __________
10. *DENT/I, DENT/O* __________
11. *DIVERT/I* __________
12. *DUODEN/I, DUODEN/O* __________
13. *ENTER/O* __________
14. *ESOPHAG/O* __________
15. *FREN/O* __________
16. *GASTR/O* __________

17. *GINGIV/O* ____________________

18. *HEPAT/O* ____________________

19. *HIAT/O* ____________________

20. *ILE/O* ____________________

21. *INTESTIN/O* ____________________

22. *JEJUN/O* ____________________

23. *LABI/O* ____________________

24. *LINGU/O* ____________________

25. *PANCREAT/O* ____________________

26. *PARIET/O* ____________________

27. *PROCT/O* ____________________

28. *PYLOR/O* ____________________

29. *RECT/O* ____________________

30. *RUG/O* ____________________

31. *SIAL/O* ____________________

32. *SIGMOID/O* ____________________

33. *-STALSIS* ____________________

34. *UVUL/O* ____________________

35. *VISCER/O* ____________________

DEFINITIONS

Circle the letter next to the correct answer.

1. ________________, also known as swallowing, is the action that moves the food bolus from the mouth into the pharynx and on into the esophagus.
   a) Deglutition
   b) Insalivation
   c) Mastication
   d) Peristalsis

2. The _______________ salivary glands are located on the face in front of, and slightly lower than, each ear.
   a) maxillary
   b) parotid
   c) sublingual
   d) submandibular

3. The _______________ are posterior teeth that are used for grinding and chewing.
   a) canines
   b) molars
   c) premolars
   d) b and c

4. The liver removes excess _______________ from the bloodstream.
   a) bilirubin
   b) glucose
   c) glycogen
   d) lipase

5. The gallbladder stores and concentrates _______________ for later use.
   a) bile
   b) glycogen
   c) hydrochloric acid
   d) pepsin

6. The duodenum is part of the _______________.
   a) cecum.
   b) large intestine.
   c) small intestine.
   d) stomach.

7. _______________ is the process of breaking down body cells or substances.
   a) Anabolism
   b) Catabolism
   c) Defecation
   d) Deglutition

8. Each _______________, which is located on the tongue, contains the receptors for the sense of taste.
   a) frenum
   b) papilla
   c) ruga
   d) villa

9. Each tooth is surrounded by its own _______________ ligament, which cushions it and holds it in place.
   a) alveolar
   b) gingival
   c) mucosal
   d) periodontal

10. _______________ is/are responsible for the chemical changes that break foods down into simpler forms that can be utilized by the body.
    a) Chyme
    b) Emulsification
    c) Enzymes
    d) Metabolism

MISSING WORDS

Write the missing word on the line.

1. ________________________ , also known as stools, are the solid body wastes that are expelled through the rectum.
2. The _______________ colon is the third major part of the large intestine.
3. The _______________ sphincter controls the flow from the stomach to the duodenum.
4. Bile travels down the _______________ duct when it leaves the liver.
5. The _______________, also known as the gullet, is a collapsible tube that leads from the pharynx to the stomach.
6. The _______________ is the last division of the large intestine.
7. _______________, also known as icterus, is a yellow discoloration of the skin and other tissues caused by greater than normal amounts of bilirubin in the blood.
8. _______________ are the folds in the mucosa lining the stomach.
9. The _______________ is the part of the small intestine that lies between the duodenum and the ileum.
10. A/an _______________ hernia occurs when a small loop of bowel protrudes through a weak place in the lower abdominal wall or groin.
11. A/an _______________ is an abnormal opening between two organs or from an organ through the skin.
12. _______________ stomatitis, also known as canker sores, is an inflammation of the mouth.

13. Esophageal _______________ are enlarged and swollen veins at the lower end of the esophagus.
14. _______________ is the return of swallowed food to the mouth.
15. The visceral _______________ surrounds the internal organs of the abdominal cavity.

SPELLCHECK

Select the correct spelling and write it on the line.

1. The _______________________, which hangs from the free edge of the soft palate, helps in producing sounds and speech.
   uvula
   uvulo
   youvuela
2. The cecum is connected to the ileum by the _______________ sphincter.
   ileocecal
   iliocecal
   iliocecol
3. _______________ is an acute bacterial infection of the small intestine.
   Cholera
   Cholira
   Colera
4. _______________ is the surgical joining of two parts to allow flow from one to the other.
   Anastomosis
   Anastomusis
   Anatomosis
5. _______________ is an inflammation of the liver caused by a virus or by damage from toxic substances.
   Hepatitis
   Hepatitus
   Hepetitus
6. _______________ is the lack or loss of the appetite for food.
   Anoresia
   Anoresis
   Anorexia
7. _______________ is loose or watery stools and an increase in bowel movements.
   Diarhhea
   Diarrhea
   Dierhear

8. _______________ is an inflammation of the colon.
   Colitis
   Coloitis
   Colonitis

9. _______________ is the sensation that leads to the urge to vomit.
   Nausea
   Nausia
   Nawsia

10. _______________ is a loss of the body's normal water content, which can affect both physical and mental function.
   Dehydration
   Dehydroation
   Dihydration

CASE STUDIES

Write the correct answer on the line.

1. James Ridgeview suffers from _______________________ which is a chronic degenerative disease of the liver.
2. Chang Hoon suffers from _______________ which is an inflammation of the stomach.
3. Geraldine Davenport has difficulty in swallowing. This is called _______________
4. During his trip to the jungle Mike Kilgore contracted _______________ _______________ that is an inflammation of the intestine which is characterized by frequent loose stools flecked with blood and mucus.
5. A/an _______________ was performed on Mr. Gonzalez to create an opening between the colon and the body surface.
6. Mr. Volmer underwent a/an _______________ for the partial removal of the liver.
7. Catherine Baldwin's presenting symptom was _______________ which is the passage of black stools containing digested blood.
8. As part of his physical examination, Mr. Adams underwent a/an _______________ which is the direct visual examination of the interior of the sigmoid colon.
9. Jason Norton suffers from _______________ labialis, which is also known as cold sores.
10. Her dentist informed Lisa Ortega that she has _______________ which is an inflammation of the gums.
11. The Anderson baby was born with a/an _______________ _______________which is also known as palatoschisis.
12. After eating Mr. Warren often suffers from _______________ which is also known as heartburn.

13. Richard Grovenor was admitted to the hospital for _______________ which is the vomiting of blood.

14. Mr. Strauss underwent _______________ for the surgical repair of the rectum.

15. The stool specimen was tested for _______________ (hidden) blood.

WORD BUILDING

Write the correct word or word part on the line.

1. Enlarged liver
   a) The combining form _______________ means liver.
   b) The combing form _______________ means large or great.
   c) The term _______________ means an enlargement of the liver.

2. Inflammation of the stomach and intestine
   a) The combining form _______________ means stomach.
   b) The combining form _______________ means small intestine.
   c) The suffix _______________ means inflammation.
   d) The term _______________ means an inflammation of the stomach and small intestine.

3. Intubation
   a) The combining form _______________ means nose.
   b) The combining form _______________ means stomach.
   c) The term _______________ intubation means the placement of a tube through the nose and into the stomach.

4. Polyps
   a) The combining form _______________ means colon.
   b) The combining form _______________ means rectum.
   c) The term _______________ polyps means small growths that protrude from the mucous membrane lining of the colon and rectum.

5. Surgical repair of the esophagus
   a) The combining form _______________ means esophagus
   b) The suffix _______________ means surgical repair.
   c) The term _______________ means the surgical repair of the esophagus.

LABELING EXERCISES

Identify the numbered items on this diagram.

1. ______________________________
2. ______________________________ sphincter
3. ______________________________
4. ______________________________ sphincter
5. ______________________________

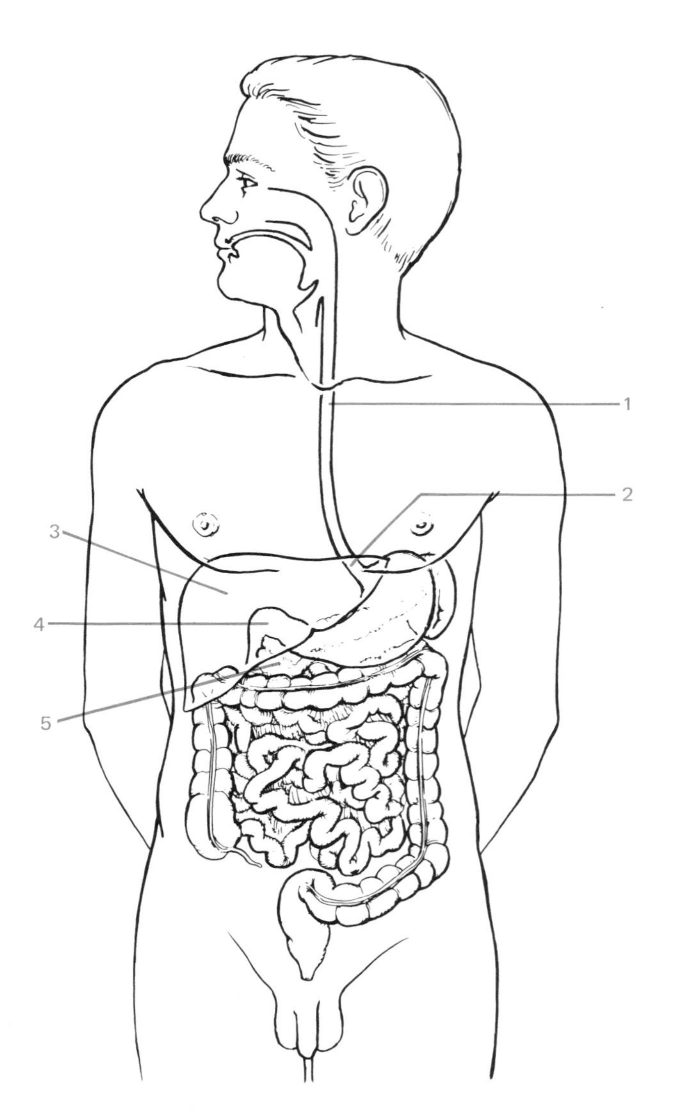

9

THE URINARY SYSTEM

LEARNING GOALS

In this chapter you will learn to:

- describe the functions and structures of the urinary system.
- state how urine is formed.
- recognize and define the terms related to the diagnosis, pathology and treatment of disorders of the urinary system.

STRUCTURES AND FUNCTIONS OF THE URINARY SYSTEM

The major function of the urinary system is to remove urea and other waste materials from the bloodstream. (**Urea** (you-**REE**-ah) is the major end-product of protein metabolism within the body.)

Another important function of the urinary system is to maintain the proper balance of water, salts and acids in the body fluids.

The urinary system, which excretes most of the liquid waste products, consists of two kidneys, two ureters, one bladder and a urethra.

The combining forms *URIN/O* and *UR/O* both mean urine or pertaining to the urinary organs. The combining forms *REN/O* and *NEPHR/O* both mean kidney.

THE KIDNEYS

The kidneys are located one on each side of the vertebral column below the diaphragm in the **retroperitoneal space** (**ree**-troh-**per**-ih-toh-**NEE**-al), which is located between the peritoneum and the muscles of the back. (The combining form *RETR/O* means behind.)

The **renal hilum** (**HIGH**-lum) is the notch in the bean-shape of the kidney where the blood vessels, nerves, and the renal pelvis enter and exit the kidney. (The combining form *HIL/O* means hilum or notch.)

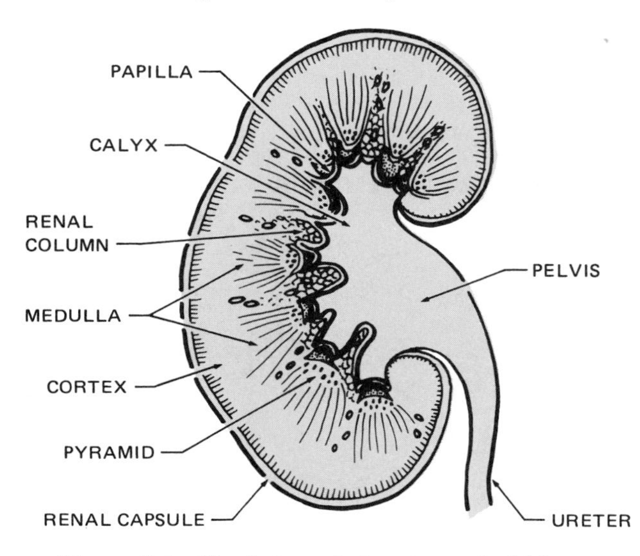

Figure 9-1 The internal structure of a kidney.

Each kidney consists of two layers that surround the renal pelvis. The outer, granular layer is called the **cortex** (**KOR**-tecks). (The combining form *CORTIC/O* means cortex or outer region.)

The **medulla** (meh-**DULL**-ah) is the inner layer and contains millions of microscopic units called nephrons. (The combining form *MEDULL/O* means middle or inner portion.)

Nephrons

The nephrons (**NEF**-rons) are shaped like a funnel with a long, twisted tail. **Bowman's capsule** is the expanded cup-like top of the funnel and it surrounds the glomerulus.

The **glomerulus** (glow-**MER**-you-lus) is a tiny ball of very small, coiled and intertwined capillaries. (The combining form *GLOMERUL/O* means glomerulus.) (Plural, **glomeruli.**)

The Bowman's capsule is joined to the convoluted **renal tubule** that forms the tail of the nephron. This tubule twists and descends to form **Henle's loop,** which is surrounded by **peritubular capillaries.** The distal portion of the convoluted tubule joins a straight collecting tubule, which eventually empties into the **calyces** (**KAL**-ih-seez) (Singular, **calyx.**)

The nephrons are supported by triangular-shaped wedges called **renal pyramids.** These pyramids are separated and supported by inward extensions of cortical material called the **renal columns.** The bases of the renal pyramids are toward the cortex.

The **renal papillae** (pah-**PILL**-ee), which are the narrower tops of these pyramids, empty into cavities called calyces. (The combining forms *PAPILL/I* and *PAPILL/O* mean nipple-like.) (Singular, **papilla.**)

Urine drains from the renal papillae into the calyces which are cup-like extensions of the renal pelvis. (The combining forms *CALI/O* and *CALIC/O* mean cup or calyx.)

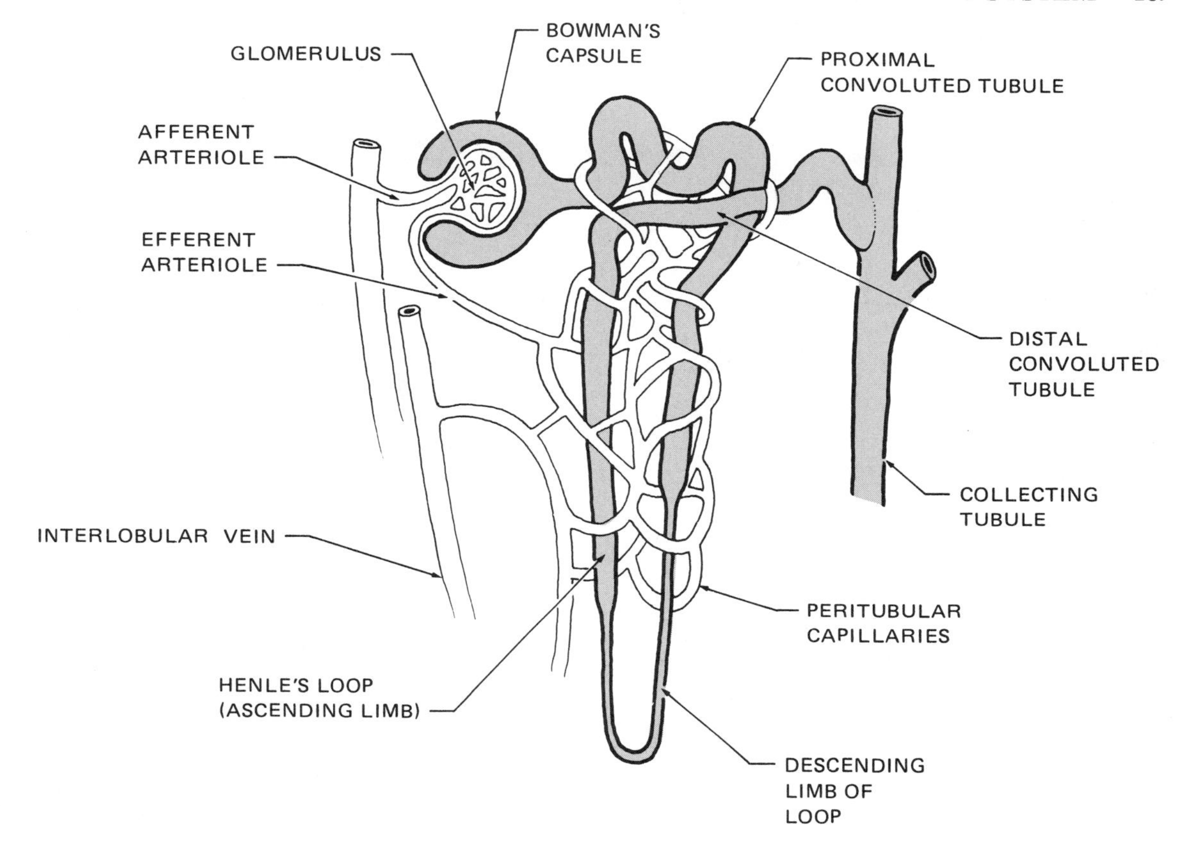

Figure 9-2 The structure of a nephron.

The **renal pelvis** is actually the upper end of the ureter. It is enlarged inside the medulla of the kidney into a funnel-shaped structure that receives urine from the calyces. (The combining form *PYEL/O* means renal pelvis or bowl of the kidney.)

THE URETERS

The ureters (you-**REE**-ters) are narrow tubes, each about ten to twelve inches long. Each ureter carries urine from a kidney to the urinary bladder. (The combining form *URETER/O* means ureter.)

THE URINARY BLADDER

The urinary bladder is a hollow muscular organ that serves as a reservoir for urine. It is located in the anterior portion of the pelvic cavity. (The combining forms *CYST/O* and *VESIC/O* both mean urinary bladder.)

The exit from the bladder to the urethra is closed by sphincters that control the flow of urine from the bladder. (A **sphincter** is a ring-like muscle that closes off a passageway.)

THE URETHRA

The urethra (you-**REE**-thrah) is the tube extending from the bladder to the outside of the body. (The combining form *URETHR/O* means urethra.) **(Caution:** the spelling of the words and combining forms "ureter" and urethra" are very similar!)

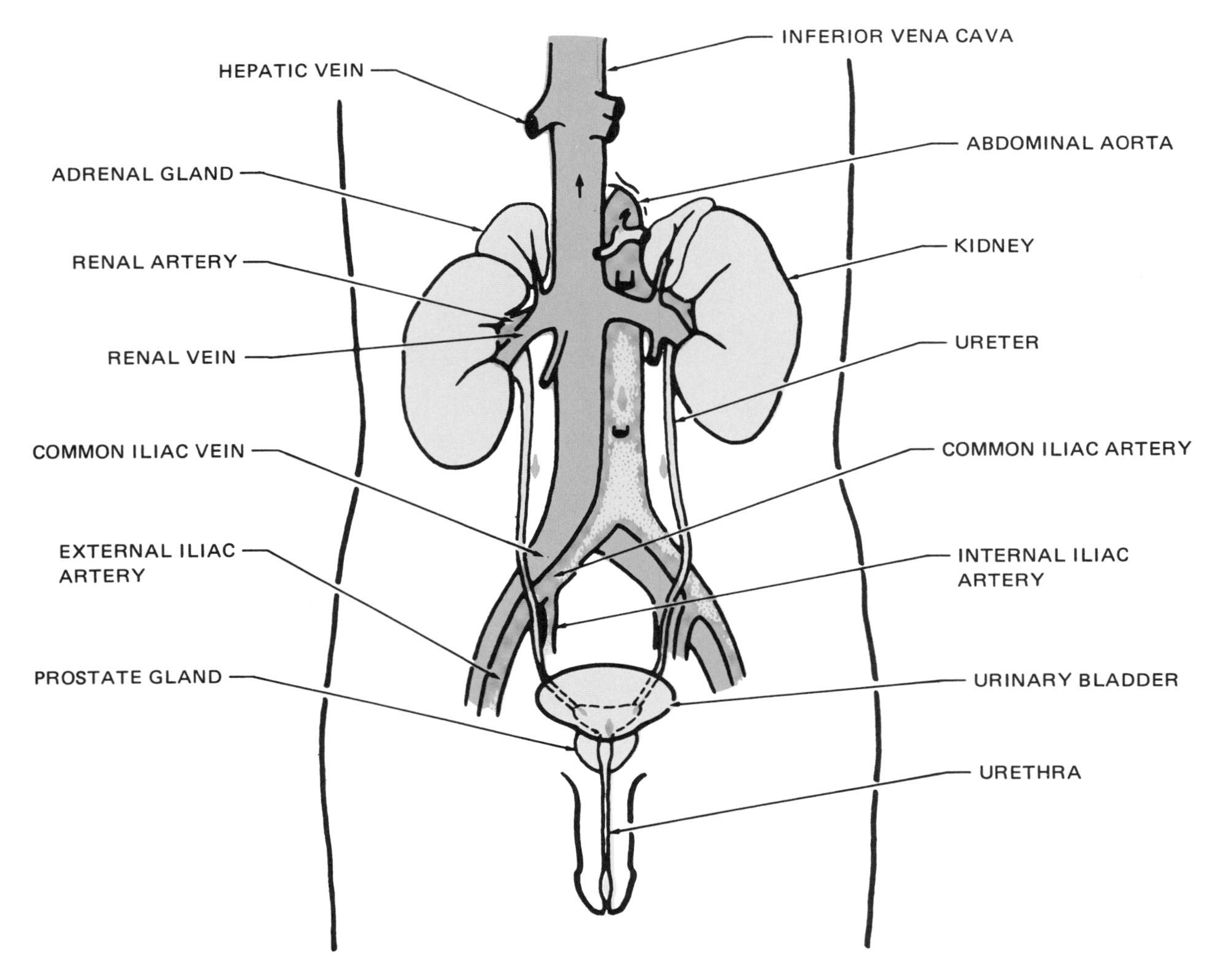

Figure 9-3 The structures of the urinary system in the male.

The **urethral meatus** (me-AY-tus), also known as the **urinary meatus,** is the external opening of the urethra. (The combining form *MEAT/O* means meatus or a passage.)

The Male Urethra

The male urethra is approximately eight inches long and is divided into the **prostatic, membranous** and **penile** sections. It conveys both urine and semen. (This function is discussed in Chapter 14.)

The Female Urethra

The female urethra is approximately one and one-half inches long. The urethral meatus is located between the clitoris and the opening of the vagina. The female urethra conveys only urine.

URINE FORMATION

Urine is formed by filtration, reabsorption and secretion within the nephrons of the kidneys.

Filtration

The glomerulus acts as a generalized filter that allows anything of a small enough size to pass through its capillaries and into the convoluted tubule.

Larger molecules such as proteins and blood cells do not normally pass through the walls of the glomerulus.

The glomerulus also takes in water and other substances that the body needs. However, only a very small percentage of this filtrate actually becomes urine. (A **filtrate** is a liquid that has passed through a filter. In this case, the filter is the walls of the glomerulus.)

This filtrate passes out of the glomerulus and into Bowman's capsule. Then it flows through the renal tubule.

Reabsorption

In the renal tubule most of the water and other useful substances are reabsorbed by the cell walls and are returned to the circulatory system through the capillaries that entwine the tubule.

Secretion

The process of secretion is the opposite of reabsorption. Secretion transports substances from the blood in the capillaries surrounding the tubules into the urine. These substances include ammonia, hydrogen ions, potassium ions and some drugs.

The urine secreted by the nephrons drops out of the tubules into the calyces, then enters the renal pelvis and continues down the ureters into the urinary bladder.

As the bladder fills up, pressure is placed on the base of the urethra and this causes the urge to urinate.

Urination, also known as **micturition** (**mick**-too-**RISH**-un) or **voiding,** is the normal process of excreting urine. (The suffix *-URIA* means urination or relating to urine.)

DIAGNOSTIC PROCEDURES RELATED TO THE URINARY SYSTEM

- **Catheterization** (**kath**-eh-ter-eye-**ZAY**-shun) is the insertion of a catheter through the urethra and into the urinary bladder to withdraw urine from the bladder.

  A **catheter** is a tube that is inserted into a body cavity to remove or to inject fluid.

- **Cystoscopy** (sis-**TOS**-koh-pee) is the visual examination of the urinary bladder using a **cystoscope.**

- An **intravenous pyelogram** (**PYE**-eh-loh-**gram**) is a diagnostic x-ray study of the renal pelvis after the injection of a contrast medium into a vein.

  This study is also known as **excretory urography.** It is so named because it traces the action of the kidney as it processes and excretes dye that has been injected into the blood stream.

- **Retrograde urography** is an x-ray of the urinary system taken after dye has been placed in the urethra and caused to flow upward through the urinary tract.

- **Cystography** (sis-**TOG**-rah-fee) is a radiographic examination of the urinary bladder following instillation of a contrast medium via a urethral catheter. The resulting film is called a **cystogram.**

- **Voiding cystourethrography** (**sis**-toh-you-ree-**THROG**-rah-fee) may be performed following cystography. In this procedure a fluoroscope may be used to examine the flow of urine from the bladder and through the urethra.

- **Nephrotomography** (**nef**-roh-toh-**MOG**-rah-fee) is the radiologic visualization of the kidney by tomography. The resulting record is called a **nephrotomogram.** (**Tomography** is an imaging technique that produces images of cross-sections of the body.)

Urinalysis

- **Urinalysis** is the examination of the physical and chemical properties of urine to determine the presence of abnormal elements.
- **Casts** are fibrous or protein materials that are thrown off into the urine in kidney disease. The forms of the casts are determined by the material of which they are made, such as pus and fats.
- The average normal **pH** range of urine is from 4.5 to 8.0. However, a pH of less than 7 indicates acid urine. A pH of above 7 indicates alkaline urine.
- The **specific gravity** of urine reflects the amount of wastes, minerals and solids in the urine. A **urinometer** (**you**-rih- **NOM**-eh-ter) or **refractometer** is an instrument used to measure the specific gravity of urine.
- **Urochrome** (**YOU**-roh-krome) is the pigment that gives urine its normal yellow color.

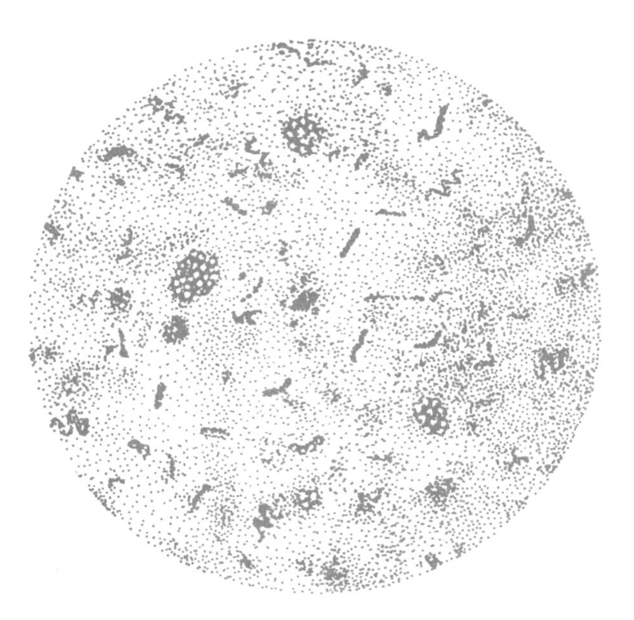

Figure 9-4 Magnified view of bacteria in urine sediment.

Specialized Results

- **Acetones** are found in small quantities in normal urine and in larger amounts in diabetic urine.
- **Albuminuria** (**al**-byou-mih-**NEW**-ree-ah) is the presence of serum protein in the urine. (The combining form *ALBUMIN/O* means albumin or protein.)
- **Bacteriuria** (back-**tee**-ree-**YOU**-ree-ah) is the presence of bacteria in the urine. (The combining form *BACTERI/O* means bacteria.)
- **Calciuria** (**kal**-sih-**YOU**-ree-ah) is the presence of calcium in the urine. (The combining form *CALC/I* means calcium.)
- **Creatinuria** (kree-**at**-ih-**NEW**-ree-ah) is an increased concentration of creatine in the urine.
- **Creatinine** is a waste product formed from the metabolism of creatine.
- **Glycosuria** (**glye**-koh-**SOO**-ree-ah) is the presence of glucose in the urine. (The combining form *GLYC/O* means glucose or sugar.)
- **Hematuria** (**hem**-ah-**TOO**-ree-ah) is the presence of blood in the urine. (The combining form *HEMAT/O* means blood.)
- **Ketonuria** (**key**-toh-**NEW**-ree-ah) is the presence of ketones in the urine. (The combining form *KET/O* means ketones.)

  Ketones are abnormal substances produced during the increased metabolism of fat.
- **Proteinuria** (**pro**-tee-in-**YOU**-ree-ah) is an excess of serum protein in the urine. (The combining form *PROT/O* means protein.)
- **Pyuria** (pye-**YOU**-ree-ah) is the presence of pus in the urine. (The combining form *PY/O* means pus.)

PATHOLOGY OF THE URINARY SYSTEM

Pathology of the Kidneys

- **Nephropathy** (neh-**FROP**-ah-thee), also called **renopathy,** is any disorder of the kidney.
- **Nephritis** (neh-**FRY**-tis) is an inflammation of the kidney.
- **Nephrosis** (neh-**FROH**-sis) is any kidney disease, but particularly diseases marked by degenerative lesions of the renal tubules.
- **Nephrotic syndrome** (neh-**FROT**-ick) is an abnormal condition of the kidney characterized by proteinuria, hypoalbuminemia and edema.
- **Hydronephrosis** (**high**-droh-neh-**FROH**-sis) is the distention of the renal pelvis and calyces of the kidney.
- **Renal calculus,** also known as a **nephrolith** (NEF-row-lith) or **kidney stone,** is a calculus (stone) in the kidney. (The combining form *LITH/O* means stone or calculus.)
- **Nephrolithiasis** (**nef**-row-lih-**THIGH**-ah-sis) is a disorder characterized by the presence of stones in the kidney.
- **Nephroma** (neh-**FROH**-mah) is a tumor of kidney tissue.
- **Nephromalacia** (**nef**-row-mah-**LAY**-she-ah) is the abnormal softening of the kidney.
- **Nephrosclerosis** (**nef**-row-sklee-**ROW**-sis) is the abnormal hardening of the kidney.
- **Nephroptosis** (**nef**-rop-**TOH**-sis) is the prolapse of the kidney. (The suffix *-PTOSIS* means drooping or dropping down.)

  Prolapse means the downward placement of a body organ.
- **Nephropyosis** (**nef**-row-pye-**OH**-sis) is suppuration of the kidney.
- **Suppuration** means the formation or discharge of pus.
- **Renal colic** is an acute pain in the kidney area that is caused by blockage during the passage of a stone.
- **Renal failure** is the inability of the kidney to excrete urine properly.
- **Glomerulonephritis** (glow-**mer**-you-low-neh-**FRY**-tis) is an inflammation of the kidney involving primarily the glomeruli.
- **Pyelitis** (**pye**-eh-**LYE**-tis) is an inflammation of the renal pelvis.
- **Pyelonephritis** (**pye**-eh-loh-neh-**FRY**-tis) is an inflammation of the renal pelvis and of the kidney.

Pathology of the Ureters

- **Ureteropathy** (you-**ree**-ter-**OP**-ah-thee) is any disease of the ureter.
- **Ureterostenosis** (you-**ree**-ter-oh-steh-**NO**-sis) is a condition of narrowing of the ureter. (The combining form *STEN/O* means a narrowing.)

  Stenosis is an abnormal narrowing or constriction of a body passage or opening.

Pathology of the Urinary Bladder and Urethra

- **Cystalgia** (sis-**TAL**-jee-ah) and **cystodynia** (**sis**-toh-**DIN**-ee-ah) both mean pain in the urinary bladder.
- **Cystitis** (sis-**TYE**-tis) is an inflammation of the bladder.
- A **cystocele** (**SIS**-toh-seel) is a hernia of the bladder into the vagina. (The suffix *-CELE* means hernia.)

  A **cystolith** (**SIS**-toh-lith) is a stone in the urinary bladder.

- **Cystorrhagia** (**sis**-toh-**RAY**-jee-ah) is hemorrhage (bleeding) from the bladder.
- **Urinary incontinence** is the inability to control the voiding of urine.

  Incontinence means being unable to control excretory functions.
- **Urethralgia** (**you**-reh-**THRAL**-jee-ah) is pain in the urethra.
- **Urethritis** (**you**-reh-**THRIGH**-tis) is an inflammation of the urethra.
- **Epispadias** (**ep**-ih-**SPAY**-dee-as), in the male, is the congenital opening of the urethra on the upper or dorsal surface of the penis.

  In the female, it is the congenital opening of the urethra in the region of the clitoris. (The combining form *SPAD/O* means draw off.)
- **Hypospadias** (**high**-poh-**SPAY**-dee-as), in the male, is the congenital opening of the urethra on the undersurface of the penis.

  In the female it is the opening of the urethra into the vagina.
- **Paraspadias** (**par**-ah-**SPAY**-dee-as) is a congenital male anomaly in which the urethra opens on one side of the penis.

  An **anomaly** is any marked deviation from the norm.

Pathology of Urination

- **Diuresis** (**dye**-you-**REE**-sis) is the increased excretion of urine.
- **Dysuria** (dis-**YOU**-ree-ah) is difficult or painful urination.
- **Oliguria** (**ol**-ih-**GOO**-ree-ah) means scanty urination. (The combining form *OLIG/O* means scanty or few.)
- **Polyuria** (**pol**-ee-**YOU**-ree-ah) means excessive urination.
- **Urinary retention** is the inability to void or empty the bladder.
- **Enuresis** (**en**-you-**REE**-sis), also known as **bed-wetting,** is a condition of involuntary discharge of urine.
- **Nocturia** (nock-**TOO**-ree-ah) is excessive urination during the night. (The combining form *NOCT/I* means night.)

Pathology of Urine Formation

- **Anuria** (ah-**NEW**-ree-ah), also known as **anuresis** (**an**-you-**REE**-sis), is the complete suppression (stopping) of urine formation by the kidneys or the inability to urinate.
- **Uremia** (you-**REE**-me-ah), also known as **uremic poisoning,** is a toxic condition caused by excessive waste products in the bloodstream due to kidney dysfunction.

PROCEDURES RELATED TO THE URINARY SYSTEM

Dialysis

- **Dialysis** (dye-**AL**-ih-sis) is the artificial filtration of waste materials from the blood and is used to replace kidney function.
- **Hemodialysis** (**he**-moh-dye-**AL**-ih-sis) uses an artificial kidney machine that filters wastes from the patient's blood.
- **Peritoneal dialysis** (**per**-ih-toh-**NEE**-al) is the removal of waste by fluid exchange through the peritoneal cavity. (**Peritoneal** is another term for the abdominal cavity.)

Procedures Related to the Kidneys and Ureters

- A **nephrectomy** (neh-**FRECK**-toh-me) is the surgical removal of a kidney.
- **Nephrolysis** (neh-**FROL**-ih-sis) is the freeing of a kidney from adhesions. It also means the destruction of kidney substance.

- **Lithotripsy** (**LITH**-oh-**trip**-see), also known as **extracorporeal shock-wave lithotripsy,** is the destruction of a kidney stone with the use of ultrasonic waves traveling through water.
- A **renal transplant**, also known as a **kidney transplant,** is the transfer of a kidney from a donor to a recipient patient.
- **Ureteroplasty** (you-**REE**-ter-oh-**plas**-tee) is the surgical repair of the ureter.

Procedures Related to the Urinary Bladder and Urethra

- **Cystectomy** (sis-**TECK**-toh-me) is the surgical removal of all or part of the urinary bladder.
- **Cystoplasty** (**SIS**-toh-**plas**-tee) is the surgical repair of the bladder.
- **Cystorrhaphy** (sis-**TOR**-ah-fee) is suturing of the bladder.
- **Litholapaxy** (lih-**THOL**-ah-**pack**-see) is a surgical procedure in which a stone is crushed within the bladder and the fragments are washed out.
- **Meatotomy** (**me**-ah-**TOT**-oh-me) is an incision of the urinary meatus to enlarge the opening.
- **Urethroplasty** (you-**REE**-throw-**plas**-tee) is the surgical repair of the urethra.

IMPORTANT TERMS: THE URINARY SYSTEM

This list will help you identify and review the major terms from this chapter.

When you work with the audio tape for this chapter, listen to the word, repeat it and then place a ✓ next to it on the list below.

- ☐ **Albuminuria** (**al**-byou-mih-**NEW**-ree-ah)
- ☐ **Anuresis** (**an**-you-**REE**-sis)
- ☐ **Anuria** (ah-**NEW**-ree-ah)
- ☐ **Bacteriuria** (back-**tee**-ree-**YOU**-ree-ah)
- ☐ **Calciuria** (**kal**-sih-**YOU**-ree-ah)
- ☐ **Calyces** (**KAL**-ih-seez)
- ☐ **Catheterization** (**kath**-eh-ter-eye-**ZAY**-shun)
- ☐ **Cortex** (**KOR**-tecks)
- ☐ **Creatinuria** (kree-**at**-ih-**NEW**-ree-ah)
- ☐ **Cystalgia** (sis-**TAL**-jee-ah)
- ☐ **Cystectomy** (sis-**TECK**-toh-me)
- ☐ **Cystitis** (sis-**TYE**-tis)
- ☐ **Cystocele** (**SIS**-toh-seel)
- ☐ **Cystodynia** (**sis**-toh-**DIN**-ee-ah)
- ☐ **Cystography** (sis-**TOG**-rah-fee)
- ☐ **Cystolith** (**SIS**-toh-lith)
- ☐ **Cystoplasty** (**SIS**-toh-**plas**-tee)
- ☐ **Cystorrhagia** (**sis**-toh-**RAY**-jee-ah)
- ☐ **Cystorrhaphy** (sis-**TOR**-ah-fee)
- ☐ **Cystoscopy** (sis-**TOS**-koh-pee)
- ☐ **Cystourethrography** (**sis**-toh-you-ree-**THROG**-rah-fee)
- ☐ **Dialysis** (dye-**AL**-ih-sis)
- ☐ **Diuresis** (**dye**-you-**REE**-sis)
- ☐ **Dysuria** (dis-**YOU**-ree-ah)
- ☐ **Enuresis** (**en**-you-**REE**-sis)
- ☐ **Epispadias** (**ep**-ih-**SPAY**-dee-as)
- ☐ **Glomerulonephritis** (glow-**mer**-you-low-neh-**FRY**-tis)
- ☐ **Glomerulus** (glow-**MER**-you-lus)
- ☐ **Glycosuria** (**glye**-koh-**SOO**-ree-ah)

- ☐ **Hematuria** (**hem**-ah-**TOO**-ree-ah)
- ☐ **Hemodialysis** (**he**-moh-dye-**AL**-ih-sis)
- ☐ **Hilum** (**HIGH**-lum)
- ☐ **Hydronephrosis** (**high**-droh-neh-**FROH**-sis)
- ☐ **Hypospadias** (**high**-poh-**SPAY**-dee-as)
- ☐ **Ketonuria** (**key**-toh-**NEW**-ree-ah)
- ☐ **Litholapaxy** (lih-**THOL**-ah-**pack**-see)
- ☐ **Lithotripsy** (**LITH**-oh-**trip**-see)
- ☐ **Meatotomy** (**me**-ah-**TOT**-oh-me)
- ☐ **Meatus** (me-**AY**-tus)
- ☐ **Medulla** (meh-**DULL**-ah)
- ☐ **Micturition** (**mick**-too-**RISH**-un)
- ☐ **Nephrectomy** (neh-**FRECK**-toh-me)
- ☐ **Nephritis** (neh-**FRY**-tis)
- ☐ **Nephrolysis** (neh-**FROL**-ih-sis)
- ☐ **Nephrolithiasis** (**nef**-row-lih-**THIGH**-ah-sis)
- ☐ **Nephromalacia** (**nef**-row-mah-**LAY**-she-ah)
- ☐ **Nephroma** (neh-**FROH**-mah)
- ☐ **Nephrons** (**NEF**-rons)
- ☐ **Nephropathy** (neh-**FROP**-ah-thee)
- ☐ **Nephropyosis** (**nef**-row-pye-**OH**-sis)
- ☐ **Nephroptosis** (**nef**-rop-**TOH**-sis)
- ☐ **Nephrosis** (neh-**FROH**-sis)
- ☐ **Nephrosclerosis** (**nef**-row-sklee-**ROW**-sis)
- ☐ **Nephrotomography** (**nef**-roh-toh-**MOG**-rah-fee)
- ☐ **Nephrotic** (neh-**FROT**-ick)
- ☐ **Nocturia** (nock-**TOO**-ree-ah)
- ☐ **Oliguria** (**ol**-ih-**GOO**-ree-ah)
- ☐ **Papillae** (pah-**PILL**-ee)
- ☐ **Paraspadias** (**par**-ah-**SPAY**-dee-as)
- ☐ **Peritoneal** (**per**-ih-toh-**NEE**-al)
- ☐ **Polyuria** (**pol**-ee-**YOU**-ree-ah)
- ☐ **Proteinuria** (**pro**-tee-in-**YOU**-ree-ah)
- ☐ **Pyelitis** (**pye**-eh-**LYE**-tis)
- ☐ **Pyelogram** (**PYE**-eh-loh-**gram**)
- ☐ **Pyelonephritis** (**pye**-eh-loh-neh-**FRY**-tis)
- ☐ **Pyuria** (pye-**YOU**-ree-ah)
- ☐ **Retroperitoneal** (**ree**-troh-**per**-ih-toh-**NEE**-al)
- ☐ **Urea** (you-**REE**-ah)
- ☐ **Uremia** (you-**REE**-me-ah)
- ☐ **Ureterostenosis** (you-**ree**-ter-oh-steh-**NO**-sis)
- ☐ **Ureteropathy** (you-**ree**-ter-**OP**-ah-thee)
- ☐ **Ureteroplasty** (you-**REE**-ter-oh-**plas**-tee)
- ☐ **Ureters** (you-**REE**-ters)
- ☐ **Urethralgia** (**you**-reh-**THRAL**-jee-ah)
- ☐ **Urethra** (you-**REE**-thrah)
- ☐ **Urethritis** (**you**-reh-**THRIGH**-tis)
- ☐ **Urethroplasty** (you-**REE**-throw-**plas**-tee)
- ☐ **Urochrome** (**YOU**-roh-krome)
- ☐ **Urinometer** (**you**-rih-**NOM**-eh-ter)

9

EXERCISES

DEFINING WORD PARTS

Write the definition for each of these word parts.

1. *ALBUMIN/O* ______
2. *BACTERI/O* ______
3. *CALC/I* ______
4. *CALI/O, CALIC/O* ______
5. *-CELE* ______
6. *CORTIC/O* ______
7. *CYST/O* ______
8. *GLOMERUL/O* ______
9. *GLYC/O* ______
10. *HIL/O* ______
11. *KET/O* ______
12. *LITH/O* ______
13. *MEAT/O* ______
14. *MEDULL/O* ______
15. *NEPHR/O* ______
16. *NOCT/I* ______

17. *PAPILL/I, PAPILL/O* ______________________________

18. *PROT/O* ______________________________

19. *-PTOSIS* ______________________________

20. *PYEL/O* ______________________________

21. *REN/O* ______________________________

22. *RETR/O* ______________________________

23. *SPAD/O* ______________________________

24. *STEN/O* ______________________________

25. *UR/O* ______________________________

26. *URETER/O* ______________________________

27. *URETHR/O* ______________________________

28. *-URIA* ______________________________

29. *URIN/O* ______________________________

30. *VESIC/O* ______________________________

DEFINITIONS

Circle the letter next to the correct answer.

1. The renal _______________ is the notch in the bean-shaped kidney.
   a) calyx
   b) cortex
   c) hilum
   d) medulla

2. The _______________ are narrow tubes that carry urine from the kidneys to the urinary bladder.
   a) glomeruli
   b) renal papillae
   c) urethras
   d) ureters

3. The _______________ is the part of the kidney that acts as a generalized filter.
   a) Bowman's capsule
   b) calyx
   c) glomerulus
   d) papilla

4. _______________ is/are the major end-product(s) of protein metabolism within the body.
   a) Albumin
   b) Creatinine
   c) Ketones
   d) Urea

5. The renal pelvis is actually the upper end of the _______________
   a) Bowman's capsule.
   b) renal papilla.
   c) ureter.
   d) urethra.

6. The exit to the urinary bladder is controlled by _______________
   a) caylces.
   b) glomeruli.
   c) papillae.
   d) sphincters.

7. The medulla of the kidney contains millions of microscopic units called _______________
   a) glomeruli.
   b) nephrons.
   c) renal pyramids.
   d) renal tubules.

8. In the renal tubule most of the water and other useful substances are _______________ by the cell walls.
   a) excreted
   b) filtrated
   c) reabsorbed
   d) secreted

9. The urethral _______________ is the external opening of the urethra.
   a) capsule
   b) meatus
   c) pelvis
   d) sphincter

10. ______________ is the complete stopping of urine formation by the kidneys.
    a) Anuria
    b) Anuresis
    c) Dysuria
    d) a and b

MISSING WORDS

Write the missing word on the line.

1. A/an ______________ is an incision of the urinary meatus to enlarge the opening.
2. A/an ______________ is a tumor of kidney tissue.
3. ______________ is the presence of ketones in the urine.
4. ______________ is the pigment that gives urine its normal yellow color.
5. An intravenous ______________ is a diagnostic x-ray study of the renal pelvis after the injection of a contrast medium into a vein.
6. Urination is also known as ______________ or voiding.
7. The ______________ syndrome is characterized by proteinuria, hypoalbuminemia and edema.
8. Renal ______________ is also known as a kidney stone.
9. ______________ is an excess of serum protein in the urine.
10. Renal ______________ is an acute pain in the kidney area that is caused by blockage during the passage of a stone.
11. ______________ means difficult or painful urination.
12. ______________ means excessive urination.
13. ______________ means the downward placement of a body organ.
14. ______________ is the abnormal softening of the kidney.
15. A/an ______________ is a marked deviation from the norm.

SPELLCHECK

Select the correct spelling and write it on the line.

1. ______________ is bleeding from the bladder.
    Cystiorrhagia
    Cystorrhagia
    Cystorrhhagia

2. _______________ uses an artificial kidney machine to filter wastes from the patient's blood.
Hemadialysis
Hemeodialysis
Hemodialysis

3. _______________ is the destruction of a kidney stone with the use of ultrasonic waves traveling through water.
Lithitrypsy
Lithotripsy
Lythotripsy

4. _______________ is the examination of the physical and chemical properties of urine to determine the presence of abnormal elements.
Urinalysis
Urinalysist
Urinoalysis

5. _______________ is the insertion of a tube into the bladder to withdraw urine.
Catherization
Catheteritization
Catheterization

6. _______________ means being unable to control excretory functions.
Incontanence
Incontinance
Incontinence

7. _______________ is also known as bed-wetting.
Anouresis
Anuresis
Enuresis

8. _______________ is the formation or discharge of pus.
Supration
Suppuration
Supuration

9. _______________ is a toxic condition caused by excessive waste products in the bloodstream due to kidney dysfunction.
Uremia
Uresia
Uroemia

10. _______________ is the artificial filtration of waste materials from the blood and is used to replace kidney function.
    Dialisis
    Dialysis
    Dielisis

11. _______________ is the presence of blood in the urine.
    Hematouria
    Hematuria
    Hemouria

12. _______________ is the presence of serum protein in the urine.
    Albinuria
    Albominuria
    Albuminuria

13. A _______________ is used to measure the specific gravity of urine.
    urinalometer
    urinometer
    urometer

14. _______________ is the presence of bacteria in the urine.
    Bacteriauria
    Bacteriuria
    Bacteruria

15. _______________ may be found abnormal amounts in diabetic urine.
    Acatones
    Acetones
    Asetones

CASE STUDIES

Write the correct answer on the line.

1. Mrs. Baldridge suffers from _______________ which is excessive urination during the night.
2. The urinalysis for Rosita LaPinta showed _______________ which is the presence of pus in the urine.
3. Doris Volk has _______________ which is an inflammation of the bladder.
4. John Danielson is being treated for _______________ which is a condition of narrowing of the ureter.
5. Norman Smith was born with the opening of the urethra on the upper (dorsal) side of the penis. This is called _______________.

6. Ralph Clark is being treated with _______________ dialysis which is the removal of waste by fluid exchange through the abdominal cavity.
7. Roberta Gridley is scheduled for _______________ to surgically repair damage to the ureter.
8. Letty Harding has _______________ which is an inflammation of the kidney involving primarily the glomeruli.
9. Mr. Morita was diagnosed as having _______________ which is an inflammation of the kidney.
10. Peter Jurgenson underwent surgery for the removal of one kidney. This is called _______________.
11. Mrs. Franklin has a kidney stone. Rather than operate, the doctor used _______________ to destroy the stone.
12. Dorothea Tyson has a/an _______________ which is a hernia of the bladder into the vagina.
13. Mr. Harmon is unable to empty his bladder. This is listed on his chart as urinary _______________.
14. The urinalysis for Andrew Parkinson indicated _______________ which is an increased concentration of creatine in the urine.
15. Jackie Martin suffers from _______________. His mother calls it bed-wetting.

WORD BUILDING

Write the correct word or word part on the line.

1. Surgical repair of the urethra
   a) The combining form _______________ means urethra.
   b) The suffix _______________ means surgical repair.
   c) The term _______________ means surgical repair of the urethra.
2. Suturing the bladder
   a) The combining form _______________ means bladder.
   b) The suffix _______________ means to suture.
   c) The term _______________ means suturing of the bladder.
3. Scanty urination
   a) The combining form _______________ means scanty or few.
   b) The suffix _______________ means pertaining to urine.
   c) The term _______________ means scanty urination.
4. Inflammation of the renal pelvis and kidney
   a) The combining form _______________ means renal pelvis.
   b) The combining form _______________ means kidney.
   c) The suffix _______________ means inflammation.
   d) The term _______________ means an inflammation of the renal pelvis and kidney.

5. Prolapsed kidney
   a) The combining form _______________ means kidney.
   b) The suffix _______________ means drooping downward or prolapsed.
   c) The term _______________ means prolapse of the kidney

LABELING EXERCISES

Identify the numbered items on this diagram.

1. _______________________
2. _______________________
3. _______________________
4. _______________________

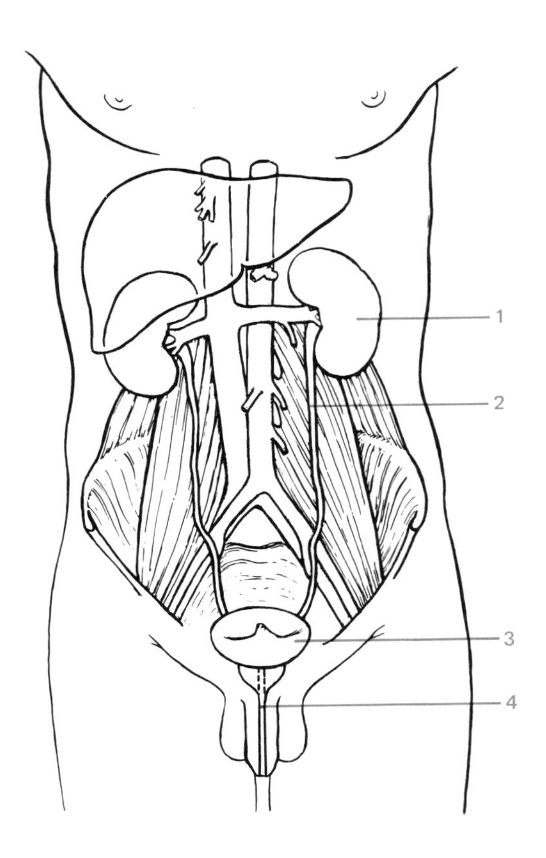

10

THE NERVOUS SYSTEM

LEARNING GOALS

In this chapter you will learn to:

- describe the structures of the nervous system including the neurons, neurotransmitters, neuroglia, myelin sheath, the meninges and cerebrospinal fluid.
- identify the three major divisions of the nervous system and describe the structures and functions of each.
- identify the major parts of the brain.
- recognize and define the terms related to the diagnosis, pathology, and treatment of disorders of the nervous system.

INTRODUCTION TO THE NERVOUS SYSTEM

The nervous system coordinates and controls all bodily activities. (The combining forms *NEUR/I* and *NEUR/O* means nerve or pertaining to nerve tissue.)

Nerves

A **nerve** is one or more bundles of impulse carrying fibers that connect the brain and the spinal cord with other parts of the body.

A **tract** is a bundle of nerve fibers located within the central nervous system.

A **ganglion (GANG-**glee-on) is a group of nerve cell bodies located outside the central nervous system. (The combining forms *GANGLI/O* and *GANGLION/O* mean ganglion.)

A **plexus (PLECK-**sus) is a network of intersecting nerves and blood or lymphatic vessels. (The combining form *PLEX/O* means plexus or network.) (Plural, **plexi.)**

Innervation is the supply of nerves to a body part. It also means the stimulation of a body part through the action of nerves.

Receptors are sensory organs (eyes, ears, skin and taste buds) that receive external stimulation and transmit it to the sensory neurons.

A **stimulus** is anything that excites or activates a nerve and causes an impulse.

An **impulse** is a wave of excitation transmitted through nerve fibers and neurons.

Neurons

Neurons are the basic cells of the nervous system. The three types of neurons are described according to their function.

Afferent neurons, also known as **sensory neurons,** emerge from the skin or sense organs and carry impulses toward the brain and spinal cord. (The prefix *AF-* means toward.)

Efferent neurons, also known as **motor neurons,** carry impulses away from the brain and spinal cord and toward the muscles and glands. (The prefix *EF-* means away from.)

Connecting neurons, also called **associative neurons,** carry impulses from one neuron to another.

Each neuron consists of a cell body, several dendrites, a single axon and terminal end fibers.

The **dendrites (DEN-**drytes) are root-like structures that receive impulses and conduct them to the cell body. (The combining form *DENDR/O* means branching or resembling a tree.)

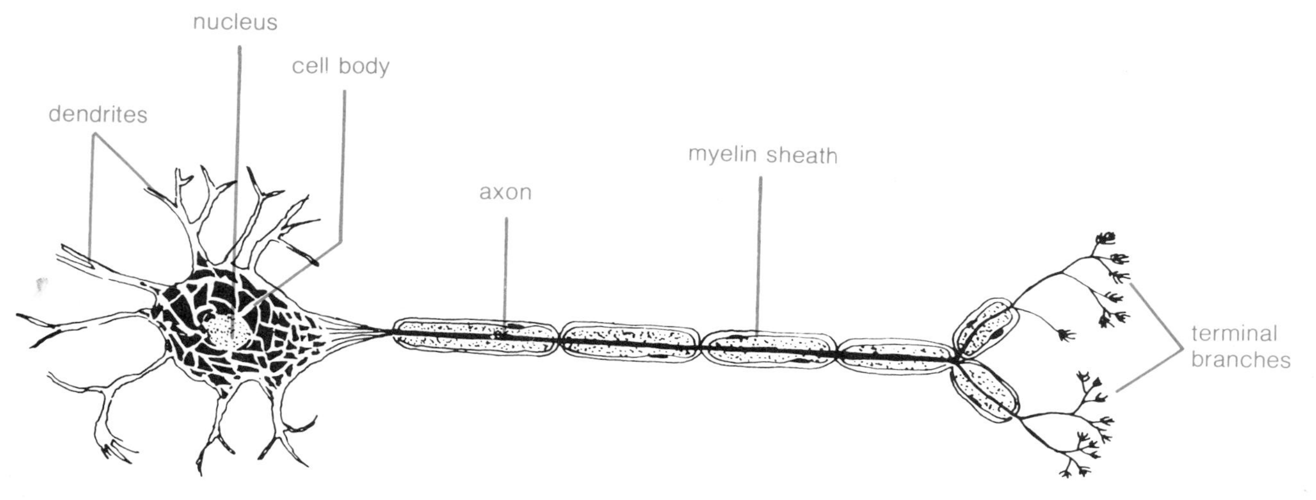

Figure 10-1 The structure of a nerve cell.

The **axon (ACK-son)** extends away from the cell body and conducts impulses away from the nerve cell. (The combining form *AX/O* means an axis or main stem.)

Some axons, but not all, are protected by a white fatty tissue covering called **myelin** (MY-eh-lin).

Terminal end fibers are the branching fibers of the neuron that lead the nervous impulse away from the axon and toward the synapse.

Neurotransmitters

A neurotransmitter is a chemical substance that makes it possible for the impulse to jump across the synapse from one neuron to another.

A **synapse (SIN-apps)** is the space between two neurons or between a neuron and a receptor organ. (The combining forms *SYNAPS/O* and *SYNAPT/O* both mean a point of contact.)

Neurohumors

A neurohumor is a chemical substance, formed and transmitted by a neuron, that is essential for the activity of adjacent neurons or nearby organs or muscles.

The Neuroglia

The neuroglia (new-**ROG**-lee-ah), also known as **glial cells,** are the supportive and connective cells of the nervous system. (The combining form *GLI/O* means glue and the neuroglia is sometimes called nerve glue.)

The Myelin Sheath

The myelin sheath is the protective covering over some nerve cells including parts of the spinal cord, the white matter of the brain, and most peripheral nerves.

The myelin sheath gives these nerve fibers a white color, and myelinated nerves are referred to as the "white matter." (**Myelinated** means having a myelin sheath.)

Nerves that do not have the myelin sheath are gray and they make up the "gray matter" of the brain and spinal cord.

The **neurilemma (new-rih-LEM-mah)**, also spelled **neurolemma,** is a membranous sheath outside the myelin sheath on the nerve cells of peripheral nerves. (The combining form *LEMM/O* means husk, peel or bark.)

DIVISIONS OF THE NERVOUS SYSTEM
The **central nervous system** consists of the brain and spinal cord.
The **peripheral nervous system** consists of the cranial nerves (extending from the brain) and the spinal nerves (extending from the spinal cord).
The **autonomic nervous system** consists of ganglia on either side of the spinal cord.

THE CENTRAL NERVOUS SYSTEM

The meninges and cerebrospinal fluid of the central nervous system protect the brain and the spinal cord.

THE MENINGES

The meninges (meh-**NIN**-jeez) are three layers of connective tissue membrane that enclose the brain and spinal cord. (The combining forms *MENING/O* and *MENINGI/O* both mean meninges.) (Singular, **meninx.**)

The Dura Mater

The dura mater (**DOO**-rah **MAY**-ter) is the thick, tough outermost membrane of the meninges. (The combining form *DUR/O* means dura mater.)

Epidural (ep-ih-DOO-ral) means located outside the dura mater. (The prefix *EPI-* means above or upon.)

The **subdural space** is located below the dura membrane and above the arachnoid membrane.

The Arachnoid Membrane

The arachnoid membrane (ah-**RACK**-noid) is the second layer surrounding the brain and spinal cord. It is loosely attached to the other meninges to allow space for fluid between the layers.

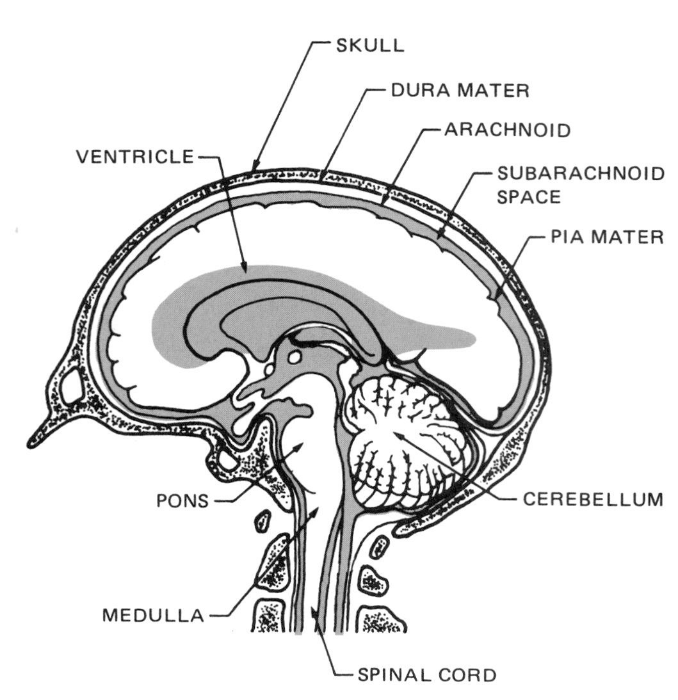

Figure 10-2 The meninges and cavities of the spinal cord and brain.

The **subarachnoid space,** which is located below the arachnoid membrane and above the pia mater, contains cerebrospinal fluid.

The Pia Mater

The pia mater, the third layer of the meninges, is located nearest to the brain and spinal cord. It consists of delicate connective tissue with a rich supply of blood vessels.

CEREBROSPINAL FLUID

Cerebrospinal fluid is a clear, colorless and watery fluid that is produced by special capillaries within the ventricles of the brain.

Cerebrospinal fluid flows throughout the brain and around the spinal cord, and its function is to cushion these organs from shock or injury.

THE BRAIN

The brain is the primary center for regulating and coordinating body activities, and each part of the brain controls different aspects of body functions. (The combining form *ENCEPHAL/O* means brain.)

The Cerebrum

The cerebrum (seh-**REE**-brum) is the largest and uppermost portion of the brain. It is responsible for all thought, judgment, memory, association and discrimination. (The combining form *CEREBR/O* means cerebrum or brain.)

The **cerebral cortex,** made up of gray matter, is the outer layer of the cerebrum and is arranged in folds. (The combining form *CORTIC/O* means cortex or outer region.)

The elevated portions or **convolutions** of the cerebral cortex are also known as **gyri** (**JIGH**-rye). (The combining form *CONVOLUT/O* means coiled and twisted. *GYR/O* means turning or folding.) (Singular, **gyrus.**)

Fissures, also known as **sulci** (**SUL**-sigh), are the normal depressions or grooves of the cerebral cortex. (The combining form *SULC/O* means groove.) (Singular, **sulcus.**)

The cerebrum is divided into left and right hemispheres and these hemispheres are divided into four lobes. Located within the middle region of the cerebrum there are four **ventricles** which contain cerebrospinal fluid. (A **ventricle** is a small cavity, such as the ventricles of the brain and of the heart.)

THE LOBES OF THE CEREBRUM
The **frontal lobe** controls motor functions.
The **parietal lobe** receives and interprets nerve impulses from the sensory receptors.
The **occipital lobe** controls eyesight.
The **temporal lobe** controls the senses of hearing and smell.

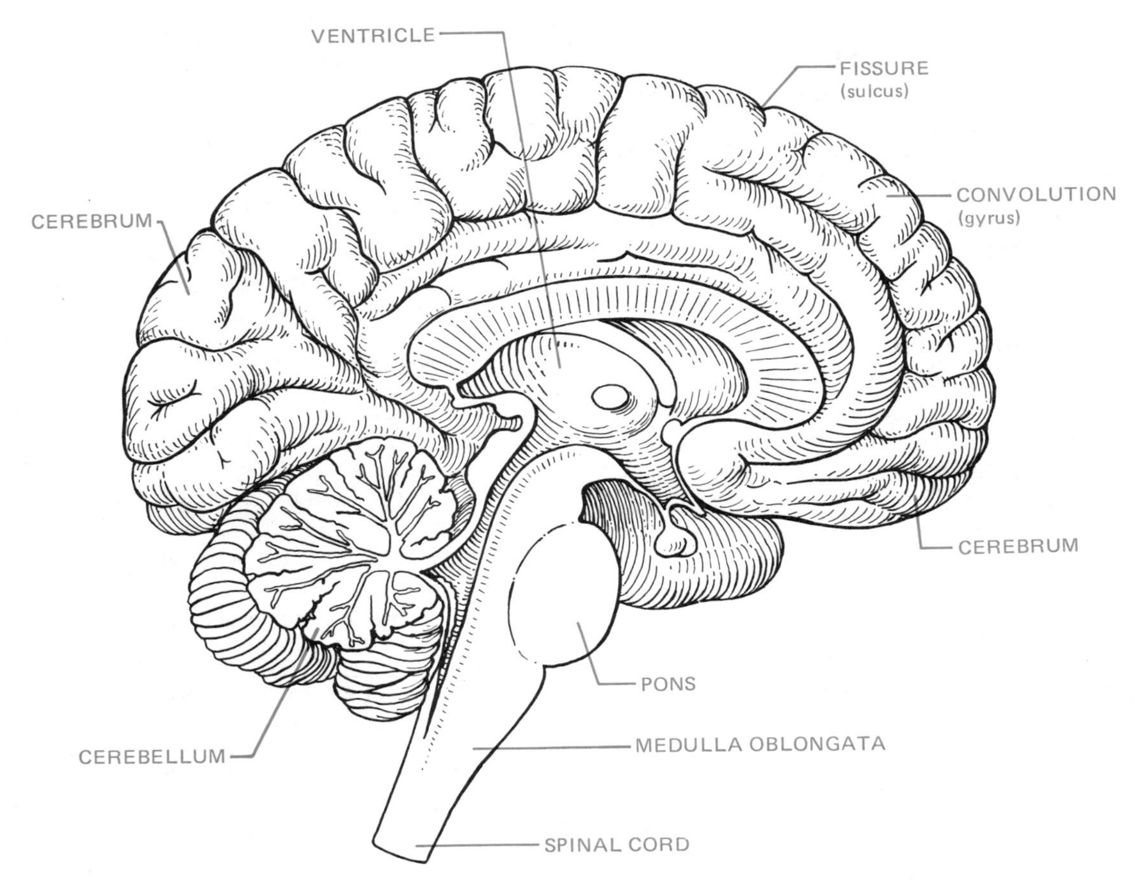

Figure 10-3 The structure of the brain.

The Thalamus

The thalamus (**THAL**-ah-mus) is located below the cerebrum. It monitors sensory stimuli by suppressing some and magnifying others. (The combining form *THALAM/O* means thalamus or inner room.)

The Hypothalamus

The hypothalamus (**high**-poh-**THAL**-ah-mus) is located below the thalamus. It has eight vital functions which include controlling the autonomic nervous system, the cardiovascular system, body temperature, appetite, water balance, the gastrointestinal system, emotional state, and sleep.

The Cerebellum

The cerebellum (**ser**-eh-**BELL**-um) is the second largest part of the brain. It is located beneath the posterior part of the cerebrum. (The combining form *CEREBELL/O* means cerebellum.)

The functions of the cerebellum are to aid in coordinating voluntary movements and to maintain balance and muscular tone.

The Pons

The pons is the part of the brain stem, situated at the base of the brain, where nerve cells cross over from one side of the brain to control the opposite side of the body.

Therefore, the nerves that control the left side of the body are found in the right side of the brain, and the nerves that control the right side of the body are found in the left side of the brain.

Because of this arrangement, damage to one side of the brain will cause paralysis on the opposite side of the body.

The Medulla Oblongata

The medulla oblongata (meh-**DULL**-ah ob-long-**GAH**-tah) is located at the lowest part of the brain stem. It contains vital centers that control the muscles of respiration, the rate of the heart beat and the blood pressure. (The combining form *MEDULL/O* means inner section.)

THE SPINAL CORD

The spinal cord carries all the nerves that affect the limbs and lower part of the body and is the pathway for impulses going to and from the brain. (The combining form *MYEL/O* means spinal cord. It also means bone marrow.)

Like the brain, the spinal cord is protected by cerebrospinal fluid and is surrounded by the three meninges. The gray matter in the spinal cord (which is not protected by a myelin sheath) is located in the internal section. The myelinated white matter composes the outer portion of the spinal cord.

THE PERIPHERAL NERVOUS SYSTEM

The peripheral nervous system includes the cranial nerves and the spinal nerves.

The Cranial Nerves

The 12 pairs of cranial nerves originate from the undersurface of the brain and are arranged in identical pairs so that both nerves of a pair are identical in function and structure.

The cranial nerves are generally named for the area or function they serve and are identified with Roman numerals.

I	**Olfactory Nerves** conduct impulses from receptors in the nose to the brain and are sensory in function.
II	**Optic Nerves** conduct impulses from receptors in the eyes to the brain and are sensory in function.
III	**Oculomotor Nerves** send motor impulses to four of the external eye muscles, as well as to certain internal eye muscles.
IV	**Trochlear Nerves** send motor impulses to one external eye muscle of each eye.
V	**Trigeminal Nerves** each divide into three branches. The **ophthalmic** branches go to the eyes and forehead. The **maxillary** branches go to the upper jaw. The **mandibular** branches go to the lower jaw.
VI	**Abducens Nerves** innervate the muscles that turn the eye to the side.
VII	**Facial Nerves** innervate the facial muscles, salivary glands, lacrimal glands, and the sensation of taste on the anterior two-thirds of the tongue.
VIII	**Acoustic Nerves** each divide into two branches. The **cochlear** branches are concerned with the sense of hearing. The **vestibular** branches are concerned with the sense of balance.
IX	**Glossopharyngeal Nerves** innervate the parotid glands, the sense of taste on the posterior third of the tongue and part of the pharynx.
X	**Vagus Nerves** innervate part of the pharynx, the larynx and vocal cords and parts of the thoracic and abdominal viscera.

continued ...

XI	**Spinal Accessory Nerves** innervate the shoulder muscles. Some of the fibers of these nerves arise from the spinal cord.
XII	**Hypoglossal Nerves** primarily innervate the muscles concerned with movements of the tongue.

The Spinal Nerves

The thirty-one pairs of spinal nerves are usually named after the artery they accompany or the body part they innervate.

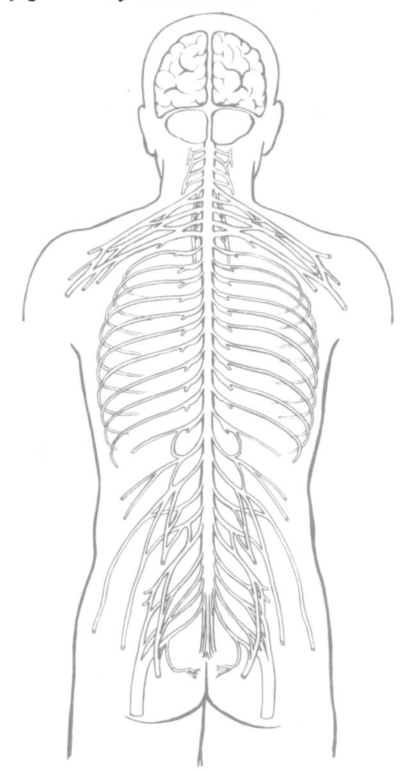

Figure 10-4 The spinal cord and the nerves emerging from it.

THE AUTONOMIC NERVOUS SYSTEM

The autonomic nervous system is sometimes described as being part of the peripheral nervous system because it is composed primarily of fibers from spinal nerves.

The autonomic nervous system is subdivided into two divisions. Each division balances the activity of the other to keep the body in a state of homeostasis. (**Homeostasis** is the process of maintaining the constant internal environment of the body.)

The Sympathetic Nervous System

The sympathetic division of the autonomic nervous system is concerned with body functions under stress. Receptors in the sympathetic nervous system are classified as being alpha or beta receptors.

Alpha receptors are found primarily in the smooth muscle tissue of peripheral blood vessels and in the sphincters of the gastrointestinal and genitourinary tracts.

Stimulation of the alpha receptors causes contraction of these smooth muscles, which may result in an increase in blood pressure due to constriction of peripheral blood vessels.

Beta receptors are located primarily in the muscles of the heart and in fatty tissue. Stimulation of these receptors in the heart produces a more rapid heart rate as well as more forceful heart muscle contractions.

The Parasympathetic Nervous System

The parasympathetic division of the autonomic nervous system is concerned with maintaining bodily functions during ordinary circumstances that are not stressful emotionally or physically.

This division is sometimes called the **cholinergic nervous system (koh-lin-ER-jick).**

DIAGNOSTIC PROCEDURES RELATED TO THE NERVOUS SYSTEM

- **Electroencephalography** (ee-**leck**-troh-en-**sef**-ah-**LOG**-rah-fee), also known as EEG, is the process of recording brain-wave activity. The resulting record is called an **electroencephalogram.**

- **Echoencephalography (eck-**oh-en-sef-ah-**LOG-**rah-fee) is a diagnostic technique in which pulses of ultrasonic waves are beamed through the head from both sides. (The combining form *ECH/O* means sound.)

- **Encephalography** (en-**sef**-ah-**LOG**-rah-fee) is an x-ray study demonstrating the intracranial fluid-containing spaces of the brain. The resulting film is called an **encephalogram.**

- **Ventriculography** (ven-**trick**-you-**LOG**-rah-fee), a form of encephalography, is a procedure for the radiographic visualization of the head after the injection of air or another contrast medium into the cerebral ventricles.

  Ventriculography also describes a radiographic study of a ventricle of the heart after the injection of a contrast medium.

PATHOLOGY OF THE NERVOUS SYSTEM

Pathology of the Nerves

- **Neuropathy** (new-**ROP**-ah-thee) is any disease of the nervous system.

- **Neuralgia** (new-**RAL**-jee-ah) is pain in a nerve or nerves.

- **Neuritis** (new-**RYE**-tis) is an inflammation of a nerve or nerves. (The terms neuritis and neuralgia are often used interchangeably.)

- **Polyneuritis (pol**-ee-new-**RYE**-tis) is an inflammation affecting many nerves.

- **Herpes zoster (HER**-peez **ZOS**-ter), also known as **shingles,** is an acute viral infection which is characterized by painful skin eruptions that follow the underlying route of the inflamed nerve.

- **Causalgia** (kaw-**ZAL**-jee-ah) is an intense burning pain following an injury to a sensory nerve. (The combining forms *CAUS/O* and *CAUST/O* mean burning.)

- **Hyperesthesia (high**-per-es-**THEE**-zee-ah) means a condition of excessive sensitivity to stimuli. (The suffix *-ESTHESIA* means sensation or feeling.)

- **Paresthesia (par**-es-**THEE**-zee-ah) is an abnormal sensation, such as burning, tingling or numbness, for no apparent reason.

- **Bell's palsy** is paralysis of the facial (seventh cranial) nerve that causes a unilateral distortion of the affected side of the face.

- **Trigeminal neuralgia,** also known as **tic douloureux** (**TICK** doo-loo-**ROO**) or **trifacial neuralgia,** is an inflammation of the trigeminal (fifth cranial) nerve. It is characterized by sudden, intense, sharp pain on one side of the face.

- **Sciatica** (sigh-**AT**-ih-kah) is an inflammation of the sciatic nerve that may result in pain along the course of the nerve through the thigh and leg.

Pathology of the Brain, Head and Spinal Cord

- **Meningopathy (men**-in-**GOP**-ah-thee) is any disease of the meninges.

- **Meningitis (men**-in-**JIGH**-tis) is an inflammation of the meninges of the spinal cord or brain.

- **Encephalopathy** (en-**sef**-ah-**LOP**-ah-thee) is any degenerative disease of the brain.

- **Encephalitis (en**-sef-ah-**LYE**-tis) is an inflammation of the brain.

- **Macrocephaly (mak**-roh-**SEF**-ah-lee) is a condition in which the head is abnormally large.

- **Microcephaly (my**-kroh-**SEF**-ah-lee) is a condition in which the head is abnormally small.

- **Hydrocephalus** (high-droh-**SEF**-ah-lus) is an abnormally increased amount of cerebrospinal fluid within the brain. (The prefix *HYDRO-* means water.)

- A **craniocele (KRAY-nee-oh-seel)** is the herniation of brain substance through the skull. (The suffix *-CELE* means hernia.)

- A **concussion,** also called a brain concussion or cerebral concussion, is a violent shaking up or jarring of the brain caused by a direct blow or explosion. (The combining form *CONCUSS/O* means shaken together.)

- A **cerebral contusion** (kon-**TOO**-zhun) is the bruising of brain tissue as a result of a head injury. (The combining form *CONTUS/O* means bruise.)

- A **cranial hematoma** is a collection of blood trapped in the tissues of the brain.

  Named for their location, the types of hematoma include: **epidural hematoma, subdural hematoma** and **intracerebral hematoma.**

  A **cerebrovascular accident** (**ser**-eh-broh-**VAS**-kyou-lar), also known as a **stroke** or **apoplexy** (**AP**-oh-**pleck**-see), is the general term used to indicate that the blood supply to a portion of the brain has been suddenly shut off.

- **Amnesia** (am-**NEE**-zee-ah) is partial or total memory loss usually due to brain injury, illness, or psychological disturbances.

- **Aphasia** (ah-**FAY**-zee-ah) is the loss, due to brain damage, of the ability to speak or write or to comprehend the written or spoken word. (The suffix *-PHASIA* means speak.)

- **Dysphasia** (dis-**FAY**-zee-ah) is an impairment of speech due to a brain lesion. (A **lesion** is an injury or pathological change in the tissue.)

- **Apraxia** (ah-**PRACK**-see-ah) is an impairment in the ability to perform purposeful acts or to properly use familiar objects. (The suffix *-PRAXIA* means action.)

- **Cephalalgia (sef**-ah-**LAL**-jee-ah) and **cephalodynia (sef**-ah-loh-**DIN**-ee-ah) both mean headache or pain in the head.

- A **migraine headache** is a syndrome characterized by sudden, severe, sharp headache that is usually present only on one side.

- **Syncope** (**SIN**-koh-pee), also known as **fainting,** is the brief loss of consciousness caused by transient cerebral hypoxia.

  Hypoxia is a lack of cellular oxygen.

- **Cerebral anoxia** is an abnormal condition in which oxygen is deficient in brain tissue. If this condition continues for more than 4 to 6 minutes, irreversible brain damage may occur.

  Anoxia is an abnormal condition characterized by the lack of oxygen.

- **Myelitis** (**my**-eh-**LYE**-tis) is an inflammation of the spinal cord.

- **Poliomyelitis** (**poh**-lee-oh-**my**-eh-**LYE**-tis) is a viral infection of the gray matter of the spinal cord that may result in paralysis. (The combining form *POLI/O* means gray matter of the brain and spinal cord.)

- **Multiple sclerosis** is a progressive disease characterized by scattered patches of demyelination of nerve fibers of the brain and spinal cord.

  Demyelinization is the destruction or loss of the myelin sheath from myelinated fibers.

Neoplasms of the Nervous System

- A **neuroma** (new-**ROH**-mah) is a benign neoplasm made up of neurons and nerve fibers.

- A **neuroblastoma** (**new**-roh-blas-**TOH**-mah) is a sarcoma of nervous system origin.

  A **neuroblast** is an embryonic cell that develops into nerve tissue.

- A **glioma** (glee-**OH**-mah) is a primary tumor of the brain composed of malignant glial cells.

- A **meningioma** (meh-**nin**-jee-**OH**-mah) is a tumor of the meninges that originates in the arachnoidal tissue.

General Pathology of the Nervous System

- **Paralysis** is the loss of muscle function or the loss of sensation, or the loss of both function and sensation. (Plural, **paralyses**.)

- **Paraplegia** (**par**-ah-**PLEE**-jee-ah) means the paralysis of both legs and the lower part of the body. (The suffix *-PLEGIA* means paralysis.)

- **Hemiplegia** (**hem**-ee-**PLEE**-jee-ah) means paralysis of one side of the body. (The prefix *HEMI-* means half.)

- **Quadriplegia** (**kwad**-rih-**PLEE**-jee-ah) means the paralysis of all four extremities. (The combining forms *QUADR/I* and *QUADR/O* mean four.)

- **Hemiparesis** (**hem**-ee-**PAR**-ee-sis) means slight paralysis of one side of the body. (The suffix *-PARESIS* means slight, not total, paralysis.)

- A **coma** is a profound (deep) state of unconsciousness characterized by the absence of spontaneous eye movements, response to painful stimuli and vocalization.

  Comatose refers to one who is in a coma.

- A **stupor** is a state of lethargy and unresponsiveness in which a person seems unaware of his surroundings.

  Lethargy is a state of being indifferent, apathetic, or sluggish.

- **Narcolepsy** (**NAR**-koh-**lep**-see) is a syndrome characterized by recurrent uncontrollable seizures of drowsiness and sleep. (The combining form *NARC/O* means numbness or stupor.)

- **Somnolence** means sleepiness and also an unnatural drowsiness. A somnolent person can usually be aroused by verbal stimuli. (The combining forms *SOMN/I* and *SOMN/O* both means sleep.)

- **Somnambulism** (som-**NAM**-byou-lizm), also known as **noctambulism** or **sleepwalking**, is the condition of walking without awakening. (The combining form *NOCT/I* means night. *AMBUL/O* and *AMBULAT/O* mean to walk.)

- A **seizure**, also known as a **convulsion**, is a sudden, violent, involuntary contraction of a group of muscles. It may be accompanied by a loss of consciousness.

- **Epilepsy** (**EP**-ih-**lep**-see) is a group of neurologic disorders characterized by recurrent episodes of convulsive seizures and related disturbances characterized by petit mal or grand mal seizures.

  A **petit mal seizure** (peh-**TEE MAHL**) is a sudden, momentary loss of consciousness. A **grand mal seizure** involves generalized involuntary muscular spasms.

- **Alzheimer's disease** (**ALTZ**-high-merz), also known as **presenile dementia**, is characterized by variable degrees of confusion, memory failure and other cognitive defects.

  Cognition is the mental process characterized by knowing, thinking, learning and judging.

- **Amyotrophic lateral sclerosis** (ah-**my**-oh-**TROH**-fick) also known as **Lou Gehrig's disease**, is a degenerative disease of the motor neurons.

- **Cerebral palsy** is a motor function disorder caused by a permanent, non-progressive brain defect or lesion present at birth or shortly thereafter. It is characterized by spasticity, athetosis, tremors and loss of muscle tone.

Spasticity refers to uncontrolled contractions of the skeletal muscles. (The combining forms *SPASM/O* and *SPASMOD/O* both mean involuntary muscular tightening or cramping.)

Athetosis (ath-eh-**TOH**-sis) is a condition of constant involuntary movements (usually of the upper extremities) that are slow, irregular, and snake-like. (The combining form *ATHET/O* means uncontrolled.)

A **tremor** is involuntary shaking or trembling of the body or of any of its parts. (The combining form *TREM/O* means shaking or trembling.)

- **Parkinson's disease** is a slowly progressive, degenerative, neurologic disorder characterized by stiffness, slowed movements and rhythmic fine tremors.
- **Tetanus** (**TET**-ah-nus), also known as **lockjaw,** is an acute and potentially fatal infection of the central nervous system caused by the tetanus bacillus.

PROCEDURES RELATED TO THE NERVOUS SYSTEM

- **Trephination (tref**-ih-**NAY**-shun) is the process of cutting a hole in the skull using a trephine.

  A **trephine** (treh-**FINE**) is a circular, saw-like instrument used to remove pieces of bone or tissue, usually from the skull.
- A **lobotomy** (loh-**BOT**-oh-me) is a procedure in which nerve fibers are severed in the frontal lobe of the brain.
- A **prefrontal lobotomy** is a procedure in which the connecting fibers between the prefrontal lobes of the brain and the thalamus are severed.
- A **neurectomy** (new-**RECK**-toh-me) is the surgical removal of a nerve.
- **Neuroplasty** (**NEW**-roh-**plas**-tee) is the surgical repair of a nerve or nerves.
- **Neurorrhaphy** (new-**ROR**-ah-fee) means to suture the ends of a severed nerve.
- **Neurotomy** (new-**ROT**-oh-me) is a surgical incision or the dissection of a nerve.
- **Sympathectomy (sim**-pah-**THECK**- toh-me) is the surgical interruption of part of the sympathetic nerve pathways.

IMPORTANT TERMS: THE NERVOUS SYSTEM

This list will help you identify and review the major terms from this chapter.

When you work with the audio tape for this chapter, listen to the word, repeat it and then place a ✓ next to it on the list below.

- □ **Alzheimer's** (**ALTZ**-high-merz)
- □ **Amyotrophic** (ah-**my**-oh-**TROH**-fick)
- □ **Aphasia** (ah-**FAY**-zee-ah)
- □ **Apraxia** (ah-**PRACK**-see-ah)
- □ **Arachnoid** (ah-**RACK**-noid)
- □ **Athetosis (ath**-eh-**TOH**-sis)
- □ **Causalgia** (kaw-**ZAL**-jee-ah)
- □ **Cephalalgia (sef**-ah-**LAL**-jee-ah)
- □ **Cephalodynia (sef**-ah-loh-**DIN**-ee-ah)
- □ **Cerebellum (ser**-eh-**BELL**-um)
- □ **Cerebrum** (seh-**REE**-brum)
- □ **Cholinergic(koh**-lin-**ER**-jick)
- □ **Contusion** (kon-**TOO**-zhun)
- □ **Craniocele (KRAY**-nee-oh-**seel)**
- □ **Dura mater (DOO**-rah **MAY**-ter)
- □ **Dysphasia** (dis-**FAY**-zee-ah)

- ☐ **Echoencephalography** (**eck**-oh-en-sef-ah-**LOG**-rah-fee)
- ☐ **Electroencephalography** (ee-**leck**-troh-en-**sef**-ah-**LOG**-rah-fee)
- ☐ **Encephalitis**(**en**-sef-ah-**LYE**-tis)
- ☐ **Encephalography** (en-**sef**-ah-**LOG**-rah-fee)
- ☐ **Encephalopathy** (en-**sef**-ah-**LOP**-ah-thee)
- ☐ **Epidural** (**ep**-ih-**DOO**-ral)
- ☐ **Epilepsy** (**EP**-ih-**lep**-see)
- ☐ **Ganglion** (**GANG**-glee-on)
- ☐ **Glioma** (glee-**OH**-mah)
- ☐ **Gyri** (**JIGH**-rye)
- ☐ **Hemiparesis** (**hem**-ee-**PAR**-ee-sis)
- ☐ **Hemiplegia** (**hem**-ee-**PLEE**-jee-ah)
- ☐ **Herpes zoster** (**HER**-peez **ZOS**-ter)
- ☐ **Hydrocephalus** (high-droh-**SEF**-ah-lus)
- ☐ **Hyperesthesia** (**high**-per-es-**THEE**-zee-ah)
- ☐ **Hypothalamus** (**high**-poh-**THAL**-ah-mus)
- ☐ **Macrocephaly** (**mak**-roh-**SEF**-ah-lee)
- ☐ **Medulla oblongata** (meh-**DULL**-ah **ob**-long-**GAH**-tah)
- ☐ **Meninges** (meh-**NIN**-jeez)
- ☐ **Meningitis** (**men**-in-**JIGH**-tis)
- ☐ **Meningioma** (meh-**nin**-jee-**OH**-mah)
- ☐ **Meningopathy** (**men**-in-**GOP**-ah-thee)
- ☐ **Microcephaly** (**my**-kroh-**SEF**-ah-lee)
- ☐ **Myelin** (**MY**-eh-lin)
- ☐ **Myelitis** (**my**-eh-**LYE**-tis)
- ☐ **Narcolepsy** (**NAR**-koh-**lep**-see)
- ☐ **Neuralgia** (new-**RAL**-jee-ah)
- ☐ **Neurectomy** (new-**RECK**-toh-me)
- ☐ **Neurilemma** (**new**-rih-**LEM**-mah)
- ☐ **Neuritis** (new-**RYE**-tis)
- ☐ **Neuroblastoma** (**new**-roh-blas-**TOH**-mah)
- ☐ **Neuroglia** (new-**ROG**-lee-ah)
- ☐ **Neuroma** (new-**ROH**-mah)
- ☐ **Neuropathy** (new-**ROP**-ah-thee)
- ☐ **Neuroplasty** (**NEW**-roh-**plas**-tee)
- ☐ **Neurorrhaphy** (new-**ROR**-ah-fee)
- ☐ **Neurotomy** (new-**ROT**-oh-me)
- ☐ **Paraplegia** (**par**-ah-**PLEE**-jee-ah)
- ☐ **Paresthesia** (**par**-es-**THEE**-zee-ah)
- ☐ **Plexus** (**PLECK**-sus)
- ☐ **Poliomyelitis** (**poh**-lee-oh-**my**-eh-**LYE**-tis)
- ☐ **Polyneuritis** (**pol**-ee-new-**RYE**-tis)
- ☐ **Quadriplegia** (**kwad**-rih-**PLEE**-jee-ah)
- ☐ **Sciatica** (sigh-**AT**-ih-kah)
- ☐ **Somnambulism** (som-**NAM**-byou-lizm)
- ☐ **Sulci** (**SUL**-sigh)
- ☐ **Sympathectomy** (**sim**-pah-**THECK**-toh-me)
- ☐ **Synapse** (**SIN**-apps)
- ☐ **Syncope** (**SIN**-koh-pee)
- ☐ **Thalamus** (**THAL**-ah-mus)
- ☐ **Tic douloureux** (**TICK** doo-loo-**ROO**)
- ☐ **Trephination** (**tref**-ih-**NAY**-shun)
- ☐ **Ventriculography** (ven-**trick**-you-**LOG**-rah-fee)

EXERCISES

DEFINING WORD PARTS

Write the definition for each of these word parts.

1. *AF-* ______
2. *AX/O* ______
3. *CAUS/O, CAUST/O* ______
4. *CEREBELL/O* ______
5. *CEREBR/O* ______
6. *CONCUSS/O* ______
7. *CONVOLUT/O* ______
8. *DENDR/O* ______
9. *DUR/O* ______
10. *EF-* ______
11. *ENCEPHAL/O* ______
12. *-ESTHESIA* ______
13. *GANGLI/O, GANGLION/O* ______
14. *GLI/O* ______
15. *MENING/O, MENINGI/O* ______
16. *MYEL/O* ______

17. *NARC/O* ______________________________

18. *NEUR/I, NEUR/O* ______________________________

19. *-PARESIS* ______________________________

20. *-PHASIA* ______________________________

21. *-PLEGIA* ______________________________

22. *POLI/O* ______________________________

23. *SULC/O* ______________________________

24. *SYNAPS/O, SYNAPT/O* ______________________________

25. *THALAM/O* ______________________________

DEFINITIONS

Circle the letter next to the correct answer.

1. A ______________ is the space between two neurons or between a neuron and a receptor.
   a) dendrite
   b) ganglion
   c) plexus
   d) synapse

2. The ______________ sheath is the protective covering over some nerve cells including parts of the spinal cord, the white matter of the brain and most peripheral nerves.
   a) glial
   b) myelin
   c) neurilemma
   d) pia mater

3. The ______________ are the root-like structures of a nerve that receive impulses and conduct them to the cell body.
   a) dendrites
   b) plexi
   c) synapses
   d) terminal end fibers

4. The ______________ is the third layer of the meninges and is located nearest the brain and spinal cord.
   a) arachnoid membrane
   b) dura mater
   c) meninx
   d) pia mater

5. The functions of the _______________ include controlling body temperature, appetite and water balance.
   a) cerebrum
   b) hypothalamus
   c) pons
   d) thalamus

6. The _______________ division of the autonomic nervous system is concerned with body functions under stress.
   a) cranial
   b) parasympathetic
   c) peripheral
   d) sympathetic

7. A _______________ is a network of intersecting nerves and blood or lymphatic vessels.
   a) ganglion
   b) plexus
   c) synapse
   d) tract

8. The peripheral nervous system includes the _______________
   a) brain.
   b) cranial nerves.
   c) spinal nerves.
   d) b and c.

9. The _______________ are the three layers of connective tissue membrane that enclose the brain and spinal cord.
   a) encephalomeninges
   b) meninges
   c) neurilemma
   d) neurolemma

10. _______________ neurons carry impulses away from the brain and spinal cord and toward the muscles and glands.
    a) Afferent
    b) Efferent
    c) Motor
    d) b and c

MISSING WORDS

Write the missing word on the line.

1. ______________________ is the process of maintaining the constant internal environment of the body.
2. A/an ______________________, also known as an EEG, is the record of brain-wave activity.
3. The fifth cranial nerves are called the ______________________ nerves and they divide into three parts.
4. ______________________, also known as sulci, are the normal grooves of the cerebral cortex.
5. The occipital lobe of the ______________________ controls eyesight.
6. A cranial ______________________ is a collection of blood trapped in the tissues of the brain.
7. ______________________ is an abnormally increased amount of cerebrospinal fluid within the brain.
8. ______________________ is an abnormal sensation, such as burning, tingling or numbness, for no apparent reason.
9. ______________________ means the paralysis of both legs and the lower part of the body.
10. ______________________ means the paralysis of one side of the body.
11. A/an ______________________ is a profound state of unconsciousness characterized by the absence of spontaneous eye movement, response to painful stimuli and vocalization.
12. The ______________________, or gyri, are the elevated portions of the cerebral cortex.
13. The ______________________ ______________________ is located at the lowest part of the brain stem and contains vital centers which control the muscles of respiration the rate of the heart beat and blood pressure.
14. The ______________________ lobe of the cerebrum controls motor functions.
15. A/an ______________________ is a chemical substance that makes it possible for a nerve impulse to jump across the synapse from one neuron to another.

SPELLCHECK

Select the correct spelling and write it on the line.

1. ______________________ is the loss, due to brain damage, of the ability to speak or write or to comprehend the written or spoken word.
   Aphasia
   Aphazia
   Aphesia

2. A ______________________ is a violent shaking up or jarring of the brain caused by a direct blow or explosion.
   cancussion
   concusion
   concussion

3. ______________________ is partial or total memory loss usually due to brain injury, illness, or psychological disturbances.
   Ammenesia
   Amnesia
   Amnisia

4. ______________________ is also known as fainting.
   Syncope
   Synicope
   Synkope

5. ______________________ means paralysis of all four extremities.
   Quadraplegia
   Quadrapligea
   Quadriplegia

6. A ______________________ headache is characterized by sudden, severe, sharp headache that is usually present only on one side.
   miagraine
   migraine
   migrain

7. ______________________ is a state of being indifferent, apathetic, or sluggish.
   Lethargy
   Lethergy
   Lethurgy

8. ______________________ is the mental process characterized by knowing, thinking, learning and judging.
   Cognetion
   Cognision
   Cognition

9. Multiple ______________________ is a progressive disease characterized by scattered patches of demyelination of nerve fibers of the brain and spinal cord.
   scleroses
   sclerosis
   sclirosis

10. ______________________ is the loss of muscle function of the loss of sensation, or the loss of both function and sensation.
    Paralysis
    Parelysis
    Parilyses

11. ______________________ disease is characterized by variable degrees of confusion, memory failure and other cognitive defects.
    Alsheimer's
    Altzheimer's
    Alzheimer's

12. A ______________________ is involuntary shaking of the body or of any of its parts.
    tremor
    tremour
    tremur

13. A ______________________, also known as a convulsion, is a sudden, violent, involuntary contraction of a group of muscles.
    seazure
    seezure
    seizure

14. ______________________ refers to uncontrolled contractions of the skeletal muscles.
    Spacitity
    Spaciticity
    Spasticity

15. ______________________ disease is a slowly progressive, degenerative, neurological disorder.
    Parkenson's
    Parkington's
    Parkinson's

CASE STUDIES

Write the correct answer on the line.

1. After he stepped on a rusty nail, Newton Jennings went to the doctor for an injection to prevent ______________________, which is also known as lockjaw.
2. The Baily baby was born with ______________________ ______________________. This birth defect is characterized by spasticity, athetosis, tremors and loss of muscle tone.
3. After the auto accident, Anthony DeNatali required ______________________ to suture the ends of a severed nerve in his hand.

4. Jeff Wacker suffers from ______________________ which is also known as noctambulism or sleepwalking.

5. Following the drug overdose, John Doe was in a/an ______________________ in which he was in a state of lethargy and unresponsiveness and was unaware of his surroundings.

6. Mr. Woo was diagnosed as having a/an ______________________ which is a benign tumor made up of neurons and nerve fibers.

7. George Houghton suffered a/an ______________________ accident, which is also known as a stroke.

8. Richard Cook's head injury was diagnosed as being a/an ______________________ ______________________ which is bruising of the brain tissue.

9. Mrs. Deighton suffers from a very painful viral infection which her doctor calls ______________________ ______________________. She refers to it as shingles.

10. Mary Beth Cawthorn was vaccinated against ______________________, also known as polio, which is a viral infection of the gray matter of the spinal cord that may result in paralysis.

11. After the near-drowning accident, Bryan Harper suffered from cerebral ______________________ which is an abnormal condition in which oxygen is deficient in brain tissue.

12. Mildred Carson suffers from ______________________ which is also called neuralgia.

13. Jeff Unger has ______________________ which is an inflammation of the meninges of the spinal cord or brain.

14. Warren Phillips has ______________________ which is an inflammation of a nerve that results in pain along the course of the nerve through the thigh and leg.

15. Jill Beck has epilepsy. The sudden momentary loss of consciousness that she experiences is called a ______________________ mal seizure.

WORD BUILDING

Write the correct word or word part on the line.

1. Degenerative disease of the brain
   a) The combining form ______________________ means brain.
   b) The suffix ______________________ means disease.
   c) The term ______________________ is any degenerative disease of the brain.

2. Hernia of the brain
   a) The combining form ______________________ means skull.
   b) The suffix ______________________ means hernia.
   c) The term ______________________ means the herniation of brain substance through the skull.

3. Burning pain
   a) The combining form ______________________ means burning.
   b) The suffix ______________________ means pain.
   c) The term ______________________ means burning pain following an injury to a sensory nerve.

4. Excessive sensitivity
   a) The prefix ______________________ means above or increased.
   b) The suffix ______________________ means sensation or feeling.
   c) The term ______________________ means a condition of excessive sensitivity to stimuli.

5. An x-ray study of the brain
   a) The combining form ______________________ means brain.
   b) The suffix ______________________ means process of recording.
   c) The term ______________________ is an x-ray study of the brain.

LABELING EXERCISES

Identify the numbered items on this diagram.

1. ______________________
2. ______________________
3. ______________________
4. ______________________
5. ______________________

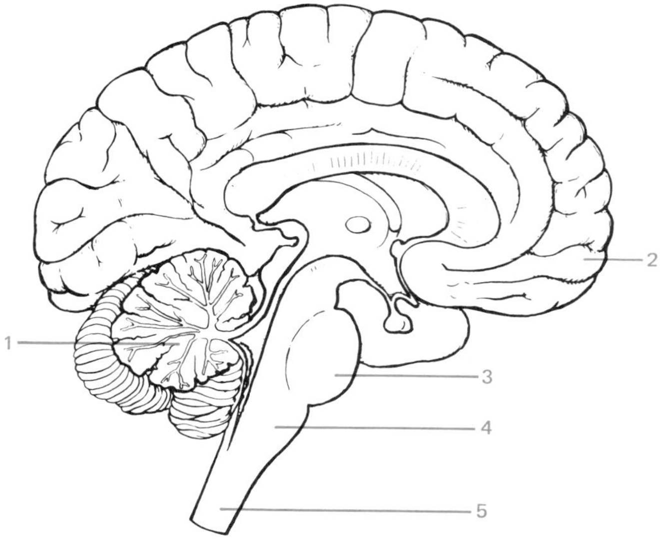

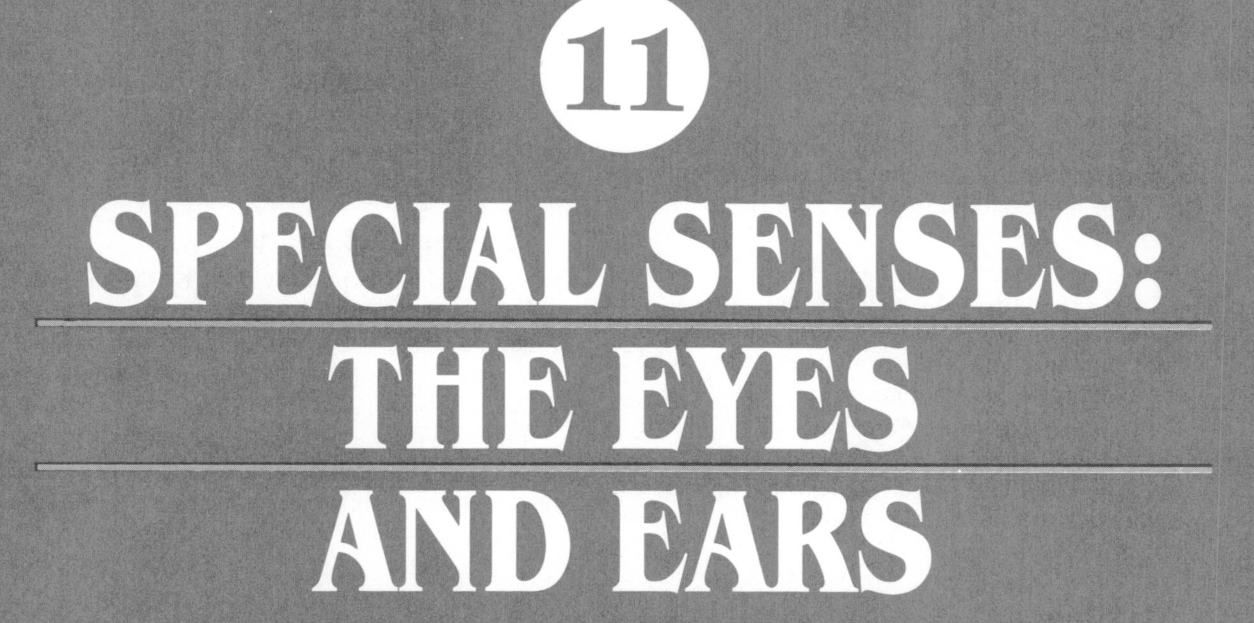

11 SPECIAL SENSES: THE EYES AND EARS

LEARNING GOALS

In this chapter you will learn to:

- describe the eyes and their related structures.
- describe the structures of the ears.
- recognize and define the terms related to the pathology, diagnostic procedures and treatment of disorders of the eyes.
- recognize and define the terms related to the pathology, diagnostic procedures and treatment of disorders of the ears.

THE EYES

The eyes are the receptor organs for the sense of sight. The term **optic** means pertaining to the eye or sight. (The combining forms *OPT/I, OPT/O, OPTIC/O* and *OPHTHALM/O* all mean eye or vision.)

Ocular (OCK-you-lar) also pertains to the eye. (The combining form *OCUL/O* means eye.) **Extraocular** means on the outside of the eye and **intraocular** means within the eye.

The **adnexa (ad-NECK-sah)** of the eye include the orbit, the muscles of the eye, the eyelids, the conjunctiva and the lacrimal apparatus. (**Adnexa** refers to the appendages or accessory structures of an organ.)

The Orbit

The orbit is the bony cavity of the skull that contains and protects the eyeball and its associated muscles, blood vessels and nerves.

The Eyelids

Each eye has a pair of eyelids that protect the eyeball from foreign matter, excessive light and impact. (The combining form *BLEPHAR/O* means eyelid.)

The **canthus (KAN-thus)** is the angle where the upper and lower eyelids meet. (The combining form *CANTH/O* means corner of the eye.) (Plural, **canthi.**)

The **epicanthus (ep-ih-KAN-thus)** is a vertical fold of skin on either side of the nose, sometimes covering the inner canthus.

The edges of the eyelids contain **cilia (SILL-ee-ah)**, also known as **eyelashes,** and oil-producing sebaceous glands.

(The combining form *TARS/O* means the edge of the eyelid; however, it also means ankle and instep.) (The combining form *CILI/O* means eyelashes.)

The Conjunctiva

The conjunctiva **(kon-junk-TYE-vah)** is the mucous membrane that lines the underside of each eyelid and continues to form a protective covering of the exposed surface of the eyeball. (The combining form *CONJUNCTIV/O* means conjunctiva.)

The Lacrimal Apparatus

The lacrimal apparatus **(LACK-rih-mal)** consists of the structures that produce, store and remove tears. (The combining forms *LACRIM/O* and *DACRY/O* both mean tear, tear duct or lacrimal duct.)

The **lacrimal glands** are located above the outer corner of each eye. These glands secrete **lacrimal fluid,** also known as **tears,** onto the surface of the conjunctiva of the upper lid. **Lacrimation (lack-rih-MAY-shun)** is the normal continuous secretion of tears by the lacrimal glands.

The **lacrimal canaliculi (kan-ah-LICK-you-lee)** are the ducts at the inner corner of each eye that collect tears and drain them into the lacrimal sac. (Singular, **canaliculus.**)

The **lacrimal sac,** also known as the **dacryocyst (DACK-ree-oh-sist)** or tear sac, is an enlargement of the upper portion of the lacrimal duct.

The **lacrimal duct,** also known as the **nasolacrimal duct,** is the passageway that drains lacrimal fluid into the nose.

STRUCTURES OF THE EYE

The Eyeball

The eyeball is a sphere about 1 inch in diameter. It is a hollow structure with walls made up of three layers: the sclera, the choroid and the retina.

The Sclera and Cornea

The **sclera (SKLEE-rah),** also known as the **white of the eye,** is a fibrous tissue that maintains the shape of the eye and protects the delicate inner layers of tissue. (The combining form *SCLER/O* means sclera, white of eye, or hard.)

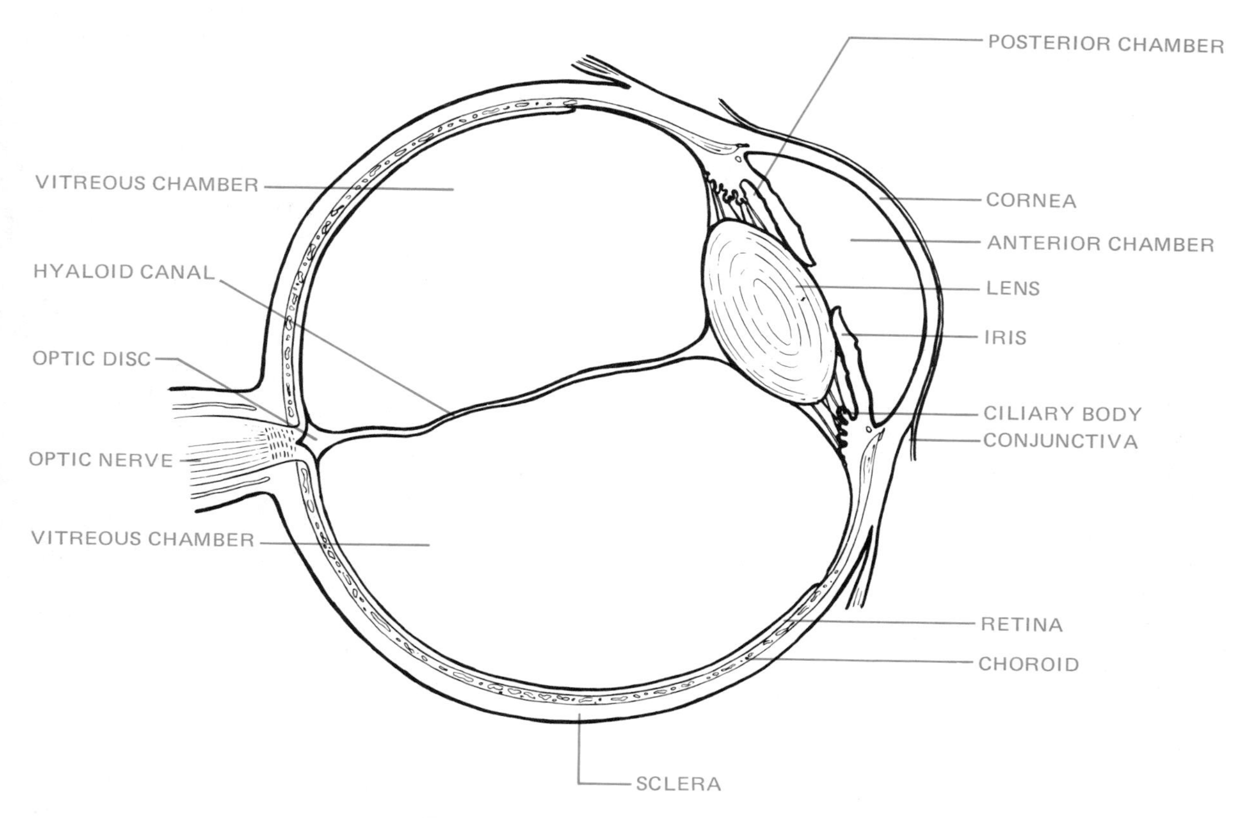

Figure 11-1 Structures of the eye.

The **cornea (KOR-**nee-ah) is the transparent anterior portion of the sclera. (The combining forms *CORNE/O* and *KERAT/O* both mean cornea; however, *KERAT/O* also means hard or horny and is used in relation to the epidermis, hair and nails.)

The Choroid, Pupil and Iris

The **choroid (KOH-**roid), also known as the **choroid layer** or **choroid coat,** is the middle layer of the eyeball. (The combining form *CHOROID/O* means choroid.)

The choroid is opaque and contains many blood vessels. (**Opaque** means that light cannot pass through this substance.)

The **pupil** is the circular opening in the front of the choroid. (The combining form *PUPILL/O* means pupil.)

The **iris** is the colored muscular layer that surrounds the pupil. (The combining forms *IR/I, IR/O, IRID/O* and *IRIT/O* all refer to the iris of the eye.)

The amount of light that is permitted to enter the eye is controlled by two sets of muscles within the iris that change the size of the pupil. To decrease the amount of light, the muscles contract the pupil (make it smaller). To increase the amount of light, the muscles dilate the pupil (make it larger).

The Lens and Related Structures

The lens is the flexible and curved structure located behind the iris and pupil. (The combining form *PHAC/O* means lens of the eye.)

The **ciliary muscles,** located within the **ciliary body** of the choroid, adjust the shape and thickness of the lens.

Chambers of the Eye

The **ocular chamber** lies in front of the lens. This chamber is subdivided by the iris into the **anterior** and **posterior chambers.**

The **ocular chamber** is filled with a watery substance called **aqueous humor.** (A **humor** is any clear body liquid or semifluid substance. The combining form *AQUE/O* means water.)

The **vitreous chamber (VIT**-ree-us) is the large region behind the lens. It is filled with a soft jelly-like material, the **vitreous humor.** (The combining form *VITRE/O* means glassy.)

The Retina

The retina **(RET**-ih-nah) is the sensitive inner nerve layer of the eye. It is located between the posterior chamber and the choroid layer at the back of the eye. (The combining form *RETIN/O* means retina or a net.)

The retina contains specialized light-sensitive cells called **rods** and **cones** that initiate nerve impulses that travel from the eye to the brain via the **optic nerve.**

The **optic disk,** also known as the **blind spot,** is the region in the eye where the nerve endings of the retina gather to form the optic nerve. It is called the blind spot because it does not contain any rods or cones.

The **macula lutea (MACK**-you-lah **LOO**-tee-ah) is a yellow spot in the center of the retina. (The combining form *MACUL/O* means spot and the combining form *LUTE/O* means yellow.)

The **fovea centralis (FOH**-vee-ah sen-**TRAH**-lis) is a pit located within the macula lutea. This section of the retina is the area of sharpest vision. (The combining form *FOVE/O* means pit.)

The Action of the Eye

Light rays enter the eye through the cornea, pass through the lens and travel to the retina. The image focused there is transmitted to the brain.

Refraction is the ability of the lens to bend the light rays to help them focus on the retina. This term is also used to describe an eye examination to determine and correct refractive errors of the eye.

Accommodation is the process whereby the eyes make adjustments for seeing objects at various distances. Accommodation includes constriction or dilation of the pupil, movement of the eyes and changes in the shape of the lens.

Emmetropia (em-eh-**TROH**-pee-ah) is the normal relationship between the refractive power of the eye and the shape of the eye which enables light rays to focus correctly on the retina.

Convergence (kon-**VER**-jens) is the movement of the two eyes toward fixation of the same near point.

THE EAR

The ear is a sensory organ that enables us to hear and helps us to maintain our balance. The term **auditory** means pertaining to the sense of hearing. (The combining forms *AUDI/O* and *AUDIT/O* both mean ear, hearing and the sense of hearing.)

The term **acoustic** means relating to sound or hearing. (The combining form *ACOUS/O* and *ACOUST/O* both mean hearing or related to hearing.)

The term **otic** means pertaining to the ear, and the combining form *OT/O* means ear or hearing. The ear is divided into three separate regions. These are the outer ear, middle ear and inner ear.

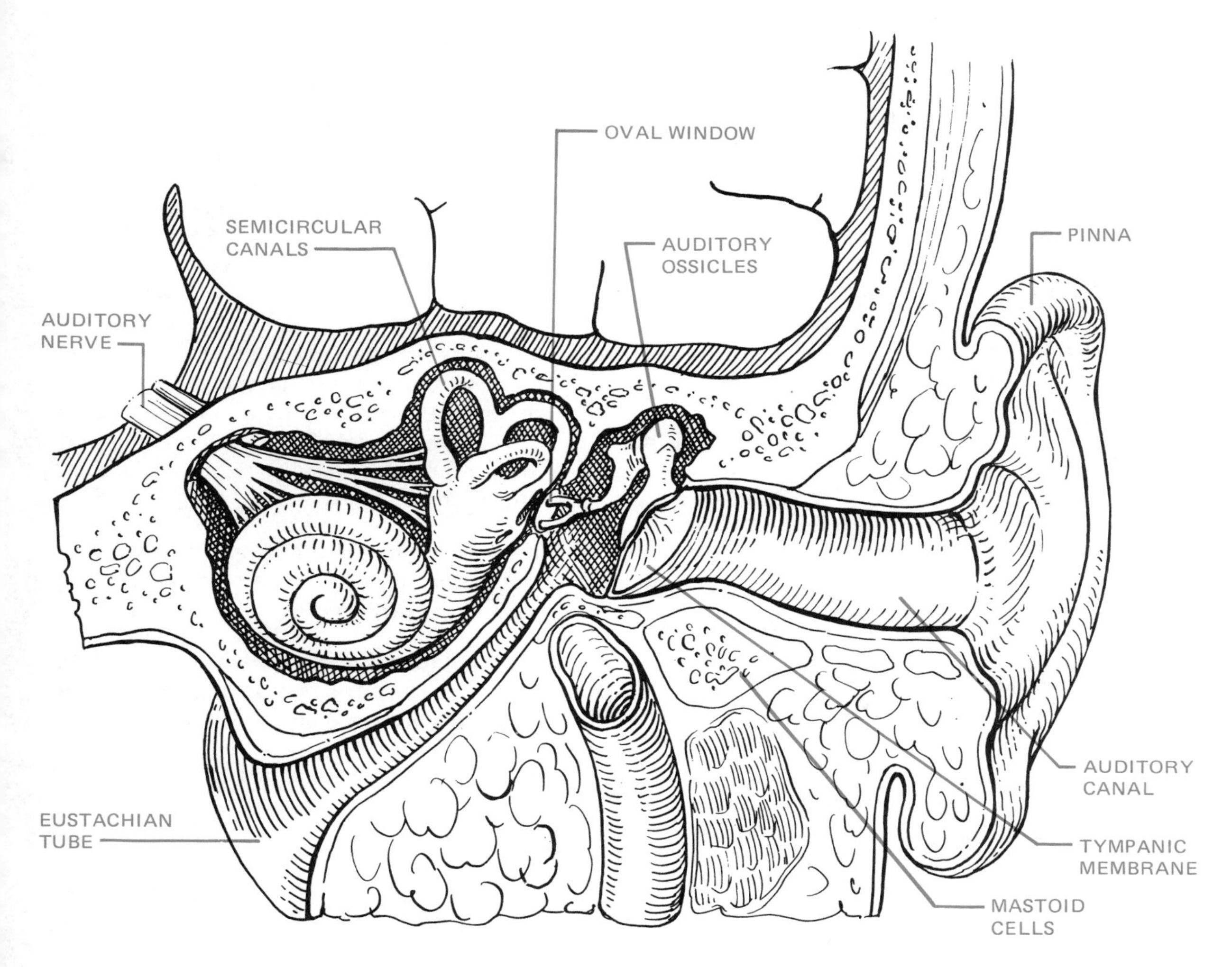

Figure 11-2 The structure of the ear.

The Outer Ear

The **pinna (PIN-**nah), also known as the **auricle,** is the external portion of the ear. (The combining forms *AUR/I* and *AUR/O* both mean ear or hearing. The combining form *PINN/I* means external ear.)

The **auditory canal** leads from the pinna to the middle ear. **Cerumen** (seh-**ROO-**men), also known as ear wax, is secreted by glands which line the auditory canal.

The Middle Ear

The **tympanic membrane** (tim-**PAN-**ick), also known as the **eardrum,** is located between the middle and outer ear. (The combining forms *TYMPAN/O* and *MYRING/O* both mean tympanic membrane.)

The middle ear is surrounded by the **mastoid cells** which are hollow air spaces located in the mastoid process of the temporal bone. (The combining form *MASTOID/O* means mastoid process.)

The three small bones found in the middle ear are the **malleus** (MAL-ee-us) also known as the hammer, **incus** (ING-kus) also known as the anvil, and **stapes** (STAY-peez) which is also known as the stirrup. Together they are known as the **auditory ossicles.**

The **eustachian tube** (you-STAY-key-an) is a narrow tube leading from the middle ear to the pharynx. It equalizes the air pressure in the middle ear with that of the outside atmosphere.

The Inner Ear

The inner ear, also known as the **labyrinth** (LAB-ih-rinth), contains the sensory receptors for hearing and balance. (The combining form *LABYRINTH/O* means a maze, labyrinth, and the inner ear.)

The **oval window** is a membrane which separates the middle from the inner ear. The **cochlea** (KOCK-lee-ah) is the spiral-shaped passage that leads from the oval window. (The combining form *COCHLE/O* means a snail or spiral.)

The **cochlear duct,** located within the cochlea, is filled with fluid that vibrates when the sound waves strike it.

The **organ of Corti,** also located within the cochlea, receives these vibrations and relays them to the **auditory nerve fibers** which transmit them to the auditory center of the cerebral cortex, where they are interpreted and "heard."

The three **semicircular canals,** which are also located within the inner ear, contain **endolymph** (a liquid) and sensitive hair-like cells. The bending of these cells in response to the movements of the head sets up impulses in nerve fibers.

The nerve fibers transmit this information to the brain and the brain sends messages to muscles in all parts of the body to assure that equilibrium is maintained. (**Equilibrium** is the state of balance.)

The Action of the Ear

Sound waves enter the ear through the pinna, travel through the auditory canal and strike a tympanic membrane between the outer and middle ear. This is called **air conduction.**

As the eardrum vibrates it moves the ossicles which conduct the sound waves through the middle ear. This is called **bone conduction.**

Sound vibrations reach the inner ear via the oval window. The structures of the inner ear receive the sound waves and relay them to the brain. This is called **sensorineural conduction.**

DIAGNOSTIC PROCEDURES RELATED TO SPECIAL SENSES

- An **ophthalmoscope** (ahf-**THAL**-moh-skope) is an instrument for examining the interior of the eye. It includes a light, a mirror with a single hole through which the examiner may look, and a dial holding several lenses of varying strengths.
- An **otoscope** (**OH**-toh-skope) is an instrument used to visually examine the external ear and the eardrum.
- An **audiometer** (**aw**-dee-**OM**-eh-ter) is an electric device for testing hearing and for measuring bone and air conduction.

PATHOLOGY OF THE EYE

Pathology of the Adnexa

- **Blepharitis** (**blef**-ah-**RYE**-tis), also known as **tarsitis** is an inflammation of the edges of the eyelids.
- **Blepharoptosis** (**blef**-ah-roh-**TOH**-sis) is a drooping of the upper eyelid. (The suffix *-PTOSIS* means drooping or sagging.)
- **Ectropion** (eck-**TROH**-pee-on) is the eversion of an eyelid. (**Eversion** means turned outward.)
- **Entropion** (en-**TROH**-pee-on) is the inversion of an eyelid. (**Inversion** means turned inward.)
- **Tarsadenitis** (**tahr**-sad-eh-**NIGH**-tis) is an inflammation of the edge of the eyelid.

- A **hordeolum** (hor-**DEE**-oh-lum), also known as a **sty** or **stye,** is an infection of one or more of the glands at the border of the eyelid.
- A **chalazion** (kah-**LAY**-zee-on) is a small localized swelling of the eyelid resulting from obstruction of one of the sebaceous follicles of the eyelid.
- **Dacryoma** (**dack**-ree-**OH**-mah) is a tumor-like swelling due to obstruction of the lacrimal duct.
- **Conjunctivitis** (kon-**junk**-tih-**VYE**-tis), also known as **pinkeye,** is an inflammation of the conjunctiva.

General Pathology of the Eye

- **Ophthalmia** (ahf-**THAL**-me-ah) is a severe inflammation of the eye.
- **Xenophthalmia** (**zen**-ahf-**THAL**-me-ah) is an inflammation caused by foreign material in the eye. (The combining form *XEN/O* means strange or foreign.)
- **Hemophthalmos** (**he**-mahf-**THAL**-mos) is extravasation of blood into the eye. (**Extravasation** is the escape of blood from a vessel into the tissue.)
- **Nystagmus** (nis-**TAG**-mus) is an involuntary, constant, rhythmic movement of the eyeball.
- **Scleritis** (sklee-**RYE**-tis) is an inflammation of the sclera.
- **Keratitis** (**ker**-ah-**TYE**-tis) is an inflammation of the cornea.
- **Trachoma** (trah-**KOH**-mah) is a contagious disease of the conjunctiva and cornea.
- **Iritis** (eye-**RYE**-tis) is an inflammation of the iris.
- **Synechia** (sigh-**NECK**-ee-ah) is an adhesion of the iris to the cornea or lens. (Plural, **synechiae.**)
- **Aphakia** (ah-**FAY**-kee-ah), also known as **aphacia,** is the absence of the lens of an eye.
- A **cataract** is a clouding of the lens, causing partial or total blindness.
- **Cycloplegia** (**sigh**-kloh-**PLEE**-jee-ah), also known as **paralysis of accommodation,** is paralysis of the ciliary muscle.

Pathology of the Retina

- **Retinopathy** (**ret**-ih-**NOP**-ah-thee) is any disease of the retina.
- **Retinitis** (**ret**-ih-**NIGH**-tis) is an inflammation of the retina.
- **Retinal detachment,** also known as a **detached retina,** is the separation of the retina from the choroid in the back of the eye.
- **Diabetic retinopathy** is a disorder of the blood vessels in the retina that may develop as a complication of diabetes.
- A **retinoblastoma** (**ret**-ih-no-blas-**TOH**-mah) is a malignant tumor arising from cells of the retina.
- **Papilledema** (**pap**-ill-eh-**DEE**-mah), also known as **choked disk,** is edema of the optic disk.
- **Macular degeneration** is the deterioration of the macula lutea of the retina.
- **Glaucoma** (glaw-**KOH**-mah) is a group of diseases characterized by increased intraocular pressure that causes damage to the optic disk.

Pathology of the Function of the Eye

- **Agnosia** (ag-**NO**-zee-ah) is the inability to recognize sensory impressions. This includes the eyes and other sensory organs.

- **Diplopia** (dih-**PLOH**-pee-ah), also known as **double vision,** is the perception of two images of a single object. (The combining form *DIPL/O* means double.)
- **Blindness** is the lack or loss of the ability to see.
- **Hemianopia** (**hem**-ee-ah-**NO**-pee-ah) is defective vision or blindness in half of the visual field.
- **Amblyopia** (**am**-blee-**OH**-pee-ah) is a dimness of vision or the partial loss of sight without detectable organic lesion of the eye. (The combining form *AMBLY/O* means dim or dull.)
- **Scotoma** (skoh-**TOH**-mah) is an area of absent or depressed vision surrounded by an area of normal vision. (The combining form *SCOT/O* means darkness.)
- **Esophoria** (**es**-oh-**FOH**-ree-ah), also known as **cross-eye,** is the deviation of the visual axis of one eye toward that of the other eye. (The prefix *ESO-* means inward.)
- **Exophoria** (eck-soh-**FOH**-ree-ah) is a deviation of the visual axis of one eye away from that of the other eye. (The prefix *EXO-* means outward.)
- **Myopia** (my-**OH**-pee-ah), also known as **nearsightedness,** is a defect in vision in which parallel rays come to a focus in front of the retina.
- **Hyperopia** (**high**-per-**OH**-pee-ah), known as **hypermetropia** (**high**-per-me-**TROH**-pee-ah) or **farsightedness,** is a defect in vision in which light rays come to a focus beyond the retina.
- **Presbyopia** (**pres**-bee-**OH**-pee-ah) is the lessening of the accommodation of the lens occurring normally with aging. (The combining form *PRESBY/O* means old age.)
- **Strabismus** (strah-**BIZ**-mus), also known as a **squint,** is a disorder in which the optic axes of the eyes cannot be directed to the same object. (The combining form *STRAB/I* means squint-eyed.)
- **Esotropia** (**es**-oh-**TROH**-pee-ah) is a type of strabismus characterized by an inward deviation of one eye in relation to the other.
- **Exotropia** (**eck**-soh-**TROH**-pee-ah) is strabismus characterized by the outward deviation of one eye relative to the other.
- **Anisocoria** (**an**-ih-so-**KOH**-ree-ah) is a condition in which the pupils are unequal in size. (The combining form *ANIS/O* means unequal.)
- **Ametropia** (**am**-eh-**TROH**-pee-ah) is a defect in the refractive powers of the eye in which images fail to come to focus on the retina. (The combining form *AMETR/O* means out of proportion.)
- **Astigmatism** (ah-**STIG**-mah-tizm) is a defect in the refractive powers of the eye in which light rays are not sharply focused on the retina.
- **Nyctalopia** (**nick**-tah-**LOH**-pee-ah), also known as **night blindness,** is a condition in which the individual has difficulty seeing at night. (The combining form *NYCTAL/O* means night.)
- **Monochromatism**, also known as **color blindness,** is the lack of the ability to distinguish colors. (The prefix *MONO-* means one and the combining form *CHROM/O* means color.)

PATHOLOGY OF THE EAR

Pathology of the Outer Ear

- **Otopathy** (oh-**TOP**-ah-thee) is any disease of the ear.

- **Otalgia** (oh-**TAL**-gee-ah), also known as **otodynia** or **earache,** is pain in the ear.
- **Otorrhea** (**oh**-toh-**REE**-ah) is a discharge from the ear. (The suffix *-RRHEA* means discharge or flow.)
- **Otopyorrhea** (**oh**-toh-**pye**-**oh**-**REE**-ah) is the flow of pus from the ear. The combining form *PY/O* means pus.)
- **Otomycosis** (**oh**-toh-my-**KOH**-sis) is a fungus infection of the external auditory canal. (The combining form *MYC/O* means fungus.)
- **Macrotia** (mack-**ROH**-she-ah) means abnormally large ears.
- **Microtia** (my-**KROH**-she-ah) means abnormally small ears.
- An **acoustic neuroma** is a progressively enlarging, benign tumor of the auditory canal arising from the acoustic nerve. (The combining form *NEUR/O* means nerve and the suffix *-OMA* means tumor.)

Pathology of the Middle Ear

- **Eustachitis** (**you**-stay-**KYE**-tis) is an inflammation of the eustachian tube.
- **Patulous eustachian tube** is distention of the eustachian tube.

  Patulous (**PAT**-you-lus) means extended spread wide open.
- **Mastoidalgia** (**mas**-toy-**DAL**-jee-ah) is pain in the mastoid region.
- **Mastoiditis** (**mas**-toy-**DYE**-tis) is an inflammation of the mastoid process.
- **Myringitis** (**mir**-in-**JIGH**-tis) is an inflammation of the tympanic membrane.
- **Otitis media** (oh-**TYE**-tis **ME**-dee-ah), also known as **tympanitis,** is an inflammation of the middle ear. (**Otitis** means an inflammation of the ear.)
- **Otosclerosis** (**oh**-toh-sklee-**ROH**-sis) is ankylosis of the bones of the middle ear that results in a conductive hearing loss. (**Ankylosis** means fused together.)

Pathology of the Inner Ear

- **Labyrinthitis** (**lab**-ih-rin-**THIGH**-tis) is an inflammation of the labyrinth resulting in vertigo.

  Vertigo (**VER**-tih-go) is a sense of whirling, dizziness and the loss of balance.
- **Meniere's disease** (**men**-ee-**AYRZ**) is a chronic disease of the inner ear characterized by recurrent episodes of vertigo, progressive unilateral nerve deafness and tinnitus.

Pathology of the Sense of Hearing

- **Deafness** is the complete or partial loss of the ability to hear. It may range from the inability to hear sounds of a certain pitch or intensity to a complete loss of hearing.
- A **conductive hearing loss** is one in which the outer or middle ear does not conduct sound vibrations to the inner ear normally.
- A **sensorineural hearing loss,** also known as **nerve deafness,** is a symptom of problems affecting the inner ear.
- **Presbycusis** (**pres**-beh-**KOO**-sis) is a progressive hearing loss occurring in old age.
- **Tinnitus** (tih-**NIGH**-tus) is a ringing sound in the ears.

PROCEDURES INVOLVING THE EYE

- **Enucleation** (**ee**-**new**-klee-**AY**-shun) is the process of removing an entire organ or other mass intact from its supporting tissues. For example, removing an eyeball from its orbit.
- **Orbitotomy** (**or**-bih-**TOT**-oh-me) is a surgical incision into the orbit.

- **Tarsorrhaphy** (tahr-**SOR**-ah-fee) is the suture of a portion of the entire upper and lower eyelids together.
- **Conjunctivoplasty** (**kon**-junk-**TYE**-voh-**plas**-tee) is the surgical repair of the conjunctiva.
- **Corneal transplant** is the surgical process of transferring the cornea from a donor to a patient.
- **Keratoplasty** (**KER**-ah-toh-**plas**-tee) is the surgical repair of the cornea.
- **Keratotomy** (**ker**-ah-**TOT**-oh-me) is a surgical incision into the cornea.
- An **iridectomy** (**ir**-ih-**DECK**-toh-me) is the surgical removal of a portion of the iris.
- **Iridotasis** (**ir**-ih-**DOT**-ah-sis) is the surgical stretching of the iris in treatment of glaucoma.

PROCEDURES INVOLVING THE EAR

- **Otoplasty** (**OH**-toh-**plas**-tee) is the surgical repair of the pinna of the ear.
- **Myringectomy** (**mir**-in-**JECK**-toh-me) is the surgical excision of the tympanic membrane.
- **Myringoplasty** (mih-**RING**-go-**plas**-tee) is the surgical repair of the tympanic membrane.
- **Myringotomy** (**mir**-in-**GOT**-oh-me) is the surgical incision of the eardrum.
- **Tympanectomy** (**tim**-pah-**NECK**-toh-me) is the surgical removal of the tympanic membrane.
- **Tympanoplasty** (**tim**-pah-no-**PLAS**-tee) is the surgical reconstruction of the tympanic membrane.
- **Tympanocentesis** (**tim**-pah-no-sen-**TEE**-sis) is the surgical puncture of the tympanic membrane to remove fluid.
- **Stapedectomy** (**stay**-peh-**DECK**-toh-me) is the surgical removal of the stapes.
- **Mastoidectomy** (**mas**-toy-**DECK**-toh-me) is the surgical removal of the mastoid cells.
- **Fenestration** (**fen**-es-**TRAY**-shun) is a surgical procedure in which a new opening is made in the labyrinth of the inner ear to restore hearing.
- **Labyrinthectomy** (**lab**-ih-rin-**THECK**-toh-me) is the surgical removal of the labyrinth.
- **Labyrinthotomy** (**lab**-ih-rin-**THOT**-oh-me) is the surgical incision of the labyrinth of the inner ear.

IMPORTANT TERMS: THE SPECIAL SENSES

This list will help you identify and review the major terms from this chapter.

When you work with the audio tape for this chapter, listen to the word, repeat it and then place a ✓ next to it on the list below.

- ☐ **Adnexa** (ad-**NECK**-sah)
- ☐ **Agnosia** (ag-**NO**-zee-ah)
- ☐ **Amblyopia** (**am**-blee-**OH**-pee-ah)
- ☐ **Ametropia** (**am**-eh-**TROH**-pee-ah)
- ☐ **Anisocoria** (**an**-ih-so-**KOH**-ree-ah)
- ☐ **Aphakia** (ah-**FAY**-kee-ah)
- ☐ **Astigmatism** (ah-**STIG**-mah-tizm)
- ☐ **Audiometer** (**aw**-dee-**OM**-eh-ter)
- ☐ **Blepharitis** (**blef**-ah-**RYE**-tis)
- ☐ **Blepharoptosis** (**blef**-ah-roh-**TOH**-sis)
- ☐ **Canaliculi** (**kan**- ah-**LICK**-you-lee)
- ☐ **Canthus** (**KAN**-thus)
- ☐ **Cerumen** (seh-**ROO**-men)

- ☐ **Chalazion** (kah-**LAY**-zee-on)
- ☐ **Choroid** (**KOH**-roid)
- ☐ **Cilia** (**SILL**-ee-ah)
- ☐ **Cochlea** (**KOCK**-lee-ah)
- ☐ **Conjunctivoplasty** (**kon**-junk-**TYE**-voh-**plas**-tee)
- ☐ **Conjunctivitis** (kon-**junk**-tih-**VYE**-tis)
- ☐ **Conjunctiva** (**kon**-junk-**TYE**-vah)
- ☐ **Convergence** (kon-**VER**-jens)
- ☐ **Cornea** (**KOR**-nee-ah)
- ☐ **Cycloplegia** (**sigh**-kloh-**PLEE**-jee-ah)
- ☐ **Dacryocyst** (**DACK**-ree-oh-sist)
- ☐ **Dacryoma** (**dack**-ree-**OH**-mah)
- ☐ **Diplopia** (dih-**PLOH**-pee-ah)
- ☐ **Ectropion** (eck-**TROH**-pee-on)
- ☐ **Emmetropia** (em-eh-**TROH**-pee-ah)
- ☐ **Entropion** (en-**TROH**-pee-on)
- ☐ **Enucleation** (ee-**new**-klee-**AY**-shun)
- ☐ **Epicanthus** (**ep**-ih-**KAN**-thus)
- ☐ **Esophoria** (**es**-oh-**FOH**-ree-ah)
- ☐ **Esotropia** (**es**-oh-**TROH**-pee-ah)
- ☐ **Eustachian** (you-**STAY**-key-an)
- ☐ **Eustachitis** (**you**-stay-**KYE**-tis)
- ☐ **Exophoria** (eck-soh-**FOH**-ree-ah)
- ☐ **Exotropia** (**eck**-soh-**TROH**-pee-ah)
- ☐ **Fenestration** (**fen**-es-**TRAY**-shun)
- ☐ **Fovea centralis** (**FOH**-vee-ah sen-**TRAH**-lis)
- ☐ **Glaucoma** (glaw-**KOH**-mah)
- ☐ **Hemianopia** (**hem**-ee-ah-**NO**-pee-ah)
- ☐ **Hemophthalmos** (**he**-mahf-**THAL**-mos)
- ☐ **Hordeolum** (hor-**DEE**-oh-lum)
- ☐ **Hypermetropia** (**high**-per-me-**TROH**-pee-ah)
- ☐ **Hyperopia** (**high**-per-**OH**-pee-ah)
- ☐ **Incus** (**ING**-kus)
- ☐ **Iridectomy** (**ir**-ih-**DECK**-toh-me)
- ☐ **Iridotasis** (**ir**-ih-**DOT**-ah-sis)
- ☐ **Iritis** (eye-**RYE**-tis)
- ☐ **Keratitis** (**ker**-ah-**TYE**-tis)
- ☐ **Keratoplasty** (**KER**-ah-toh-**plas**-tee)
- ☐ **Keratotomy** (**ker**-ah-**TOT**-oh-me)
- ☐ **Labyrinth** (**LAB**-ih-rinth)
- ☐ **Labyrinthectomy** (**lab**-ih-rin-**THECK**-toh-me)
- ☐ **Labyrinthitis** (**lab**-ih-rin-**THIGH**-tis)
- ☐ **Labyrinthotomy** (**lab**-ih-rin-**THOT**-oh-me)
- ☐ **Lacrimal** (**LACK**-rih-mal)
- ☐ **Lacrimation** (**lack**-rih-**MAY**-shun)
- ☐ **Macrotia** (mack-**ROH**-she-ah)
- ☐ **Macula lutea** (**MACK**-you-lah **LOO**-tee-ah)
- ☐ **Malleus** (**MAL**-ee-us)
- ☐ **Mastoidalgia** (**mas**-toy-**DAL**-jee-ah)
- ☐ **Mastoidectomy** (**mas**-toy-**DECK**-toh-me)
- ☐ **Mastoiditis** (**mas**-toy-**DYE**-tis)
- ☐ **Meniere's** (**men**-ee-**AYRZ**)
- ☐ **Microtia** (my-**KROH**-she-ah)
- ☐ **Myopia** (my-**OH**-pee-ah)

- □ **Myringectomy** (**mir**-in-**JECK**-toh-me)
- □ **Myringitis** (**mir**-in-**JIGH**-tis)
- □ **Myringoplasty** (mih-**RING**-go-**plas**-tee)
- □ **Myringotomy** (**mir**-in-**GOT**-oh-me)
- □ **Nyctalopia** (**nick**-tah-**LOH**-pee-ah)
- □ **Nystagmus** (nis-**TAG**-mus)
- □ **Ocular** (**OCK**-you-lar)
- □ **Ophthalmia** (ahf-**THAL**-me-ah)
- □ **Ophthalmoscope** (ahf-**THAL**-moh-skope)
- □ **Orbitotomy** (**or**-bih-**TOT**-oh-me)
- □ **Otalgia** (oh-**TAL**-gee-ah)
- □ **Otitis media** (oh-**TYE**-tis **ME**-dee-ah)
- □ **Otomycosis** (**oh**-toh-my-**KOH**-sis)
- □ **Otopathy** (oh-**TOP**-ah-thee)
- □ **Otoplasty** (**OH**-toh-**plas**-tee)
- □ **Otopyorrhea** (**oh**-toh-**pye**-oh-**REE**-ah)
- □ **Otorrhea** (**oh**-toh-**REE**-ah)
- □ **Otosclerosis** (**oh**-toh-sklee-**ROH**-sis)
- □ **Otoscope** (**OH**-toh-skope)
- □ **Papilledema** (**pap**-ill-eh-**DEE**-mah)
- □ **Patulous** (**PAT**-you-lus)
- □ **Pinna** (**PIN**-nah)
- □ **Presbycusis** (**pres**-beh-**KOO**-sis)
- □ **Presbyopia** (**pres**-bee-**OH**-pee-ah)
- □ **Retina** (**RET**-ih-nah)
- □ **Retinitis** (**ret**-ih-**NIGH**-tis)
- □ **Retinoblastoma** (**ret**-ih-no-blas-**TOH**-mah)
- □ **Retinopathy** (**ret**-ih-**NOP**-ah-thee)
- □ **Sclera** (**SKLEE**-rah)
- □ **Scleritis** (sklee-**RYE**-tis)
- □ **Scotoma** (skoh-**TOH**-mah)
- □ **Stapedectomy** (**stay**-peh-**DECK**-toh-me)
- □ **Stapes** (**STAY**-peez)
- □ **Strabismus** (strah-**BIZ**-mus)
- □ **Synechia** (sigh-**NECK**-ee-ah)
- □ **Tarsadenitis** (**tahr**-sad-eh-**NIGH**-tis)
- □ **Tarsorrhaphy** (tahr-**SOR**-ah-fee)
- □ **Tinnitus** (tih-**NIGH**-tus)
- □ **Trachoma** (trah-**KOH**-mah)
- □ **Tympanectomy** (**tim**-pah-**NECK**-toh-me)
- □ **Tympanic** (tim-**PAN**-ick)
- □ **Tympanocentesis** (**tim**-pah-no-sen-**TEE**-sis)
- □ **Tympanoplasty** (**tim**-pah-no-**PLAS**-tee)
- □ **Vertigo** (**VER**-tih-go)
- □ **Vitreous** (**VIT**-ree-us)
- □ **Xenophthalmia** (**zen**-ahf-**THAL**-me-ah)

EXERCISES

DEFINING WORD PARTS

Write the definition for each of these word parts.

1. *ACOUS/O, ACOUST/O* ______
2. *AMBLY/O* ______
3. *AMETR/O* ______
4. *AQUE/O* ______
5. *AUDI/O, AUDIT/O* ______
6. *AUR/I, AUR/O* ______
7. *BLEPHAR/O* ______
8. *CANTH/O* ______
9. *CHOROID/O* ______
10. *CILI/O* ______
11. *COCHLE/O* ______
12. *CONJUNCTIV/O* ______
13. *CORNE/O* ______
14. *DACRY/O* ______
15. *DIPL/O* ______
16. *ESO-* ______

17. *EXO-* ______________________________

18. *FOVE/O* ______________________________

19. *IR/I, IR/O, IRID/O, IRIT/O* ______________________________

20. *KERAT/O* ______________________________

21. *LABYRINTH/O* ______________________________

22. *LACRIM/O* ______________________________

23. *LUTE/O* ______________________________

24. *MACUL/O* ______________________________

25. *MASTOID/O* ______________________________

26. *MYRING/O* ______________________________

27. *NYCTAL/O* ______________________________

28. *OCUL/O* ______________________________

29. *OPHTHALM/O* ______________________________

30. *OPT/I, OPT/O* ______________________________

31. *OPTIC/O* ______________________________

32. *OT/O* ______________________________

33. *PHAC/O* ______________________________

34. *PINN/I* ______________________________

35. *PRESBY/O* ______________________________

36. *-PTOSIS* ______________________________

37. *PUPILL/O* ______________________________

38. *RETIN/O* ______________________________

39. *-RRHEA* ______________________________

40. *SCLER/O* ______________________________

41. *SCOT/O* ______________________________

42. *STRAB/I* ______________________________

43. *TARS/O* ______________________________

44. *TYMPAN/O* ______________________________

45. *VITRE/O* ______________________________

DEFINITIONS

Circle the letter next to the correct answer.

1. The _______________, also known as the white of the eye, is a fibrous tissue that maintains the shape of the eye and protects the delicate inner layers of tissue.
   a) choroid
   b) conjunctiva
   c) cornea
   d) sclera

2. The _______________ is a spiral-shaped passage that leads from the oval window of the inner ear.
   a) cochlea
   b) eustachian tube
   c) organ of Corti
   d) semilunar canal

3. The _______________ is a yellow spot in the center of the retina.
   a) fovea centralis
   b) macula lutea
   c) optic disk
   d) optic nerve

4. The _______________ is a membrane that separates the middle from the inner ear.
   a) mastoid
   b) oval window
   c) pinna
   d) tympanic

5. The _______________ duct is the passageway that drains tear fluid into the nose.
   a) adnexa
   b) canthus
   c) lacrimal
   d) optic

6. _______________ is the state of balance.
   a) Equilibrium
   b) Hemostasis
   c) Vertigo
   d) a and b

7. The _______________ is a vertical fold of skin on either side of the nose.
   a) canthus
   b) cilia
   c) epicanthus
   d) lacrimal fold

8. The _______________ is the colored muscular layer of the eye that surrounds the pupil.
   a) cornea
   b) choroid
   c) iris
   d) lens

9. The inner ear is also known as the _______________
   a) cochlea.
   b) labyrinth.
   c) organ of Corti.
   d) semicircular canal.

10. _______________ is the normal relationship between the refractive power of the eye and the shape of the eye that enables light rays to focus correctly on the retina.
   a) Convergence
   b) Emmetropia
   c) Esophoria
   d) Esotropia

MISSING WORDS

Write the missing word on the line.

1. Sound vibrations reach the inner ear via the oval window. This is called nerve or _______________________ conduction.

2. The _______________________ muscles, located within the choroid of the eye, adjust the shape and thickness of the lens.

3. The _______________________ canal leads from the pinna to the middle ear.

4. The _______________________ _______________________, also known as the blind spot, is the region of the eye where the nerve endings of the retina gather to form the optic nerve.

5. The term _______________________ means turned outward.

6. The term _______________________ means turned inward.

7. The _______________________, which is also known as the auricle, is the outer ear.

8. The _______________________ glands secrete tears.

9. The term ______________________ means that light cannot pass through a substance.

10. The ______________________ layer or coat is the middle layer of the eyeball.

SPELLCHECK

Select the correct spelling and write it on the line.

1. The ______________________ tubes lead from the middle ear to the pharynx.
   euctachian
   eustachian
   eustation

2. An ______________________ is an instrument for examining the interior of the eye.
   ophthalmoscope
   ophthalmascope
   opthalmoscope

3. ______________________, also known as ear wax, is secreted by glands which line the auditory canal.
   Cerumen
   Cerunem
   Seerumen

4. The ______________________ is the transparent anterior portion of the sclera of the eye.
   cornea
   cornia
   coronea

5. An ______________________ is a defect in the refractive powers of the eye in which light rays are not sharply focused on the retina.
   astegmatism
   astigmatism
   astigomatism

6. The ______________________ is the sensitive inner nerve layer of the eye.
   retana
   retena
   retina

7. ______________________ is the movement of the two eyes toward fixation of the same near point.
   Convergance
   Convergence
   Convergience

8. ______________________ is a group of diseases characterized by increased intraocular pressure that causes damage to the optic disk.
   Glakoma
   Glaucoma
   Glawcoma

9. A ______________________ is the surgical incision of the eardrum.
   myergotomy
   myringiotomy
   myringotomy

10. ______________________ is also known as nearsightedness.
    Myeopia
    Myopea
    Myopia

11. ______________________ is the surgical procedure in which a new opening is made in the labyrinth of the inner ear.
    Fenestration
    Fenistration
    Finestration

12. ______________________ is a sense of whirling, dizziness and the loss of balance.
    Vertago
    Vertigo
    Virtigo

13. ______________________ is the surgical incision of the labyrinth of the inner ear.
    Labryinthectomy
    Labryinthomy
    Labyrinthotomy

14. ______________________ is also known as pinkeye.
    Canjunctivitis
    Conjunctivitis
    Conjunctovitis

15. A ______________________ is small localized swelling of the eyelid resulting from obstruction of one of the sebaceous follicles of the eyelid.
    chalasion
    chalision
    chalazion

CASE STUDIES

Write the correct answer on the line.

1. Following the fight, Jack Lawson required ____________________ to repair the pinna of his injured ear.

2. Sheila Valladares suffers from a/an ____________________ hearing loss because the middle ear does not conduct sound vibrations to the inner ear normally.

3. Edward Jankowski has a/an ____________________ which is a malignant tumor arising from cells of the retina.

4. After the blow on the head, Margo Wilkins complained of ____________________ or double vision.

5. Mr. Eisner suffers from ____________________ which is a progressive hearing loss that occurs in old age.

6. Clara Dixon suffers from diabetic ____________________ as a complication of diabetes.

7. The doctor diagnosed Jimmy Smith's earache as being ____________________ ____________________. The doctor might have called it tympanitis.

8. Adrianne Jacobus suffers from ____________________ which is also known as night blindness.

9. Mr. Unger's was diagnosed as having a/an ____________________ ____________________ which is a progressively enlarging, benign tumor of the auditory canal.

10. His eye examination revealed that Paul Ogelthorpe is color blind. This diagnosis was listed on his chart as ____________________.

11. Maude Colson is troubled by ____________________ which is a ringing sound in her ears.

12. William Hillman complained of problems with balance and hearing. After performing several tests, the doctor diagnosed that Mr. Hillman is suffering from ____________________ disease.

13. Carlos Montoya's hearing loss was diagnosed as being ____________________ which is caused by ankylosis of the bones of the middle ear.

14. Donna Baldwin's condition required ____________________ which is the surgical repair of the cornea.

15. The other children tease Tommy Nolan about his abnormally large ears. A doctor would say that Tommy has ____________________.

WORD BUILDING

Write the correct word or word part on the line.

1. Discharge from the ear
   a) The combining form ______________________ means ear.
   b) The suffix ______________________ means discharge or flow.
   c) The term ______________________ means discharge (flow) from the ear.

2. Surgical repair of the eardrum
   a) The combining form ______________________ means eardrum.
   b) The suffix ______________________ means surgical repair.
   c) The term ______________________ means surgical repair of the eardrum.

3. Fluid removal
   a) The combining form ______________________ means tympanic membrane or eardrum.
   b) The suffix ______________________ means surgical puncture to remove fluid.
   c) The term ______________________ means the surgical puncture of the tympanic membrane to remove fluid.

4. Pus from the ear
   a) The combining form ______________________ means ear.
   b) The combining form ______________________ means pus.
   c) The suffix ______________________ means discharge or flow.
   d) The term ______________________ means the flow of pus from the ear.

5. Inflammation of the mastoid process
   a) The combining form ______________________ means mastoid process.
   b) The suffix ______________________ means inflammation.
   c) The term ______________________ means an inflammation of the mastoid process.

LABELING EXERCISES

Identify the numbered items on this diagram.

1. ______________________ or auricle
2. ______________________ membrane
3. ______________________ ossicles
4. ______________________ tube
5. ______________________ canals

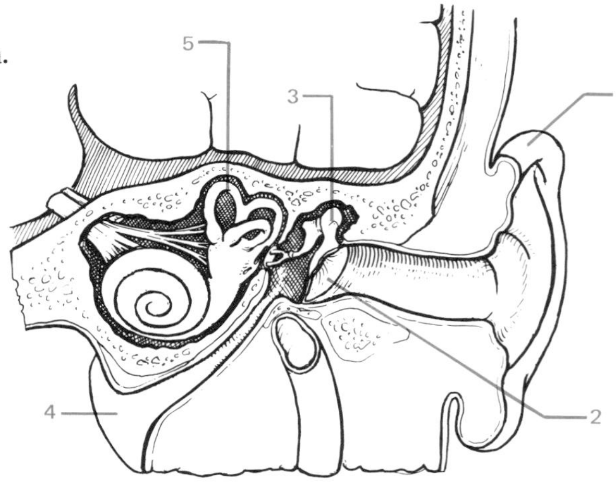

12

THE INTEGUMENTARY SYSTEM

LEARNING GOALS

In this chapter you will learn to:

- define the major terms related to the structures of the integumentary system.
- recognize and define terms used to describe the diagnosis, pathology and procedures related to disorders of the skin.
- recognize and define terms used to describe the diagnosis, pathology and procedures related to disorders of the hair, nails and the sebaceous glands.

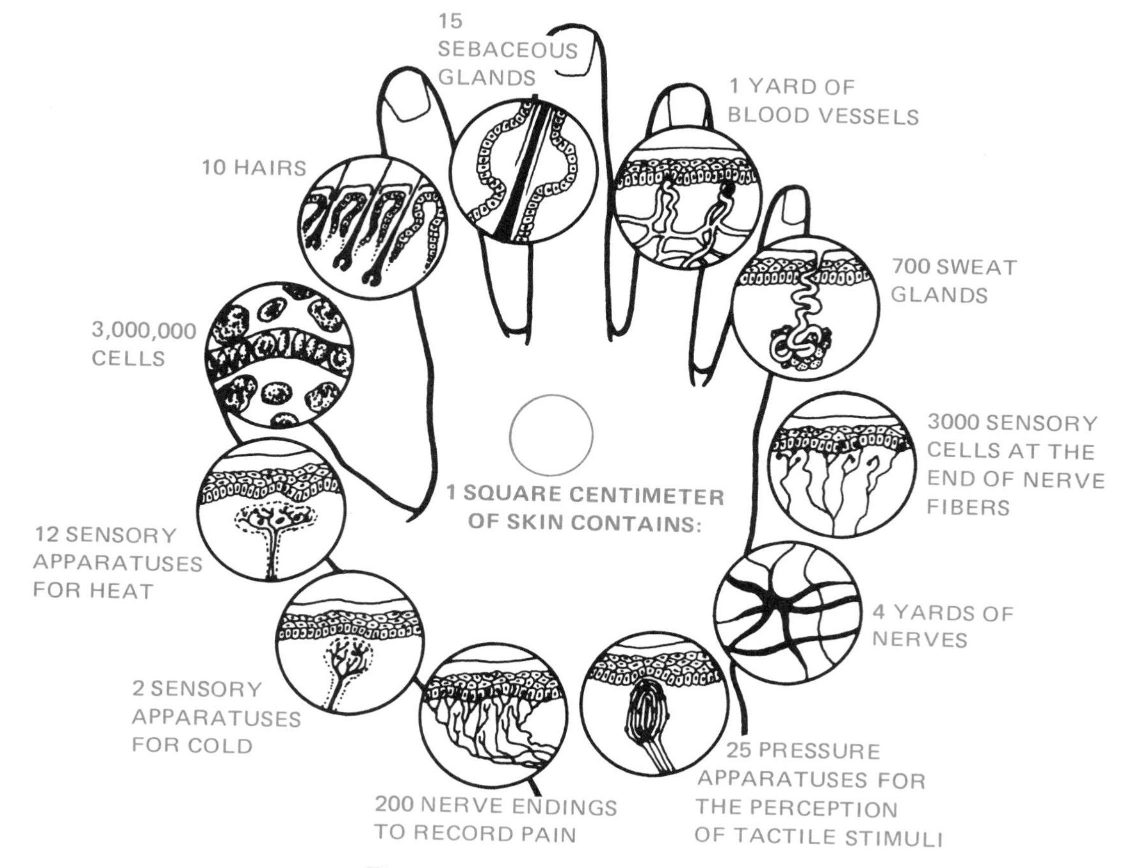

Figure 12-1 Structure of the skin.

STRUCTURES OF THE INTEGUMENTARY SYSTEM

The integumentary system consists of the skin and its associated structures, which are the sweat glands, sebaceous glands, hair and nails.

The important functions of the integumentary system are to protect the body and control body temperature; to serve as the sense organ of touch; and to be active in absorption and excretion.

THE LAYERS OF THE SKIN

The skin, which forms the outer covering of the body, is a complex system of specialized tissues. The terms **cutaneous** (kyou-**TAY**-nee-us) and **derma** are both used to describe the skin. (The combining forms *CUTANE/O, DERMAT/O* and *DERM/O* all mean skin.)

The skin is made up of three layers. These are the epidermis, dermis or corium and subcutaneous layers.

The Epidermis

The **epidermis** (**ep**-ih-**DER**-mis) is the outermost layer of the skin. (The prefix *EPI-* means upon and the root word **dermis** means true skin.) The epidermis is made up of squamous epithelium.

Epithelium (**ep**-ih-**THEE**-lee-um) is the specialized cellular tissue that covers all of the internal and external surfaces of the body.

The **squamous epithelium** that makes up the epidermis consists of flat, plate-like cells arranged in several layers. It is also known as **stratified epithelium.**

The epidermis does not contain any blood vessels or connective tissue and is dependent upon the lower layers for nourishment.

The deepest layer of the epidermis is called the **basal layer.** The cells of this layer multiply and push upward. As the cells move toward the surface, they die and become filled with keratin.

Keratin (KER-ah-tin), a fibrous protein, is the primary component of the epidermis, hair and nails. (The combining form *KERAT/O* means horny or hard. This same combining form also refers to the cornea of the eye.)

The basal layer also contains special cells called **melanocytes (MEL-**ah-no-sights) which produce and contain a black pigment called **melanin (MEL-**ah-nin). (The combining form *MELAN/O* means black or dark.)

The amount of melanin pigment determines the color of the skin. Melanin also protects the skin against some of the harmful rays of the sun.

The Dermis

The **dermis (DER-**mis), also known as the **corium (KOH-**ree-um), is the layer directly below the epidermis. It is living tissue composed of blood and lymph vessels and nerve fibers, as well as the accessory organs of the skin.

The connective tissue cells found in the dermis include fibroblasts, histiocytes and mast cells.

Fibroblasts (FIGH-broh-blasts) are the fiber producing cells of the connective tissue. Fibers in the dermis are composed primarily of collagen.

Collagen (KOL-ah-jen), which means glue, is a tough, yet flexible, fibrous protein material. In addition to being found in the skin, collagen is also found in bone, cartilage, tendons and ligaments.

Histiocytes (HISS-tee-oh-**sights)** are phagocytic cells that protect the body by engulfing foreign substances. (The combining forms *HISTI/O* and *HIST/O* both mean tissue.) (The combining form *PHAG/O* means to eat or swallow.)

Mast cells produce substances in response to injury or infection. The substances released include histamine and heparin.

Histamine (HISS-tah-meen) is released in response to allergens and produces itching.

Heparin (HEP-ah-rin) is released in response to injury and is an anticoagulant substance.

Sensitive nerve endings in the dermis receive impulses that enable the body to recognize sensations such as temperature, touch, pain, and pressure.

The term **tactile** means pertaining to touch. **Perception** is the ability to recognize sensory stimulus.

The Subcutaneous Layer

The subcutaneous layer of the skin, also a connective tissue layer, specializes in the formation of fat.

Lipocytes (LIP-oh-sights), also known as **fat cells,** are predominant in the subcutaneous layer, where they manufacture and store large quantities of fat. (The combining form *LIP/O* means fat.)

THE GLANDS OF THE SKIN

Sebaceous Glands

Sebaceous (seh-**BAY-**shus) glands are located in the dermis layer of the skin and are closely associated with hair follicles.

Sebum (SEE-bum) is the oily substance secreted by the sebaceous glands and released through ducts that open into the hair follicles. (The combining form *SEB/O* means sebum.)

The milk-producing **mammary glands,** which are modified sebaceous glands, are often classified with the integumentary system. However, they are also part of the reproductive system and in this text they are discussed with that system in Chapter 14.

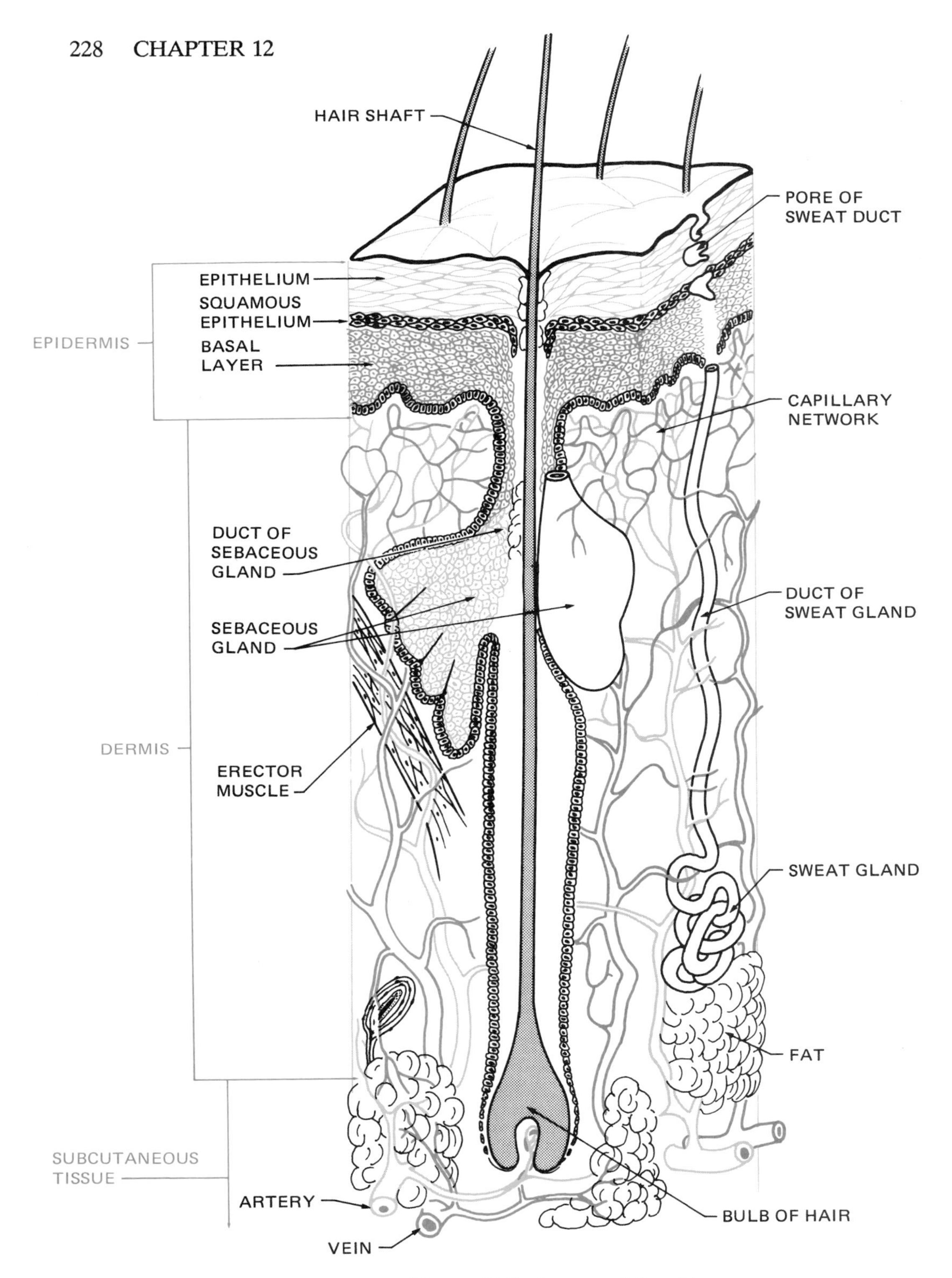

Figure 12-2 Layers of the skin.

Sweat Glands

Sweat glands are tiny, coiled glands found on almost all body surfaces. They are most numerous in the palms of the hands and the soles of the feet. The tiny opening on the surface of the skin is called a **pore.**

Sweat, or perspiration, cools the body as it evaporates into the air. The term **hidrosis** (high-**DROH**-sis) means sweat production and secretion. (The combining form *HIDR/O* means sweat.)

HAIR

Hair fibers are rod-like structures composed of tightly fused, dead protein cells called keratin. Hair grows from special cells found at the base of the hair follicles. (The combining forms *PIL/I* and *PIL/O* both mean hair.)

Hair follicles are the shafts or sacs that hold the hair fibers. The **arrector pili** (ah-**RECK**-tor **PYE**-lye), also known as the **erector muscle,** is a tiny muscle attached to the hair follicle, which causes the hair to stand erect. (See figure 12-2.)

NAILS

A nail, also known as an **unguis** (**UNG**-gwis), is the keratin plate covering the dorsal surface of the last bone of each toe and finger. (The combining form *UNGU/O* means nail.) (Plural, **Ungues.)**

Each nail consists of a root, body and free edge. The nail root fastens the nail to the finger or toe by fitting into a groove in the skin and is closely molded to the surface of the derma.

The **eponychium** (**ep**-oh-**NICK**-ee-um), also known as the **cuticle,** is a narrow band of epidermis that is attached to the surface of the nail just ahead of the root.

The **lunula** (**LOO**-new-lah) is a half-moon shaped white region at the nail root and is generally found in the thumbnail and in varying degrees in other nails. (Plural, **lunulae.)**

The **matrix,** also known as the **nail bed,** joins the body of the nail to the underlying connective tissue.

DIAGNOSTIC PROCEDURES RELATED TO THE INTEGUMENTARY SYSTEM

Biopsy Procedures

- A **biopsy** (**BYE**-op-see) is the removal of a small piece of living tissue for examination to confirm or establish a diagnosis. (The combining form *BI/O* means pertaining to life.)

- **Bioassay** (**bye**-oh-ass-**SAY**) is the analysis of a living substance derived from a specific tissue or organ.

  Assay means to determine the amount of a particular substance in a mixture.

- **Exfoliative cytology,** (ecks-**FOH**-lee-**ay**-tiv) is a form of biopsy in which cells are scraped from the tissue and examined under a microscope.

- In an **incisional biopsy,** a piece, but not all, of the tumor or lesion is removed.

- In an **excisional biopsy,** the entire tumor or lesion plus a margin of surrounding tissue are removed. (**Excision** is the complete removal of a lesion or organ.)

- In a **needle biopsy,** a needle is used to remove a core of tissue for examination.

- A **trocar** (**TROH**-kar) is a sharp, pointed rod that fits inside a tube called a **cannula** (**KAN**-you-lah).

  The trocar is used to pierce the skin and the wall of a body cavity or canal and to position the cannula. Once it is in place, the cannula may be used to aspirate fluids or to instill medication.

PATHOLOGY OF THE INTEGUMENTARY SYSTEM

Lesions

- A **lesion** (**LEE**-zhun) is a pathological change of the skin, and possibly surrounding tissues, due to disease or injury.
- A **macule** (**MACK**-youl) is a discolored, flat lesion such as a freckle or flat mole.
- A **papule** (**PAP**-youl) is a small, solid, raised skin lesion such as nonpustular acne.
- A **wheal** (**WHEEL**) is a smooth, slightly elevated, edematous (swollen) area that is redder or paler than the surrounding skin. Wheals are a large type of papule.
- **Urticaria** (**ur**-tih-**KAY**-ree-ah), also known as **hives,** is a skin condition characterized by localized areas of swelling accompanied by itching that is associated with an allergic reaction.
- A **vesicle** (**VES**-ih-kul), also known as a blister, is a circumscribed collection of clear fluid.

  Circumscribed (**SER**-kum-skryebd) means contained within a limited area.
- A **bulla** (**BULL**-ah) is a large vesicle or blister. (Plural, **bullae.**)
- A **cyst** is a closed sack or pouch containing fluid or semisolid material.
- An **ulcer** is an open sore or erosion of the skin or mucous membrane. Ulcers usually involve loss of tissue substance.
- A **fissure** of the skin is a groove or crack-like sore. (Other types of fissures, such as the folds in the brain, are normal and not an indication of pathology.)
- A **fistula** (**FIS**-tyou-lah) is an abnormal passage from an internal organ to the body surface or between two internal organs. (Plural, **fistulas** or **fistulae.**)

Infections of the Skin

- The term **purulent** (**PYOU**-roo-lent) means producing or containing pus. (The combing form *PY/O* means pus.)

  The term **suppurative** (**SUP**-you-**ray**-tiv) also means producing or containing pus. (The combining forms *SUPPUR/O* and *SUPPURAT/O* both mean to form pus.)

  Pyoderma (**pye**-oh-**DER**-mah) is any purulent skin disease.
- An **abscess** (**AB**-sess) is a localized collection of pus.
- A **pustule** (**PUS**-tyoul) is a small abscess of the skin.
- **Cellulitis** (**sell**-you-**LYE**-tis) is a diffuse infection of connective tissue with severe inflammation of the dermal and subcutaneous layers of the skin. (**Diffuse** means widespread.)
- A **furuncle** (**FYOU**-rung-kul), also known as a **boil,** is a localized skin infection originating in a gland or hair follicle.
- A **carbuncle** (**KAR**-bung-kul) is an infection of the skin and subcutaneous tissue composed of a cluster of furuncles.
- **Impetigo** (**im**-peh-**TYE**-go) is a contagious, superficial skin infection usually seen in young children.
- **Dermatomycosis** (**der**-mah-toh-my-**KOH**-sis) is a superficial fungal infection of the skin.

General Pathology of the Skin

- **Dermatosis** (**der**-mah-**TOH**-sis) is any condition of the skin that is NOT associated with inflammation.
- **Dermatitis** (**der**-mah-**TYE**-tis) is an inflammation of the skin.

- **Pruritus** (proo-**RYE**-tus), also known as **itching,** is associated with most forms of dermatitis.
- **Verrucae** (veh-**ROO**-see), also known as **warts,** are a type of papule that is caused by a virus infection.
- **Psoriasis** (so-**RYE**-uh-sis) is a chronic disease of the skin characterized by itching and by red papules covered with silvery scales.
- **Acanthosis** (**ack**-an-**THOH**-sis) is a diffuse hyperplasia and thickening of the epidermis, as seen in psoriasis.
- **Xeroderma** (zee-roh-**DER**-mah) means dry skin. (The combining form *XER/O* means dry.)
- **Erythroderma** (eh-**rith**-roh-**DER**-mah) is an abnormal redness of the skin occurring over widespread areas of the body. (The combining form *ERYTHR/O* means red.)
- **Erythema** (**er**-ih-**THEE**-mah) is a redness or inflammation of the skin such as a nervous blush or a mild sunburn. (The combining forms *ERYTHEM/O* and *ERYTHEMAT/O* both mean flushed or redness.)
- A **decubitus ulcer** (dee-**KYOU**-bih-tus), also known as a **bedsore,** is an ulcerated area resulting from prolonged pressure on a body part.
- A **laceration** is a torn, ragged wound.
- A **contusion** (kon-**TOO**-zhun) is an injury that does not break the skin and is characterized by swelling, discoloration and pain.
- An **ecchymosis** (**eck**-ih-**MOH**-sis), commonly known as a **bruise,** is a purplish patch caused by hemorrhages into the skin. (Plural, **ecchymoses.)**
- **Petechiae** (pee-**TEE**-kee-ee) are small, pinpoint hemorrhages (a smaller version of ecchymoses).
- A **polyp** (**POL**-ip) is a growth extending on a stalk, like a mushroom, from the surface of a mucous membrane.
- **Keloid** (**KEE**-loid) is an abnormally raised or thickened scar that forms after trauma or surgical incision.

  Cicatrix (sick-**AY**-tricks) is a "normal" scar left by a healed wound.
- **Tinea** (**TIN**-ee-ah), also known as **ringworm,** is a fungus that may affect the skin on different areas of the body.

  Tinea pedis, also known as **athlete's foot,** is ringworm of the foot.
- **Scabies** (**SKAY**-beez) is a skin infection caused by the itch mite.
- **Eczema** (**ECK**-zeh-mah) is an inflammatory skin disease characterized by erythema, papules, vesicles, pustules, scales, crusts and scabs alone or in combination.
- **Dyschromia** (dis-**KROH**-me-ah) is any disorder of the pigmentation of the skin or hair. (The combining form *CHROM/O* means color.)

  Melanosis (**mel**-ah-**NO**-sis) is any condition of unusual deposits of black pigment in different parts of the body. (The suffix *-OSIS* means an abnormal condition.)

  An **albino** (al-**BYE**-no) is an individual with white skin and hair because the skin is incapable of forming melanin. An albino's eyes are pink because of the absence of pigment in the normally pigmented iris of the eye. (The combining forms *ALB/O* and *ALBIN/O* both mean white.)
- **Vitiligo** (**vit**-ih-**LYE**-go) is a loss of pigment in areas of the skin, resulting in milk-white patches. (The combining form *VITI/O* means blemish or defect.)

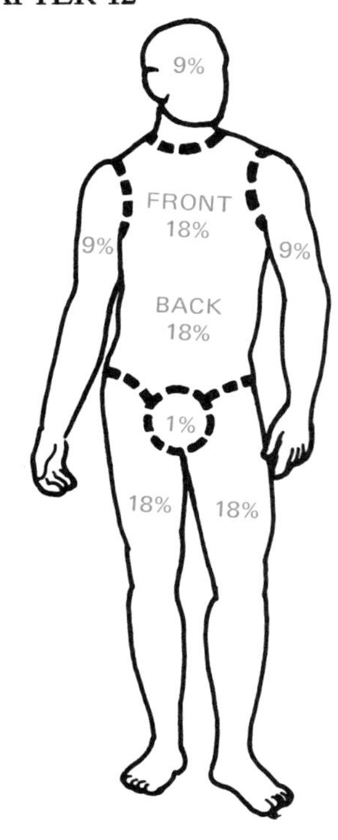

Figure 12-3 Diagram for use in calculating the percentage of body area burned.

Burns

A burn is an injury to tissues of the body caused by heat, flame, electricity, chemicals or radiation. The severity of a burn is determined by the amount of skin surface affected (more than 15% is considered serious), and the layers of skin involved.

Depending on the layer(s) of skin involved, burns may be classified into three types:

- **First degree burns,** in which there are no blisters and only superficial damage to the epidermis.
- **Second degree burns,** in which there are blisters and damage to the epidermis and corium.
- **Third degree burns,** in which the epidermis, corium and subcutaneous layers are damaged.

Neoplasms of the Skin

- A **neoplasm** (**NEE**-oh-plazm) is any abnormal growth of new tissue. It may be benign or malignant.
- A **basal cell carcinoma** (**kar**-sih-**NO**-mah) is a malignant tumor of the basal cell layer of the epidermis. It is the most frequent type of skin cancer.
- A **granuloma** is a tumor-like mass of nodular granulation tissue resulting from inflammation, injury or infection. (**Granulation tissue** is the tissue that forms during the healing of a wound.)
- A **keratosis** (**kerr**-ah-**TOH**-sis) is any benign skin condition, such as a wart or callus, in which there is overgrowth and thickening of the epidermis. (Plural, **keratoses.**)
- **Actinic keratosis** (ack-**TIN**-ick) is an abnormal skin lesion caused by excessive exposure to the sun, which may give rise to squamous cell carcinoma.
- **Leukoplakia** (**loo**-koh-**PLAY**-kee-ah) is a disease marked by the development of white, thickened patches on mucous membrane tissue of the tongue or cheek. (The combining form *LEUK/O* means white.)

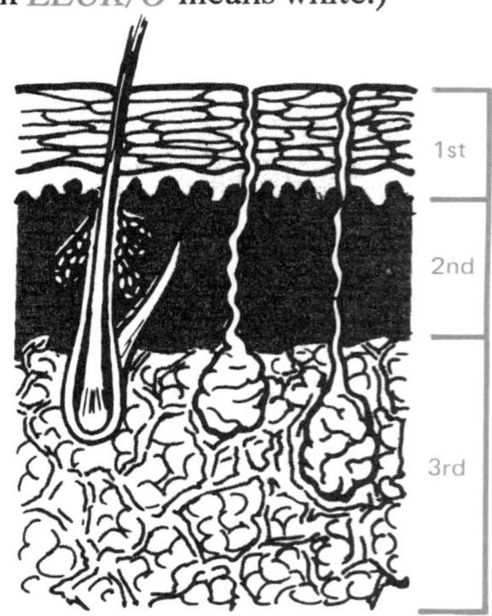

Figure 12-4 Layers of skin in relation to the degree of burn.

- A **lipoma** (lih-**POH**-mah) is a benign tumor made up of mature fat cells. (The suffix *-OMA* means tumor or mass.)
- **Malignant melanoma** (**mel**-ah-**NO**-mah) is a cancerous tumor composed of melanocytes. These tumors often metastasize (spread) to the lung, liver, and brain.
- A **nevus** (**NEE**-vus) is a benign congenital proliferation of blood vessels or pigmented cells on the skin surface. A **mole** is an example of a nevus. (Plural, **nevi.**)
- A **papilloma** (**pap**-ih-**LOH**-mah) is a benign epithelial neoplasm characterized by a branching or lobular tumor.
- A **papillary carcinoma** is a malignant neoplasm characterized by many finger-like projections.
- **Squamous cell carcinoma** is a malignant tumor of the squamous epithelial cells of the epidermis. In addition to growing on the skin, this type of tumor also grows wherever squamous epithelium is found.

Pathology of Related Glands

- **Hyperhidrosis** (**high**-per-high-**DROH**-sis) is a condition of excessive sweating.
- **Anhidrosis** (**an**-high-**DROH**-sis) is the condition of lacking or being without sweat.
- **Seborrhea** (**seb**-oh-**REE**-ah) is any of several common skin conditions in which there is an over production of sebum. (The suffix *-RRHEA* means to flow.)
- **Acne vulgaris** (**ACK**-nee vul-**GAY**-ris) is a chronic inflammatory disease characterized by pustular eruptions of the skin which usually occurs in, or near, the sebaceous glands.
- A **comedo** (**KOM**-eh-doh), known as a **blackhead,** is formed by the buildup of sebum and keratin in a pore of the skin. (Plural, **comedones.**)
- A **sebaceous cyst** is a cyst of a sebaceous gland, containing yellow, fatty material.

Pathology of the Hair

- **Pilosebaceous** (**pye**-loh-seh-**BAY**-shus) means pertaining to the hair follicles and the sebaceous glands.
- A **pilonidal cyst** (**pye**-loh-**NIGH**-dal) is a hair-containing cyst found over the sacral area of the back in the midline.
- **Hirsutism** (**HER**-soot-izm) means abnormal hairiness.
- **Alopecia** (**al**-oh-**PEE**-shee-ah), also known as **baldness,** is a partial or complete lack of hair.

  Alopecia areata is a disease of unknown cause in which there are well-defined bald patches.

  Alopecia totalis is an uncommon condition characterized by the loss of all the hair on the scalp.

  Alopecia universalis is the total loss of hair on all parts of the body.

Pathology of the Nails

- **Onychitis** (**on**-ih-**KYE**-tis) is an inflammation of the nail. (The combining form *ONYCH/O* is used to describe conditions of the nail.)
- **Onychia** (oh-**NICK**-ee-ah) is an inflammation of the nail bed, resulting in the loss of the nail.
- **Paronychia** (**par**-oh-**NICK**-ee-ah) is an infection of the fold of skin at the margin of a nail.
- **Onychomalacia** (**on**-ih-ko-mah-**LAY**-shee-ah) is an abnormal softening of the nail.
- **Onychophagia** (**on**-ih-koh-**FAY**-jee-ah) means nail biting or eating. (The suffix *-PHAGIA)* means eating.

- **Onychocryptosis** (**on**-ih-koh-krip-**TOH**-sis) means ingrown toenail. (The combining form *CRYPT/O* means hidden.)
- **Onychomycosis** (**on**-ih-koh-my-**KOH**-sis) is a fungus infection of the nail. (The combining form *MYC/O* means fungus.)
- A **subungual hematoma** (sub-**UNG**-gwal) is a collection of blood beneath a nail, usually resulting from an injury.

PROCEDURES RELATED TO THE INTEGUMENTARY SYSTEM

- **Abrasion** is scraping or rubbing away of the skin surface by friction to remove scars, tattoos or keratoses. (An abrasion may also be caused by an injury.)

  Chemabrasion (keem-ah-**BRAY**-shun), also known as **chemical peel,** is a form of abrasion that involves the use of chemicals.

  Dermabrasion (**der**-mah-**BRAY**-shun) is a form of abrasion involving the use of revolving wire brushes or sandpaper.
- **Blepharoplasty** (**BLEF**-ah-roh-**plas**-tee) is the plastic surgery of the eyelids. (The combining form *BLEPHAR/O* means eyelid.)
- **Cauterization** (**kaw**-ter-eye-**ZAY**-shun) is the destruction of tissue for therapeutic purposes.

  Electrocautery is the destruction of tissue through the use of electrical current.
- **Electrodesiccation** (ee-**leck**-troh-des-ih-**KAY**-shun), also known as **fulguration** (**ful**-goo-**RAY**-shun), is a technique in electrosurgery in which tissue is destroyed by burning with an electric spark.
- **Cryosurgery** is the destruction of tissue through the application of extreme cold. (The combining form *CRY/O* means cold.)
- **Debridement** is the removal of dirt, foreign objects, damaged tissue, and cellular debris from a wound to prevent infection and to promote healing.
- **Incision and drainage** involves incision (cutting open) a lesion, such as an abscess, and draining the contents.
- **Lipectomy** (lih-**PECK**-toh-me), also known as **adipectomy** (**ad**-ih-**PECK**-toh-me), is the surgical removal of fat beneath the skin.
- **Marsupialization** (mar-**soo**-pee-al-eye-**ZAY**-shun) is surgically changing a closed cavity, such as a cyst, into an open pouch to encourage drainage and healing.
- **Plication** (plih-**KAY**-shun) is the surgical procedure of taking tucks in a structure to shorten it. (The combining form *PLIC/O* means fold or ridge.)
- **Rhytidectomy** (**rit**-ih-**DECK**-toh-me), also known as a **face lift,** is the surgical removal of excess skin for the elimination of wrinkles. (The combining form *RHYTID/O* means wrinkle.)
- **Percutaneous treatment** (**per**-kyou-**TAY**-nee-us) means a procedure performed through the skin. For example, a needle passed through the skin is used to aspirate fluid from a space below the skin.
- **Transdermal delivery** is a method of applying a drug to unbroken skin via a patch worn on the patient's skin. (The prefix *TRANS-* means across or through.)
- **Transcutaneous electronic nerve stimulation** (TNS) is a method of pain control by the application of electronic impulses to the nerve endings through the skin.

IMPORTANT TERMS: THE INTEGUMENTARY SYSTEM

This list will help you identify and review the major terms from this chapter.

When you work with the audio tape for this chapter, listen to the word, repeat it and then place a ✓ next to it on the list below.

- □ **Abscess** (**AB**-sess)
- □ **Acanthosis** (**ack**-an-**THOH**-sis)
- □ **Acne vulgaris** (**ACK**-nee vul-**GAY**-ris)
- □ **Actinic** (ack-**TIN**-ick)
- □ **Adipectomy** (**ad**-ih-**PECK**-toh-me)
- □ **Albino** (al-**BYE**-no)
- □ **Alopecia** (**al**-oh-**PEE**-shee-ah)
- □ **Anhidrosis** (**an**-high-**DROH**-sis)
- □ **Arrector pili** (ah-**RECK**-tor **PYE**-lye)
- □ **Bioassay** (**bye**-oh-ass-**SAY**)
- □ **Biopsy** (**BYE**-op-see)
- □ **Blepharoplasty** (**BLEF**-ah-roh-**plas**-tee)
- □ **Bulla** (**BULL**-ah)
- □ **Cannula** (**KAN**-you-lah)
- □ **Carbuncle** (**KAR**-bung-kul)
- □ **Carcinoma** (**kar**-sih-**NO**-mah)
- □ **Cauterization** (**kaw**-ter-eye-**ZAY**-shun)
- □ **Cellulitis** (**sell**-you-**LYE**-tis)
- □ **Chemabrasion** (keem-ah-**BRAY**-shun)
- □ **Cicatrix** (sick-**AY**-tricks)
- □ **Circumscribed** (**SER**-kum-skryebd)
- □ **Collagen** (**KOL**-ah-jen)
- □ **Comedo** (**KOM**-eh-doh)
- □ **Contusion** (kon-**TOO**-zhun)
- □ **Corium** (**KOH**-ree-um)
- □ **Cutaneous** (kyou-**TAY**-nee-us)
- □ **Decubitus** (dee-**KYOU**-bih-tus)
- □ **Dermabrasion** (**der**-mah-**BRAY**-shun)
- □ **Dermatitis** (**der**-mah-**TYE**-tis)
- □ **Dermatosis** (**der**-mah-**TOH**-sis)
- □ **Dermatomycosis** (**der**-mah-toh-my-**KOH**-sis)
- □ **Dermis** (**DER**-mis)
- □ **Dyschromia** (dis-**KROH**-me-ah)
- □ **Ecchymosis** (**eck**-ih-**MOH**-sis)
- □ **Eczema** (**ECK**-zeh-mah)
- □ **Electrodesiccation** (ee-**leck**-troh-des-ih-**KAY**-shun)
- □ **Epidermis** (**ep**-ih-**DER**-mis)
- □ **Epithelium** (**ep**-ih-**THEE**-lee-um)
- □ **Eponychium** (**ep**-oh-**NICK**-ee-um)
- □ **Erythema** (**er**-ih-**THEE**-mah)
- □ **Erythroderma** (eh-**rith**-roh-**DER**-mah)
- □ **Exfoliative** (ecks-**FOH**-lee-**ay**-tiv)
- □ **Fibroblasts** (**FIGH**-broh-blasts)
- □ **Fistula** (**FIS**-tyou-lah)
- □ **Fulguration** (**ful**-goo-**RAY**-shun)
- □ **Furuncle** (**FYOU**-rung-kul)
- □ **Heparin** (**HEP**-ah-rin)
- □ **Hidrosis** (high-**DROH**-sis)
- □ **Hirsutism** (**HER**-soot-izm)
- □ **Histamine** (**HISS**-tah-meen)

- □ **Histiocytes** (**HISS**-tee-oh-**sights**)
- □ **Hyperhidrosis** (**high**-per-high-**DROH**-sis)
- □ **Impetigo** (**im**-peh-**TYE**-go)
- □ **Keloid** (**KEE**-loid)
- □ **Keratin** (**KER**-ah-tin)
- □ **Keratosis** (**kerr**-ah-**TOH**-sis)
- □ **Lesion** (**LEE**-zhun)
- □ **Leukoplakia** (**loo**-koh-**PLAY**-kee-ah)
- □ **Lipectomy** (lih-**PECK**-toh-me)
- □ **Lipocytes** (**LIP**-oh-sights)
- □ **Lipoma** (lih-**POH**-mah)
- □ **Lunula** (**LOO**-new-lah)
- □ **Macule** (**MACK**-youl)
- □ **Marsupialization** (mar-**soo**-**pee**-**al**-**eye**-**ZAY**-shun)
- □ **Melanocytes** (**MEL**-ah-no-sights)
- □ **Melanoma** (**mel**-ah-**NO**-mah)
- □ **Melanosis** (**mel**-ah-**NO**-sis)
- □ **Neoplasm** (**NEE**-oh-plazm)
- □ **Nevus** (**NEE**-vus)
- □ **Onychia** (oh-**NICK**-ee-ah)
- □ **Onychitis** (**on**-ih-**KYE**-tis)
- □ **Onychocryptosis** (**on**-ih-koh-krip-**TOH**-sis)
- □ **Onychomycosis** (**on**-ih-koh-my-**KOH**-sis)
- □ **Onychomalacia** (**on**-ih-ko-mah-**LAY**-shee-ah)
- □ **Onychophagia** (**on**-ih-koh-**FAY**-jee-ah)
- □ **Papilloma** (**pap**-ih-**LOH**-mah)
- □ **Papule** (**PAP**-youl)
- □ **Paronychia** (**par**-oh-**NICK**-ee-ah)
- □ **Percutaneous** (**per**-kyou-**TAY**-nee-us)
- □ **Petechiae** (pee-**TEE**-kee-ee)
- □ **Pilonidal** (**pye**-loh-**NIGH**-dal)
- □ **Pilosebaceous** (**pye**-loh-seh-**BAY**-shus)
- □ **Plication** (plih-**KAY**-shun)
- □ **Polyp** (**POL**-ip)
- □ **Pruritus** (proo-**RYE**-tus)
- □ **Psoriasis** (so-**RYE**-uh-sis)
- □ **Purulent** (**PYOU**-roo-lent)
- □ **Pustule** (**PUS**-tyoul)
- □ **Pyoderma** (**pye**-oh-**DER**-mah)
- □ **Rhytidectomy** (**rit**-ih-**DECK**-toh-me)
- □ **Scabies** (**SKAY**-beez)
- □ **Seborrhea** (**seb**-oh-**REE**-ah)
- □ **Sebum** (**SEE**-bum)
- □ **Subungual** (sub-**UNG**-gwal)
- □ **Suppurative** (**SUP**-you-**ray**-tiv)
- □ **Tinea** (**TIN**-ee-ah)
- □ **Trocar** (**TROH**-kar)
- □ **Unguis** (**UNG**-gwis)
- □ **Urticaria** (**ur**-tih-**KAY**-ree-ah)
- □ **Verrucae** (veh-**ROO**-see)
- □ **Vesicle** (**VES**-ih-kul)
- □ **Vitiligo** (**vit**-ih-**LYE**-go)
- □ **Wheal** (**WHEEL**)
- □ **Xeroderma** (zee-roh-**DER**-mah)

EXERCISES

DEFINING WORD PARTS

Write the definition for each of these word parts.

1. *ALB/O, ALBIN/O* ______
2. *BLEPHAR/O* ______
3. *CRYPT/O* ______
4. *CUTANE/O* ______
5. *DERM/O, DERMAT/O* ______
6. *ERYTHR/O* ______
7. *ERYTHEM/O, ERYTHEMAT/O* ______
8. *HIDR/O* ______
9. *HISTI/O, HIST/O* ______
10. *KERAT/O* ______
11. *LEUK/O* ______
12. *LIP/O* ______
13. *MELAN/O* ______
14. *MYC/O* ______
15. *ONYCH/O* ______
16. *PIL/O* ______

17. *SEB/O* ______________________________

18. *UNGU/O* ______________________________

19. *VITI/O* ______________________________

20. *XER/O* ______________________________

DEFINITIONS

Circle the letter next to the correct answer.

1. Cellulitis is a/an ______________
   a) diffuse infection of connective tissue.
   b) groove or crack-like sore.
   c) localized collection of pus.
   d) open sore or erosion of the skin.

2. Blepharoplasty is plastic surgery ______________
   a) for a face lift.
   b) for fat removal.
   c) of the eyelids.
   d) of the nose.

3. Heparin is ______________
   a) a phagocytic cell.
   b) an anticoagulant.
   c) produces itching.
   d) b and c.

4. Pruritus is commonly known as ______________
   a) baldness.
   b) dry skin.
   c) itching.
   d) pus.

5. A/an ______________ is an abnormal skin lesion caused by excessive exposure to the sun.
   a) actinic keratosis
   b) basal cell carcinoma
   c) nevus
   d) papilloma

6. An ecchymosis is commonly known as a/an ______________
   a) abscess.
   b) bruise.
   c) scar.
   d) ulcer.

7. A fissure is a/an _______________
   a) groove or crack-like sore.
   b) normal fold of the brain.
   c) open sore or erosion of the skin.
   d) a and b.

8. The epidermis is _______________
   a) also known as the corium.
   b) the outermost layer of the skin.
   c) where the sebaceous glands are located.
   d) b and c.

9. Mast cells _______________
   a) are phagocytic.
   b) release histamine and heparin.
   c) are found in the subcutaneous layer.
   d) b and c.

10. The sebaceous glands are located in the _______________
    a) dermis.
    b) epidermis.
    c) keratinic layer.
    d) subcutaneous layer.

MISSING WORDS

Write the missing word on the line.

1. _______________________ and _______________________ both mean producing or containing pus.

2. A/an _______________________ is a closed sac or pouch containing fluid or semisolid material.

3. _______________________ is a skin condition in which there is an over production of sebum.

4. _______________________ treatment is performed through the skin.

5. _______________________, also known as hives, is a skin condition characterized by localized swelling associated with an allergic reaction.

6. _______________________ are cells that form and contain black pigment.

7. _______________________ is commonly known as a face lift.

8. _______________________ is the destruction of tissue through the application of extreme cold.

9. The primary component of hair and nails is the fibrous protein called _______________________.

10. The _______________________ is commonly known as the cuticle of a fingernail or toenail.

11. ______________________ means dry skin.

12. ______________________ is released in response to allergens and produces itching.

13. ______________________ are small pinpoint hemorrhages.

14. The term ______________________ is used to describe a "normal" scar left by a healed wound.

15. A ______________________ is a discolored, flat lesion such as a freckle or flat mole.

SPELLCHECK

Write the correct spelling on the line.

1. ______________________ a chronic disease of the skin characterized by itching and by red papules covered with silvery scales.
   Psoriasis
   Psorosis
   Soriasis

2. ______________________ is a contagious, superficial skin infection usually seen in young children.
   Empetago
   Impetago
   Impetigo

3. A ______________________ is an area of congenital proliferation of blood vessels or pigmented cells on the skin surface.
   nevi
   neveus
   nevus

4. ______________________ is an inflammatory skin disease with erythema, papules, and scabs.
   Eczema
   Ekezma
   Eksema

5. A ______________________ cyst is a hair containing cyst found over the sacral area of the back in the midline.
   pilinidal
   pilonidal
   pylonodal

6. ______________________ is the destruction of tissue through the use of electrical current.
   Electrocautery
   Electroquartary
   Electroquatery

7. ______________________ epithelium is also known as stratified epithelium.
   Sqwaymous
   Squamious
   Squamous

8. ______________________ are phagocytic cells.
   Histeocytes
   Histiocytes
   Histocytes

9. ______________________ glands produce sebum.
   Sebaceous
   Sebaseous
   Sebayceous

10. The ______________________ is the half-moon shaped white region at the nail root.
    loonula
    lunula
    lunulla

11. An ______________________ is a localized collection of pus.
    abcess
    abscess
    absess

12. A basal cell ______________________ is a malignant tumor of the basal cell layer of the epidermis.
    carcinoma
    carsenoma
    carsinoma

13. ______________________ is an inflammation of the nail bed, resulting in the loss of the nail.
    Onychia
    Onyochia
    Oynchia

14. The ______________________ is commonly known as the cuticle.
    eponychium
    epoynchium
    epyonchium

15. ______________________ electronic nerve stimulation is commonly referred to as TNS.
    Transcutaneous
    Transcutanious
    Transqutaneous

CASE STUDIES

Write the correct answer on the line.

1. Robert Harris has a disease of unknown origin in which there are well-defined bald patches. Robert has a form of ____________________.
2. Jordan Caswell has white hair, pink eyes and very, very pale skin. Jordan is a/an ____________________.
3. Mr. Vernon has an ingrown toenail. On his chart, this diagnosis is recorded as ____________________.
4. Mary Young had an allergic reaction to penicillin. Her symptoms included large hives, which were recorded on her chart as ____________________.
5. Stan Neilsen complained that he had athlete's foot. Dr. Williams treated him for ____________________ pedis.
6. Josh Dawson had a boil on his neck. On the chart Dr. Adams listed this as incision and drainage of a/an ____________________.
7. Willie Smith was treated for a skin infection caused by the itch mite. This was entered on the chart as treatment for ____________________.
8. ____________________, involving the use of sandpaper, was used to treat Joyce Olson's severe acne scars.
9. After the surgery, Agnes Farrington's scar was abnormally raised and thickened. This condition is known as a ____________________.
10. After doing heavy yard work, Ted Jackson has a very large blister on his hand. This is called a/an ____________________.
11. Mr. Garrison's angina medication is administered via ____________________ delivery through a patch worn on his chest.
12. Norma Martin's blood disorder causes small pinpoint bruises over large areas of her body. This condition is called ____________________.
13. Mr. Vaughn has been confined to bed for a very long time and has now developed ____________________ ulcers, which are also known as bed sores.
14. Bob Thornton has a form of acne that results in ____________________ which are commonly known as blackheads.
15. Nell Solon has ____________________ which results in milk-white patches on her skin.

WORD BUILDING

Write the correct word or word part on the line.

1. A fatty tumor
   a) The combining form ______________________ means fat.
   b) The suffix ______________________ means tumor.
   c) The term ______________________ means a benign fatty tumor.
2. Sweat
   a) The combining form ______________________ means sweat.
   b) The prefix ______________________ means without.
   c) The term ______________________ means the condition of being without sweat.
3. Nail biting
   a) The combining form ______________________ means nails.
   b) The suffix ______________________ means eating.
   c) The term ______________________ means nail biting or eating.
4. Melanin
   a) The combining form ______________________ means melanin.
   b) The suffix ______________________ means an abnormal condition.
   c) The term ______________________ means an abnormal condition characterized by deposits of dark pigment.
5. Sebum
   a) The combining form ______________________ means sebum.
   b) The suffix ______________________ means to flow.
   c) The term ______________________ means excessive flow of sebum.

LABELING EXERCISES

Identify the numbered items on this diagram.

1. ______________________
2. ______________________ gland
3. ______________________
4. ______________________ tissue
5. ______________________ gland

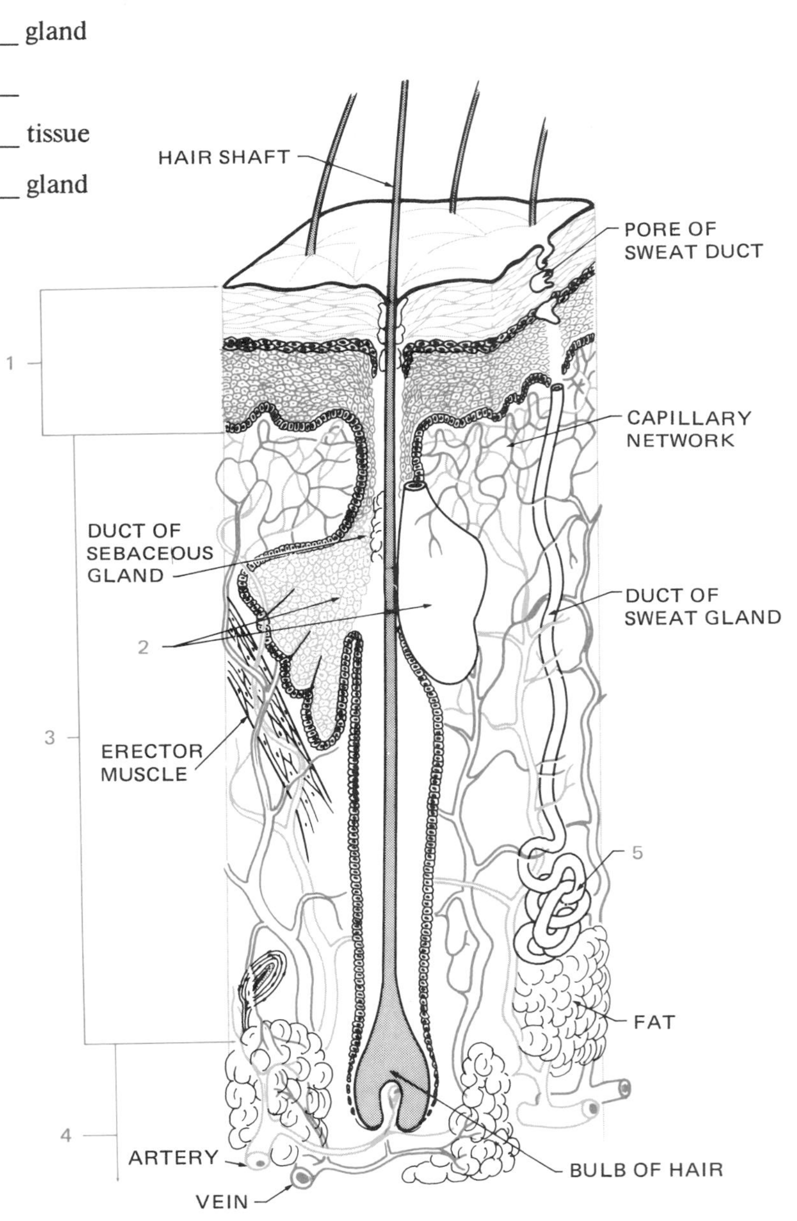

13

THE ENDOCRINE SYSTEM

LEARNING GOALS

In this chapter you will learn to:

- differentiate between endocrine and exocrine glands.
- list the glands that are included in the endocrine system.
- describe the secretions and functions of the endocrine glands.
- state the role of the endocrine system in regulating other body systems.
- recognize and define terms relating to the diagnosis, pathology and procedures related to disorders of the endocrine system.

OVERVIEW OF THE ENDOCRINE SYSTEM

Exocrine glands (**ECK**-soh-krin), such as sweat glands, secrete their chemical substances into ducts that lead either to other organs or out of the body. (The combining form *CRIN/O* means to secrete.)

Endocrine glands (**EN**-doh-krin) secrete their hormones directly into the bloodstream. The glands of the endocrine system include:

- one pituitary gland (also known as the hypophysis),
- one thyroid gland,
- four parathyroid glands,
- two adrenal glands (also known as the suprarenals),
- one pancreas,
- one thymus,
- one pineal gland and
- two gonads (ovaries in females, testes in males).

Hormones

A hormone is a chemical substance that regulates the activity of certain cells and/or organs.

The release of some hormones is controlled by nerve stimulation. Other hormones are secreted in response to the level of a particular substance in the bloodstream.

THE PITUITARY GLAND

The pituitary gland (pih-**TOO**-ih-**tair**-ee), also known as the **hypophysis** (high-**POF**-ih-sis), is a small gland located at the base of the brain. (The combining form *PITUIT/O* means pituitary.)

Many of the hormones secreted by the pituitary gland control the functions of other endocrine glands. These secretory functions of the pituitary gland are regulated by the hypothalamus of the brain.

The pituitary gland is composed of two lobes: the **anterior lobe,** also known as the **adenohypophysis** (**ad**-eh-no-high-**POF**-ih-sis), and the **posterior lobe,** also known as the **neurohypophysis** (**new**-roh-high-**POF**-ih-sis).

PITUITARY GLAND: ANTERIOR LOBE	
Hormone	**Function**
TSH **Thyroid-stimulating hormone**	Stimulates the growth and the secretion of the thyroid gland.
ACTH **Adrenocorticotropic hormone**	Stimulates the growth and the secretion of the adrenal cortex.
FSH **Follicle-stimulating hormone**	Stimulates the secretion of estrogen, growth of eggs in the ovaries and the production of sperm in the testes.
LH **Luteinizing hormone**	Stimulates ovulation and is important in maintaining pregnancy.
ICSH **Interstitial cell-stimulating hormone**	This male hormone stimulates testosterone secretion.
LTH **Lactogenic Hormone** (Also called **prolactin** or **luteotropin**)	Stimulates the secretion of milk and influences maternal behavior.
GH **Growth hormone** (Also called **somatotropin**)	Accelerates body growth.
MSH **Melanocyte-stimulating hormone**	Increases pigmentation of the skin.

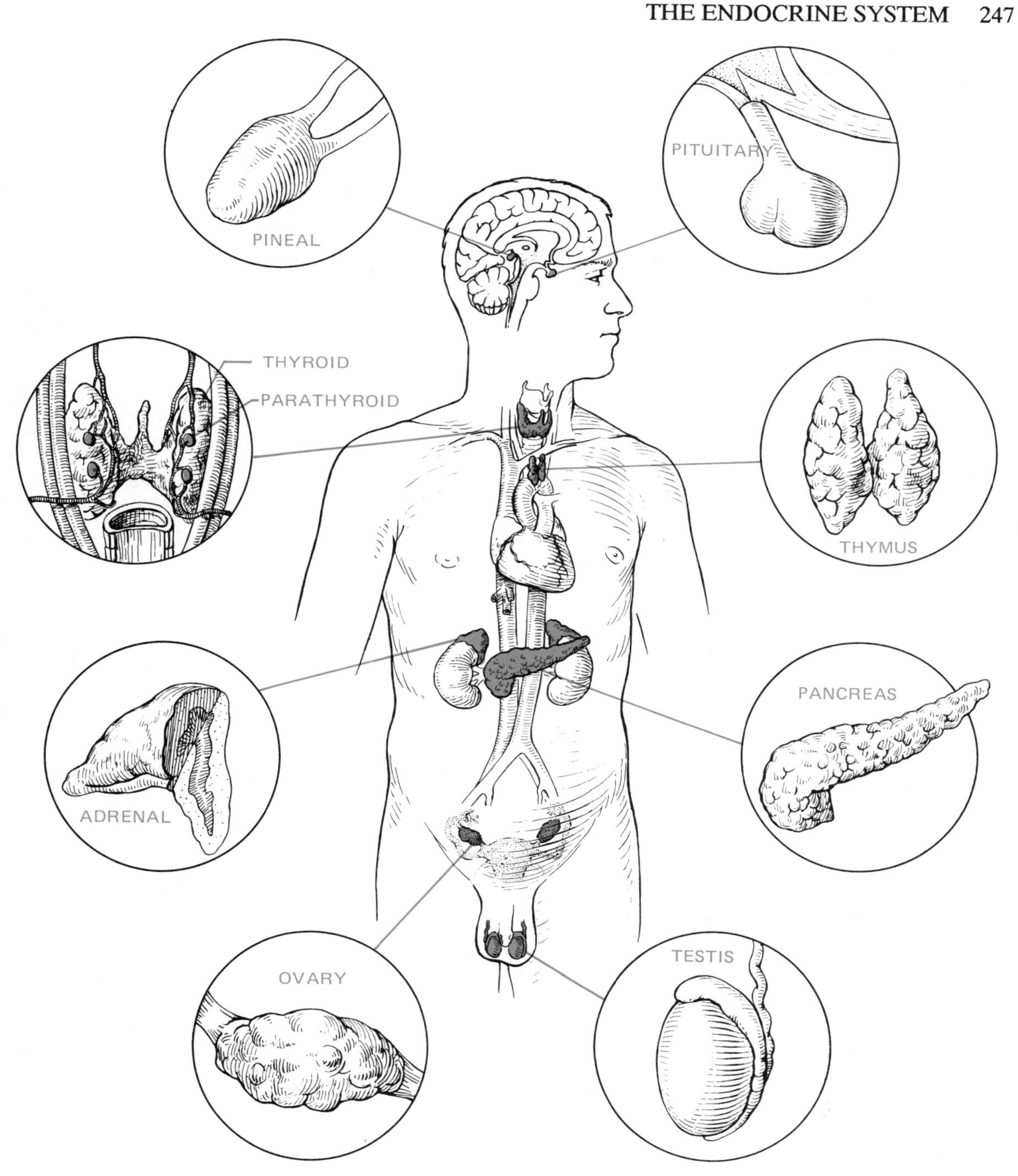

Figure 13-1 Structures of the endocrine system.

PITUITARY GLAND: POSTERIOR LOBE	
Hormone	**Function**
ADH **Antidiuretic hormone** (Also called **vasopressin)**	Maintains the body's water balance by reducing urinary output.
Oxytocin	Stimulates uterine contractions during childbirth. Also causes milk to flow from the mammary glands.

THE THYROID GLAND

The butterfly-shaped thyroid gland lies on either side of the larynx, just below the thyroid cartilage. (The combining forms *THYR/O* and *THYROID/O* both mean thyroid.)

THYROID GLAND	
Hormone	**Function**
Thyroxine and **Triiodothyronine**	Regulate the rate of metabolism and influence physical and mental development.
Calcitonin	Works with the parathyroid hormone (PTH) to regulate calcium levels in the blood and tissues.

THE PARATHYROID GLANDS

The four parathyroid glands, each of which is about the size of a grain of rice, are located on the posterior surface of the thyroid gland.

PARATHYROID GLAND	
Hormone	**Function**
PTH **Parathyroid hormone** (Also called **parathormone)**	Works with calcitonin to regulate the amount of calcium in the bloodstream.

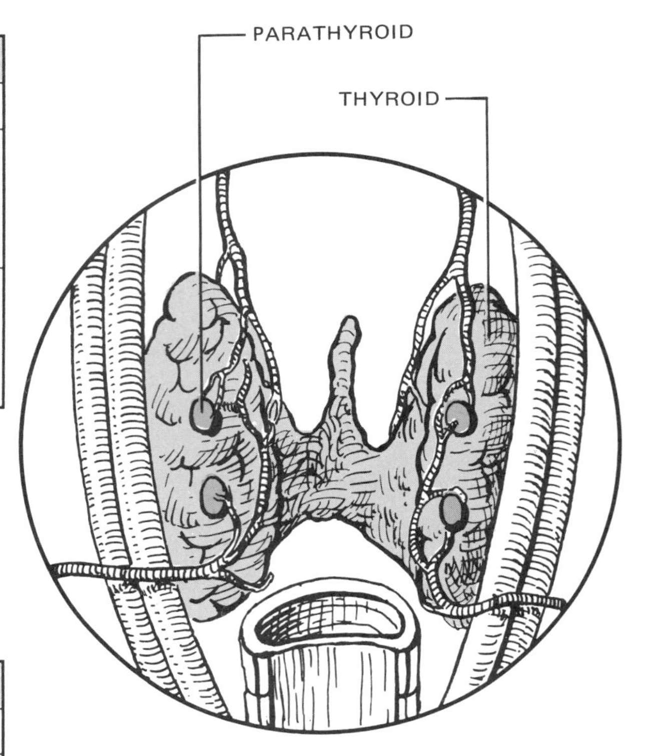

Figure 13-2 The thyroid and parathyroids.

THE ADRENAL GLANDS

The two small adrenal glands, also known as the **suprarenal glands,** are located one on top of each kidney. (The combining forms *ADREN/O* and *ADRENAL/O* both mean adrenal glands.)

Each gland consists of two parts: the **adrenal cortex,** the outer portion; and the **adrenal medulla,** which is the inner portion. (The combining form *CORTIC/O* means outer region and *MEDULL/O* means inner section.)

The adrenal cortex secretes three types of steroid hormones: **mineralocorticoids, glucocorticoids** and **androgens.**

Steroids are a group of hormonal substances with a similar basic chemical structure. A **corticosteroid (kor-**tih-koh-**STEE-**roid) is any one of the hormones associated with the adrenal cortex.

The adrenal medulla secretes two hormones within the group called **catecholamines.**

THE ADRENAL CORTEX	
Hormone	**Function**
Aldosterone	A mineralocorticoid hormone, it regulates the amount of salts in the body.
Cortisol (Also called **hydrocortisone)**	A glucocorticoid, it regulates the quantities of carbohydrate, protein, and fat in the cells. It also regulates other physiological body processes, and has an anti-inflammatory effect.
Androgens	Maintain secondary sex characteristics.

THE ADRENAL MEDULLA	
Hormone	**Function**
Epinephrine (Also called **adrenaline)**	Stimulates the sympathetic nervous system. It is a powerful vasopressor stimulating cardiac activity and increasing blood pressure.
Norepinephrine (Also called **noradrenaline)**	Stimulates the sympathetic nervous system and raises blood pressure. It acts as a vasoconstrictor, vasopressor, and neurotransmitter.

THE PANCREAS

The pancreas is located behind the stomach. (The combining form *PANCREAT/O* means pancreas.) The pancreas also functions as part of the digestive system. (See Chapter 8.)

The **islets of Langerhans** (**EYE**-lets of **LAHNG**-er-hahnz) are specialized cells in the pancreas that secrete the hormones that play a major role in the metabolism of sugars and starches in the body.

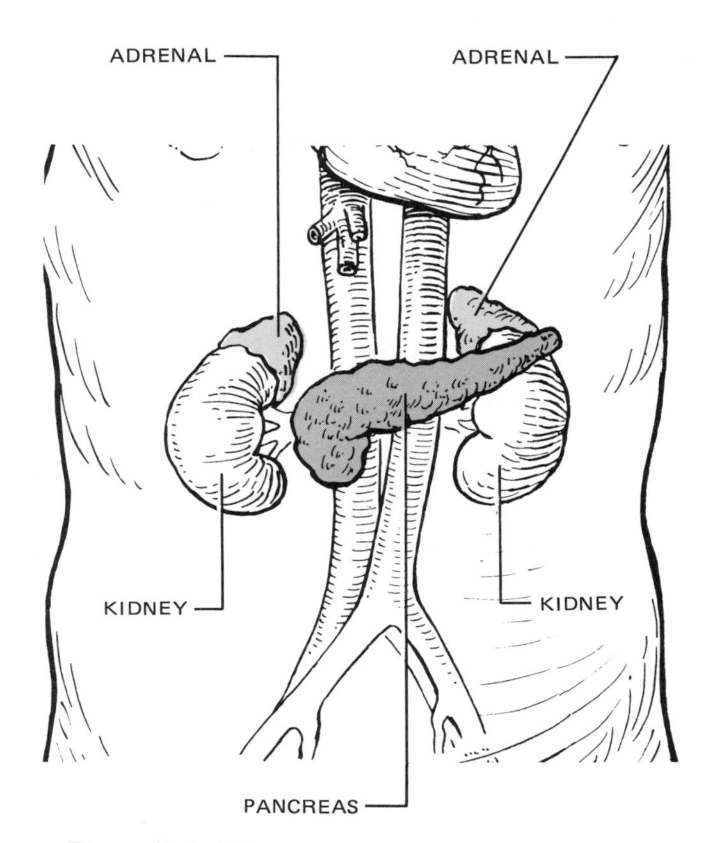

Figure 13-3 The adrenals and pancreas.

THE PANCREAS	
Hormone	**Function**
Insulin	Regulates the transport of glucose to the body cells.
Glucagon	Increases the amount of glucose in the bloodstream by stimulating the liver to convert glycogen into glucose.

THE THYMUS

The thymus (**THIGH**-mus), located behind the sternum, is fairly large in childhood but shrinks in size in adults. (The combining form *THYM/O* means thymus.)

THE THYMUS	
Hormone	**Function**
Thymosin	Secreted during infancy, it stimulates the production of antibodies against certain diseases.

THE PINEAL GLAND

The pineal gland **(PIN-ee-al)**, also known as the **pineal body**, is located in the central portion of the brain. (The combining form *PINEAL/O* means pineal gland.)

THE PINEAL GLAND	
Hormone	**Function**
Melatonin	Influences sexual maturation.
Serotonin	Acts as a neurotransmitter and vasoconstrictor. It also stimulates smooth muscles and inhibits gastric secretion.

THE GONADS

The gonads are the gamete-producing glands. These are the ovaries in females and testes in males. A **gonadotropic hormone (gon**-ah-doh-**TROP**-ick) is any hormone that stimulates the gonads.

THE OVARIES	
Hormone	**Function**
Estrogen	Is important in the development of secondary sex characteristics and regulation of the menstrual cycle. It is secreted by the ovaries.
Progesterone	Is released during the second half of the menstrual cycle by the corpus luteum in the ovary. Its function is to complete the preparations for pregnancy. If the ovum is not fertilized, secretion of this hormone ceases and is followed by the menstrual period.
HCG **Human chorionic gonadotropin**	Is secreted by the placenta which is formed when the fertilized egg is embedded in the uterus. This hormone stimulates the ovary to continue to produce progesterone and estrogen in order to maintain pregnancy.

continued ...

THE TESTES	
Hormone	**Function**
Testosterone	Stimulates the development of male secondary sex characteristics.

PATHOLOGY OF THE ENDOCRINE SYSTEM

General Pathology

- **Endocrinopathy (en**-doh-krih-**NOP**-ah-thee) is any disease due to a disorder of the endocrine system.
- **Adenosis (ad**-eh-**NO**-sis) is any disease condition of a gland.
- **Adenalgia (ad**-eh-NAL-jee-ah) is pain in a gland.
- **Hypocrinism (high**-poh-**KRY**-nism) is a condition caused by deficient secretion of any gland.
- **Adenomalacia (ad**-eh-no-mah-**LAY**-she-ah) is the abnormal softening of a gland.

- **Adenosclerosis (ad-**eh-no-sklee-**ROH-**sis) is the abnormal hardening of a gland.

Pathology of the Pituitary Gland

- **Pituitarism** (pih-**TOO-**ih-tar-izm) is any disorder of pituitary function.
- **Hypophysitis** (high-**pof-**ih-**SIGH-**tis) is an inflammation of the pituitary body.
- **Panhypopituitarism** (pan-**high-**poh-pih-**TOO-**ih-tar-izm) is a generalized insufficiency of pituitary hormones, resulting from damage to or deficiency of the gland.
- **Hyperpituitarism (high-**per-pih-**TOO-**ih-tah-rizm) is a condition due to hypersecretion of the pituitary.
- **Gigantism** is abnormal overgrowth of the body caused by hyperfunctioning of the pituitary gland before puberty.
- **Acromegaly (ack-**roh-**MEG-**ah-lee) is enlargement of the extremities (hands and feet) caused by hyperfunctioning of the pituitary gland after puberty.
- **Pituitary dwarfism** is caused by the congenital hyposecretion of somatotropin. Affected children develop normally mentally, but their bones remain small and underdeveloped.

  Achondroplastic dwarfism is a genetic defect in cartilage formation that usually results in a relatively large head and short extremities.
- **Diabetes insipidus (dye-**ah-**BEE-**teez) is a metabolic disorder characterized by extreme polydipsia and polyuria. It is caused by deficient production of the antidiuretic hormone (ADH) or by the inability of the kidneys to respond to ADH.

  Polydipsia (pol-ee-**DIP-**see-ah) is excessive thirst.

  Polyuria (pol-ee-**YOU-**ree-ah) is excessive urination.

Pathology of the Thyroid Gland

- **Thyroiditis** (thigh-roi-**DYE-**tis) is an inflammation of the thyroid gland.
- **Hyperthyroidism** is a condition caused by excessive secretion of the thyroid gland that is marked by an increased metabolic rate, goiter and disturbances in the autonomic nervous system.
- **Hypothyroidism** is a deficiency of thyroid secretion that is usually marked by decreased metabolic rate and lethargy.

  Lethargy is a condition of drowsiness or indifference.

  Myxedema (mick-seh-**DEE-**mah), also known as **nonpitting edema,** is one result of hypothyroidism. It is a condition with abnormal deposits of mucin in the skin and other tissues. (The suffix *-DEMA* means swelling.)
- **Cretinism (CREE-**tin-izm) is arrested physical and mental development due to a congenital lack of thyroid secretion.
- **Thyrotoxicosis (thy-**roh-**tock-**sih- **KOH-**sis) is a life-threatening condition resulting from overactivity of the thyroid gland.
- **Goiter (GOI-**ter), also known as **thyromegaly (thigh-**roh-**MEG-**ah-lee), is an abnormal enlargement of the thyroid gland.

  Endemic goiter is enlargement of the thyroid gland due to deficiency of iodine in the diet.

  Exophthalmic goiter, also known as **Graves' Disease, toxic goiter** and **hyperthyroidism,** is caused by excessive thyroxine secretion.

  Exophthalmos (eck-sof-**THAL-**mos), which is protrusion of the eyeballs, is one of the more common symptoms of exophthalmic goiter.

Pathology of the Parathyroid Glands

- **Hypoparathyroidism** (**high**-poh-**par**-ah-**THIGH**-roid-izm) is deficient secretion of the parathyroid glands. It is usually accompanied by **hypocalcemia,** which is abnormally low blood calcium. Severe hypoparathyroidism leads to tetany.

  Tetany (**TET**-ah-nee) is a syndrome manifested by sharp flexion (bending) of the wrist and ankle joints, muscle twitching, cramps and convulsions.

- **Hyperparathyroidism** (**high**-per-**par**-ah-**THIGH**-roid-izm) results from over secretion of parathormone and leads to hypercalcemia (excessive amounts of calcium in the blood).

  Hypercalcemia may result in the bones becoming decalcified and being susceptible to cyst formation and spontaneous fractures.

Pathology of the Adrenal Glands

- **Adrenopathy** (**ad**-ren-**OP**-ah-thee) is any disease of the adrenal gland.
- **Adrenalitis** (ah-**dree**-nal-**EYE**-tis), also known as **adrenitis,** is an inflammation of the adrenal glands.
- **Addison's disease** is a life-threatening condition caused by partial or complete failure of adrenocortical function.
- **Aldosteronism** (**al**-doh-**STER**-on-izm), also called **hyperaldosteronism,** is an abnormality of electrolyte balance caused by excessive secretion of aldosterone.

  Electrolytes are substances, such as sodium and potassium, that are found in the blood.

  Primary aldosteronism, also known as **Conn's syndrome,** is aldosteronism due to disorders of the adrenal gland.

  Secondary aldosteronism is aldosteronism due to disorders outside of the adrenal gland.

- **Cushing's disease** is a metabolic disorder of abnormally increased secretion of adrenocortical steroids.
- **Pheochromocytoma** (fee-oh-**kroh**-moh-sigh-**TOH**-mah) is a tumor occurring in the adrenal medulla.

Pathology of the Pancreas

- **Hyperinsulinism** is excessive insulin in the blood stream. This may result in insulin shock.
- An **insuloma** (**in**-soo-**LOH**-mah) is a tumor of the islets of Langerhans.

Diabetes Mellitus

Diabetes mellitus is not a single disease. Instead it is a complex metabolic disorder that is the result of inadequate insulin secretion. (Diabetes insipidus is not part of this group.)

- **Insulin-dependent diabetes mellitus,** also called **Type I** or **juvenile diabetes,** is an inability to metabolize carbohydrates that is caused by an insulin deficiency. It usually occurs in children and control is dependent upon insulin.
- **Non-insulin-dependent diabetes mellitus,** also known as **Type II** and **maturity onset diabetes,** is a form of diabetes that most frequently develops after 40 years of age. It can usually be controlled by diet and without dependence on insulin.
- **Diabetic ketoacidosis** (**key**-toh-**ah**-sih-**DOH**-sis) is acidosis accompanied by the excessive accumulation of ketone bodies (metabolic byproducts) in the body tissues and fluids. It is an acute life-threatening complication of uncontrolled diabetes mellitus.

  Acidosis is an abnormal accumulation of acid in the blood and body tissues.

Pathology of the Gonads

- **Hypergonadism** (**high**-per-**GO**-nad-izm) is the condition of excessive secretion of hormones by the sex glands.
- **Hypogonadism** (**high**-poh-**GO**-nad-izm) is the condition of deficient secretion of hormones by the sex glands.

Pathology of the Pineal Gland

- **Pinealopathy** (**pin**-ee-ah-**LOP**-ah-thee) is any disorder of the pineal gland.
- A **pinealoma** (**pin**-ee-ah-**LOH**-mah) is a tumor of the pineal body (gland).

Pathology of the Thymus Gland

- **Thymitis** (thigh-**MY**-tis) is an inflammation of the thymus gland.

PROCEDURES RELATED TO THE ENDOCRINE SYSTEM

- **Adenectomy** (**ad**-eh-**NECK**-toh-me) is the surgical removal of a gland.
- **Hypophysectomy** (high-**pof**-ih-**SECK**-toh-me) is the surgical removal of the pituitary gland.
- A **thyroidectomy** (**thigh**-roi-**DECK**-toh-me) is the surgical removal of the thyroid gland.
- A **lobectomy** (loh-**BECK**-toh-me) is the removal of one lobe of the thyroid.
- **Parathyroidectomy** (**par**-ah-**thigh**-roi-**DECK**-toh-me) is the surgical removal of one or more of the parathyroid glands.
- **Adrenalectomy** (ah-**dree**-nal-**ECK**-toh-me) is the surgical removal of one or both adrenal glands.
- **Thymectomy** (thigh-**MECK**-toh-me) is the surgical removal of the thymus gland.
- **Pinealectomy** (**pin**-ee-al-**ECK**-toh-me) is the surgical removal of the pineal body.

IMPORTANT TERMS: THE ENDOCRINE SYSTEM

This list will help you identify and review the major terms from this chapter.

When you work with the audio tape for this chapter, listen to the word, repeat it and then place a ✓ next to it on the list below.

- ☐ **Acromegaly** (**ack**-roh-**MEG**-ah-lee)
- ☐ **Adenalgia** (**ad**-eh-**NAL**-jee-ah)
- ☐ **Adenectomy** (**ad**-eh-**NECK**-toh-me)
- ☐ **Adenohypophysis** (**ad**-eh-no-high-**POF**-ih-sis)
- ☐ **Adenomalacia** (**ad**-eh-no-mah-**LAY**-she-ah)
- ☐ **Adenosclerosis** (**ad**-eh-no-sklee-**ROH**-sis)
- ☐ **Adenosis** (**ad**-eh-**NO**-sis)
- ☐ **Adrenalectomy** (ah-**dree**-nal-**ECK**-toh-me)
- ☐ **Adrenalitis** (ah-**dree**-nal-**EYE**-tis)
- ☐ **Adrenopathy** (**ad**-ren-**OP**-ah-thee)
- ☐ **Aldosteronism** (**al**-doh-**STER**-on-izm)
- ☐ **Corticosteroid** (**kor**-tih-koh-**STEE**-roid)
- ☐ **Cretinism** (**CREE**-tin-izm)
- ☐ **Diabetes** (**dye**-ah-**BEE**-teez)
- ☐ **Endocrinopathy** (**en**-doh-krih-**NOP**-ah-thee)
- ☐ **Endocrine** (**EN**-doh-krin)
- ☐ **Exocrine** (**ECK**-soh-krin)
- ☐ **Exophthalmos** (**eck**-sof-**THAL**-mos)
- ☐ **Goiter** (**GOI**-ter)
- ☐ **Gonadotropic** (**gon**-ah-doh-**TROP**-ick)

- ☐ **Hypergonadism (high-**per-**GO-**nad-izm)
- ☐ **Hyperparathyroidism (high-**per-**par-**ah-**THIGH-**roid-izm)
- ☐ **Hyperpituitarism (high-**per-pih-**TOO-**ih-tah-rizm)
- ☐ **Hypocrinism (high-**poh-**KRY-**nism)
- ☐ **Hypogonadism (high-**poh-**GO-**nad-izm)
- ☐ **Hypoparathyroidism (high-**poh-**par-**ah-**THIGH-**roid-izm)
- ☐ **Hypophysis** (high-**POF-**ih-sis)
- ☐ **Hypophysectomy** (high-**pof-**ih-**SECK-**toh-me)
- ☐ **Hypophysitis** (high-**pof-**ih-**SIGH-**tis)
- ☐ **Insuloma (in-**soo-**LOH-**mah)
- ☐ **Islets of Langerhans (EYE-**lets of **LAHNG-**er-hahnz)
- ☐ **Ketoacidosis (key-**toh-**ah-**sih-**DOH-**sis)
- ☐ **Lobectomy** (loh-**BECK-**toh-me)
- ☐ **Myxedema (mick-**seh-**DEE-**mah)
- ☐ **Neurohypophysis (new-**roh-high-**POF-**ih-sis)
- ☐ **Panhypopituitarism** (pan-**high-**poh-pih-**TOO-**ih-tar-izm)
- ☐ **Parathyroidectomy (par-**ah-**thigh-**roi-**DECK-**toh-me)
- ☐ **Pheochromocytoma** (fee-oh-**kroh-**moh-sigh-**TOH-**mah)
- ☐ **Pineal (PIN-**ee-al)
- ☐ **Pinealectomy (pin-**ee-al-**ECK-**toh-me)
- ☐ **Pinealoma (pin-**ee-ah-**LOH-**mah)
- ☐ **Pinealopathy (pin-**ee-ah-**LOP-**ah-thee)
- ☐ **Pituitary** (pih-**TOO-**ih-**tair-**ee)
- ☐ **Pituitarism** (pih-**TOO-**ih-tar-izm)
- ☐ **Polydipsia (pol-**ee-**DIP-**see-ah)
- ☐ **Polyuria (pol-**ee-**YOU-**ree-ah)
- ☐ **Tetany (TET-**ah-nee)
- ☐ **Thymectomy** (thigh-**MECK-**toh-me)
- ☐ **Thymitis** (thigh-**MY-**tis)
- ☐ **Thymus (THIGH-**mus)
- ☐ **Thyroiditis** (thigh-roi-**DYE-**tis)
- ☐ **Thyroidectomy (thigh-**roi-**DECK-**toh-me)
- ☐ **Thyromegaly (thigh-**roh-**MEG-**ah-lee)
- ☐ **Thyrotoxicosis (thy-**roh-**tock-**sih-**KOH-**sis)

13

EXERCISES

DEFINING WORD PARTS

Write the definition for each of these word parts.

1. *ADREN/O, ADRENAL/O* ______________________________
2. *CORTIC/O* ______________________________
3. *CRIN/O* ______________________________
4. *-DEMA* ______________________________
5. *MEDULL/O* ______________________________
6. *PANCREAT/O* ______________________________
7. *PINEAL/O* ______________________________
8. *PITUIT/O* ______________________________
9. *THYM/O* ______________________________
10. *THYR/O, THYROID/O* ______________________________

DEFINITIONS

Circle the letter next to the correct answer.

1. The ______________ gland secretes melatonin.
   a) adrenal
   b) parathyroid
   c) pineal
   d) thymus

2. The _______________ hormone stimulates ovulation and is important in maintaining pregnancy.
   a) follicle-stimulating
   b) growth
   c) luteinizing
   d) parathyroid

3. The _______________ gland is also known as the hypophysis.
   a) adrenal
   b) pineal
   c) pituitary
   d) thymus

4. _______________, which regulates the amount of glucose in the bloodstream, is secreted by the pancreas.
   a) Adrenaline
   b) Glucagon
   c) Serotonin
   d) Thymosin

5. _______________ stimulates the development of the male secondary sex characteristics.
   a) Aldosterone
   b) Gonadotropin
   c) Progesterone
   d) Testosterone

6. _______________ regulates the rate of metabolism and influences physical and mental development.
   a) Cortisol
   b) Norepinephrine
   c) Oxytocin
   d) Thyroxine

7. The _______________ is fairly large in childhood but shrinks in size in adults.
   a) hypophysis
   b) pineal gland
   c) thymus
   d) thyroid

8. The _______________ hormone secreted by the pituitary stimulates the growth and secretion of the adrenal cortex.
   a) adrenocorticotropic
   b) growth
   c) interstitial cell-stimulating
   d) somatotropin

9. ______________ works with the parathyroid hormone to regulate calcium levels in the blood and tissues.
   a) Calcitonin
   b) Luteotropin
   c) Prolactin
   d) Thyroxine

10. ______________ stimulates the sympathetic nervous system and raises blood pressure.
   a) Adrenaline
   b) Cortisol
   c) Norepinephrine
   d) Vasopressin

MISSING WORDS

Write the missing word on the line.

1. ______________________ is a condition of drowsiness or indifference.
2. The islets of Langerhans are located in the ______________________.
3. ______________________ are substances, such as sodium and potassium, that are found in the blood.
4. ______________________ also known as nonpitting edema, is one result of hypothyroidism.
5. ______________________ is the condition of excessive secretion of hormones by the sex glands.
6. ______________________ glands secrete their chemicals directly into the bloodstream.
7. The ______________________-stimulating hormone increases pigmentation of the skin.
8. A/an ______________________ is a chemical substance that regulates the activity of certain cells and/or organs.
9. The ______________________ gland secretes calcitonin and thyroxine.
10. The ______________________ hormone, which is also called parathormone, works with calcitonin to regulate the amount of calcium in the blood stream.
11. Norepinephrine is secreted by the ______________________ ______________________.
12. The ______________________ hormone, which is also called prolactin or luteotropin, stimulates the secretion of milk and influences maternal behavior.
13. The ______________________ hormone, also called somatotropin, accelerates body growth.
14. The ______________________ gland secretes melatonin, which influences sexual maturation.
15. The ______________________ are the male gonads.

SPELLCHECK

Select the correct spelling and write it on the line.

1. ______________________ are a group of hormonal substances with a similar basic chemical structure.
   Stereoroids
   Steriods
   Steroids

2. ______________________ insipidus is a metabolic disorder.
   Diabetes
   Diabites
   Diebetes

3. The anti-______________________ hormone maintains the body's water balance by reducing urinary output.
   diaretic
   dieretic
   diuretic

4. ______________________ is a powerful vasopressor that stimulates cardiac activity and increases blood pressure.
   Epanehprine
   Epinaphrine
   Epinephrine

5. ______________________ is another name for the hormone in question #4.
   Adraneline
   Adrenaline
   Adreniline

6. ______________________ regulates the transport of glucose to the body cells.
   Insilen
   Insolin
   Insulin

7. ______________________ regulates several physiologic body processes and has an anti-inflammatory effect.
   Hydracortisone
   Hydrocortesone
   Hydrocortisone

8. ______________________ is important in the development of female secondary sex characteristics.
   Estragen
   Estragon
   Estrogen

9. ______________________ is a syndrome manifested by sharp flexion of the wrist and ankle joints.
   Tateny
   Tetany
   Tetony

10. ______________________ is an abnormal accumulation of acid in the blood and body tissues.
    Acidaosis
    Acidiosis
    Acidosis

11. The female hormone ______________________ is released during the second half of the menstrual cycle.
    progestarone
    progesterone
    progisterone

12. The ______________________ gland is located at the base of the brain.
    patuitery
    petuitary
    pituitary

13. The ______________________ is a butterfly-shaped gland.
    thiroid
    thyroid
    tryoid

14. Thymosin is secreted by the ______________________.
    thiamus
    thimus
    thymus

15. The ______________________ are the gamete-producing glands.
    ganads
    gonads
    gonioads

CASE STUDIES

Write the correct answer on the line.

1. Theodore Sturgeon suffers from ____________________ which is an abnormal enlargement of the thyroid gland.
2. Joseph Butler complains of being thirsty all the time. The doctor listed this on his chart as ____________________ or excessive thirst.
3. Adrianne Morrison has ____________________ ____________________ which is a metabolic disorder characterized by excessive thirst and excessive urination.
4. Linda Thomas has ____________________ disease, which is a life-threatening condition caused by partial or complete failure of adrenocortical function.
5. Patty Edward, who is 7 years old, requires daily insulin injections to control her Type I (insulin-dependent) ____________________ ____________________.
6. Ronald Laws suffers from ____________________ disease, which is a metabolic disorder of abnormally increased secretion of adrenocortical steriods.
7. Bruce Ivy has ____________________ which is accompanied by abnormally low blood calcium. In a severe case this may lead to tetany.
8. Janet Mohan was rushed to the hospital with ____________________ which may lead to insulin shock.
9. Leigh Franklin has ____________________ which is characterized by extremely large hands and feet.
10. Due to a congenital lack of thyroid secretion, the Vaugh-Eames child suffers from ____________________.
11. Joyce Atkinson has ____________________ which is also called nonpitting edema.
12. Allen Jensen has been diagnosed as having ____________________ ____________________ which is also known as Conn's syndrome.
13. Raymond Grovenor is excessively tall and large. His ____________________ was caused by hyperfunction of the pituitary gland before puberty.
14. Mr. Covington underwent ____________________. This surgical procedure was performed to remove a diseased adrenal gland.
15. Iris Gilmer has a relatively large head and short extremities. Her medical records shown that she suffers from the genetic defect ____________________ dwarfism.

WORD BUILDING

Write the correct word or word part on the line.

1. Inflammation of the thymus
   a) The combining form ______________________ means thymus.
   b) The suffix ______________________ means inflammation.
   c) The term ______________________ means an inflammation of the thymus.
2. Surgical removal of the thyroid
   a) The combining form ______________________ means thyroid.
   b) The suffix ______________________ means surgical removal.
   c) The term ______________________ means surgical removal of the thyroid gland.
3. Tumor of the pineal gland
   a) The combining form ______________________ means pineal gland or body.
   b) The suffix ______________________ means tumor.
   c) The term ______________________ means a tumor of the pineal body.

LABELING EXERCISES

Identify the numbered items on this diagram.

1. ______________________
2. ______________________
3. ______________________
4. ______________________
5. ______________________
6. ______________________
7. ______________________
8. ______________________
9. ______________________

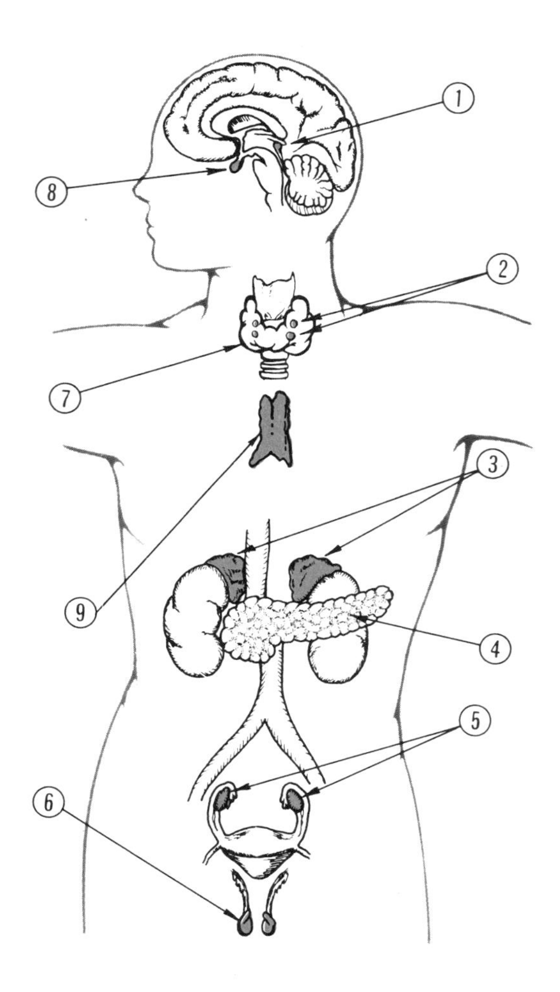

14

THE REPRODUCTIVE SYSTEMS

LEARNING GOALS

In this chapter you will learn to:

- identify the major organs and functions of the male reproductive system.
- recognize and define the terms related to the diagnosis, pathology and treatment of disorders of the male reproductive system.
- identify the major organs and functions of the female reproductive system.
- recognize and define the terms related to the diagnosis, pathology and treatment of disorders of the female reproductive system.
- describe pregnancy, childbirth and the postpartum period and the pathology and procedures related to them.

INTRODUCTION TO THE REPRODUCTIVE SYSTEMS

The major male reproductive organs, which are located outside the body, include two testes, seminal ducts, and the penis.

The major female reproductive organs are located in the pelvic cavity and are protected by the bony pelvis. They include two ovaries, two fallopian tubes, one uterus, and the vagina.

THE MALE REPRODUCTIVE SYSTEM

The Scrotum

The scrotum (**SKROH**-tum), also known as the **scrotal sac,** is an external sac that encloses and supports the testes. It is suspended from the pubic arch behind the penis and lies between the thighs.

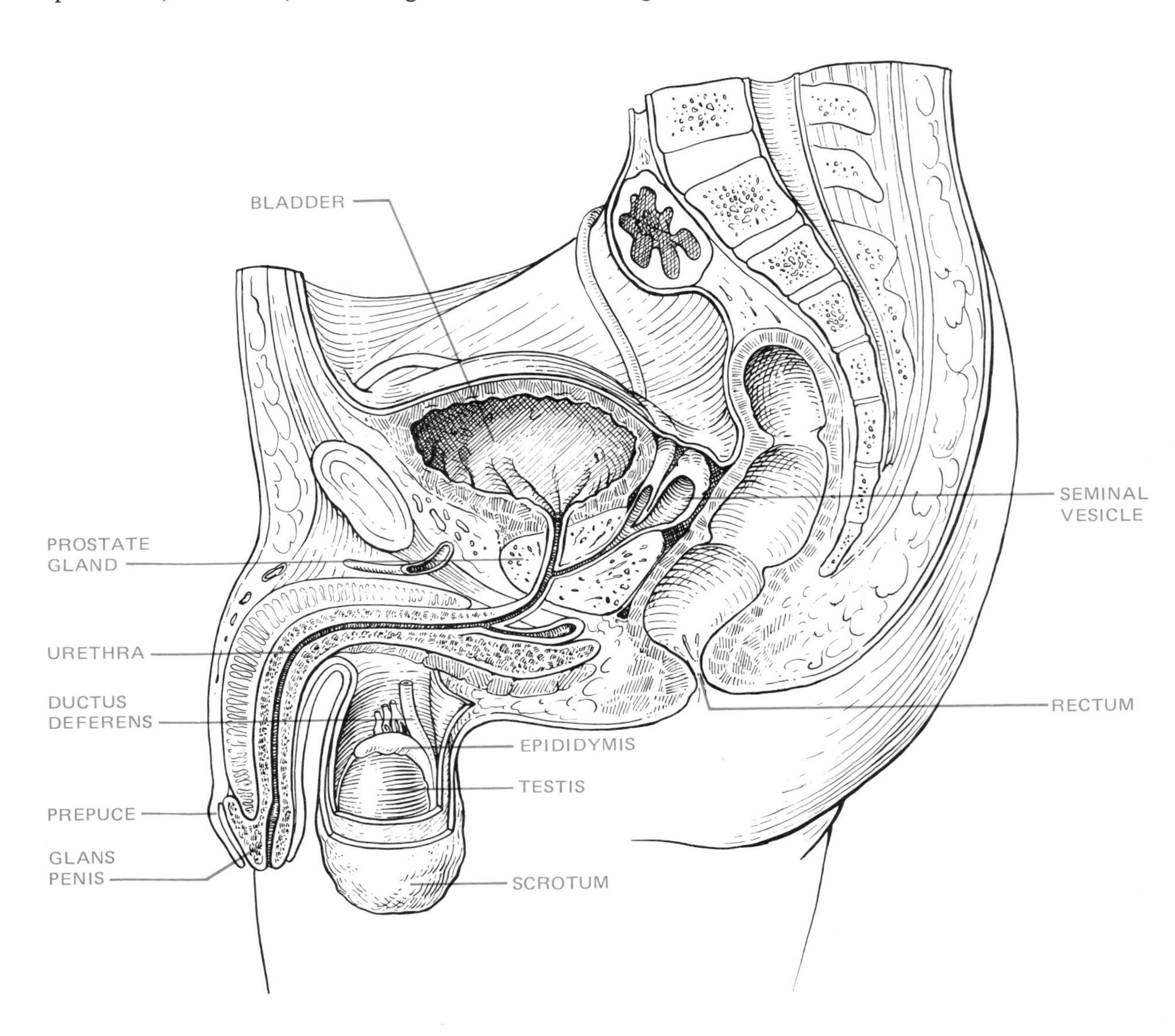

Figure 14-1 Structures of the male reproductive system.

The Spermatic Cord

The spermatic cord consists of the vas deferens plus the blood and lymph vessels and nerves that supply each testis. These are bound together by connective tissue and pass from the testes in the scrotum, through the abdominal wall (via the inguinal canal) and into the pelvic cavity.

The Testes

The testes, also known as **testicles,** are two small, ovoid glands suspended from the inguinal region by the spermatic cord and surrounded by the scrotum. (The combining forms *DIDYM/O, ORCH/O, ORCHI/O* and *ORCHID/O* all mean testes.) (Singular, **testis.**)

The testes develop within the abdomen of the male fetus and normally descend into the scrotum before birth. After puberty they produce the hormone testosterone which stimulates and promotes the growth of secondary sex characteristics in the male.

Spermatozoa

Spermatozoa (**sper**-mah-toh-**ZOH**-ah), also known as **sperm,** are the male gametes. (A **gamete** (**GAM**-eet) is a sex cell.)

Sperm are manufactured by the **seminiferous tubules** (**see**-mih-**NIF**-er-us) within the testes. (The combining forms *SPERM/O* and *SPERMAT/O* both mean spermatozoa.) (Singular, **spermatozoon.**)

The Epididymis

The epididymis (**ep**-ih-**DID**-ih-mis) is a tube at the upper part of each testis. It runs down the length of the testicle and then turns upward again and becomes a narrower tube called the vas deferens.

As sperm are formed they move through the seminiferous tubules and are collected in the epididymis where the spermatozoa become motile and are temporarily stored. (**Motile** means capable of spontaneous motion).

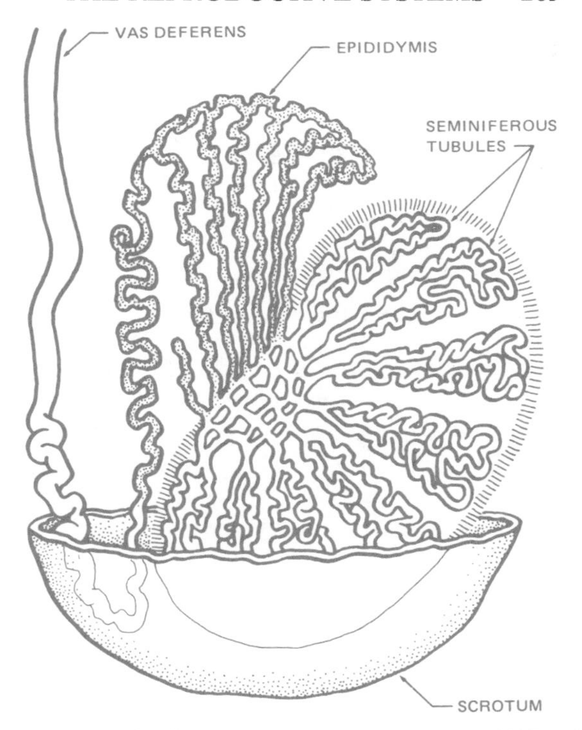

Figure 14-2 The seminiferous tubules, epididymis and vas deferens.

The Vas Deferens

The vas deferens (vas **DEF**-er-enz) carries the sperm up into the pelvic region, around the urinary bladder, and then down toward the urethra. The **ductus deferens,** at the end of the vas deferens, is the excretory duct of the testes.

The Seminal Vesicles

The seminal vesicles (**SEM**-ih-nal) are glands located at the base of the urinary bladder that open into the vas deferens as it joins the urethra. They secrete a thick, yellowish substance that nourishes the sperm cells and forms much of the volume of ejaculated semen.

The **ejaculatory duct** is one of the two final portions of the seminal vessels. It is formed by the union of the ductus deferens (from the vas deferens) and the duct from the seminal vesicle. These ducts pass through the prostate gland and enter the urethra.

Semen

Semen (**SEE**-men) is the ejaculatory fluid that contains sperm plus the secretions of the seminal vesicles, prostate gland and Cowper's glands. (The combining form *SEMIN/I* means semen or sperm.)

The Prostate Gland

The prostate gland almost encircles the upper end of the urethra in the region where the vas deferens enters the urethra. (The combining form *PROSTAT/O* means prostate gland.)

The prostate gland secretes a thick fluid that, as part of the semen, aids the motility of the sperm.

Cowper's Glands

Cowper's glands, also known as **bulbourethral glands** (**bul**-boh-you-**REE**-thral), are located on either side of the urethra just below the prostate gland, and their ducts open into the urethra.

These glands secrete a thick mucus that acts as a lubricant and that tends to flow early during sexual excitement.

The Urethra

The urethra passes through the penis to the outside of the body. It serves both the reproductive and urinary systems.

The Penis

The penis is the male sex organ that transports the sperm into the female vagina. (The combining forms *PEN/I* and *PRIAP/O* mean penis.)

At the tip of the penis there is a soft, sensitive region called the **glans penis** (glanz **PEE**-nis). The **prepuce** (**PRE**-pyous), also known as the **foreskin,** covers and protects the glans penis.

The penis is composed of erectile tissue which, during sexual stimulation, fills with blood (under high pressure) and causes an erection.

THE FEMALE REPRODUCTIVE SYSTEM

The Ovaries

The ovaries (**OH**-vah-rees) are a pair of small almond-shaped organs located in the lower abdomen, one on either side of the uterus. (The combining forms *OOPHOR/O* and *OVARI/O* both mean ovary.)

The ovaries produce the hormones estrogen and progesterone. **Estrogen** is responsible for the development and maintenance of the female secondary sex characteristics. **Progesterone** is responsible for the preparation and maintenance of the uterus in pregnancy.

The ovaries contain thousands of small sacs called **graafian follicles** (**GRAF**-ee-an **FOL**-lick-kulz). Each graafian follicle contains a single ovum.

These **ova** (**OH**-vah) are the female gametes. (The combining forms *OO/O, OV/I* and *OV/O* all mean ovum or egg.) (Singular, **ovum.**)

The Fallopian Tubes

The fallopian tubes (fal-**LOH**-pee-an), also known as **oviducts** or **uterine tubes,** are ducts that extend from the upper end of the uterus to a point near, but not attached to, each ovary. (The combining form *SALPING/O* means relating to fallopian tubes.)

The **infundibulum** (**in**-fun-**DIB**-you-lum) is the funnel-shaped opening into the fallopian tube. This opening ends in finger-like extensions called **fimbriae** (**FIM**-bree-ee) that catch the ovum when it leaves the ovary. (Singular, **fimbria.**)

The fallopian tube serves primarily as a duct to convey the ovum from the ovary to the uterus. However, it also conveys sperm traveling upward from the vagina and uterus. Fertilization actually takes place in the fallopian tube.

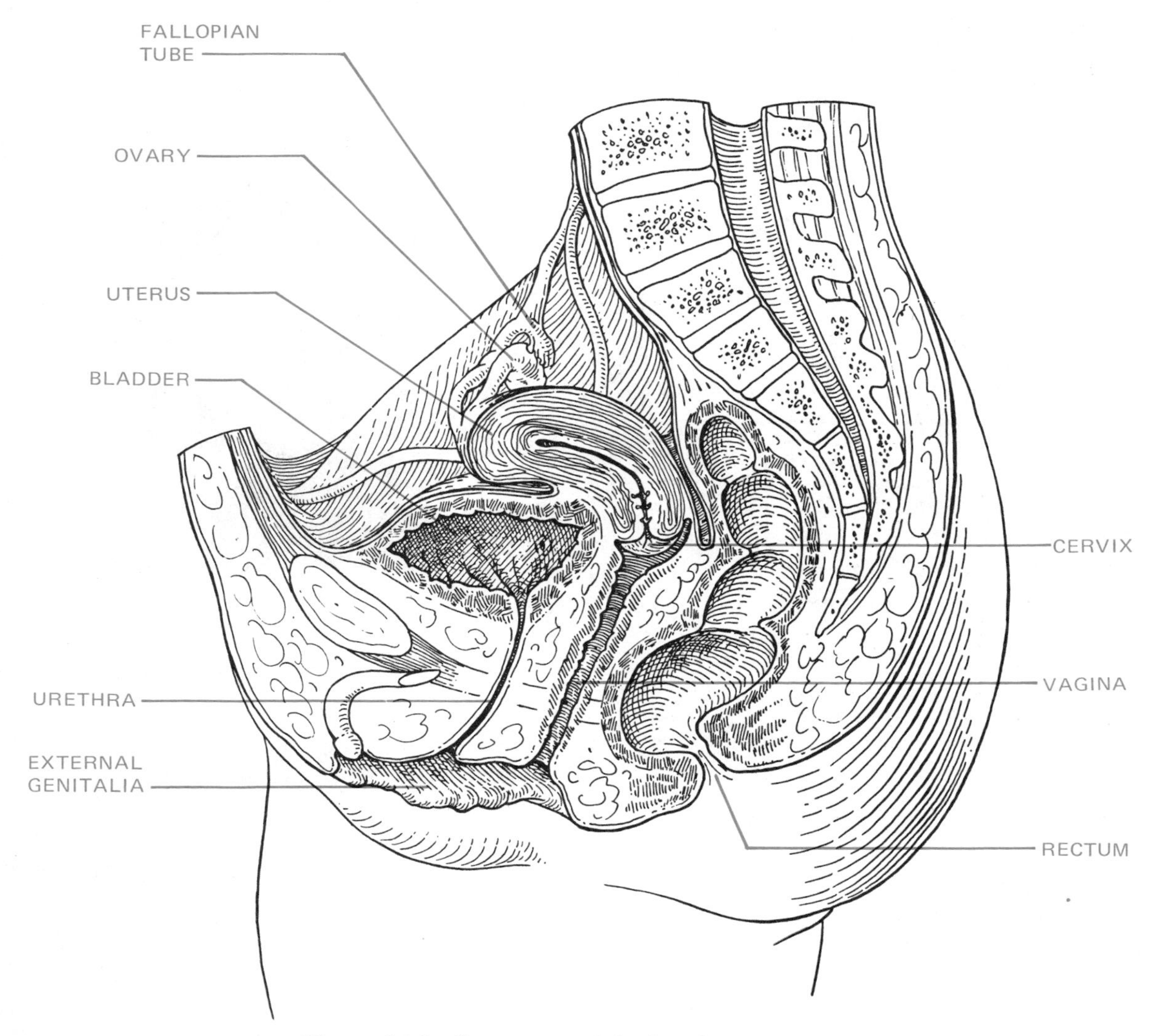

Figure 14-3 Structures of the female reproductive system.

The Uterus

The uterus (**YOU**-ter-us), also known as the **womb,** is a pear-shaped organ with muscular walls and a mucous membrane lining filled with a rich supply of blood vessels. (The combining forms *HYSTER/O, METR/O, METRI/O* and *UTER/O* all mean uterus.)

The uterus is situated between the urinary bladder and the rectum and midway between the sacrum and the pubic bone. The normal position of the uterus is bent forward in a position called **anteflexion.** (The prefix *ANTE-* means forward and the combining form *FLEX/O* means bend.)

The Parts of the Uterus
The **fundus (FUN-dus),** is the bulging rounded part above the entrance of the fallopian tubes. (The combining form *FUND/O* means base or bottom.)
The **corpus (KOR-pus),** also known as the body, is the middle portion (The combining form *CORP/U* means body.)
The **cervix (SER-vicks),** also known as the **cervix uteri,** is the lower narrow portion that extends into the vagina. (The combining form *CERVIC/O* means cervix.)

The Layers of the Uterus
The **perimetrium** (per-ih-ME-tree-um) is the membranous outer layer. (The prefix *PERI-* means surrounding.)
The **myometrium** (my-oh-ME-tree-um) is the muscular middle layer. (The combining form *MY/O* means muscle.)
The **endometrium** (en-doh-ME-tree-um) is the inner layer that consists of specialized epithelial mucosa. (The prefix *ENDO-* means within.)

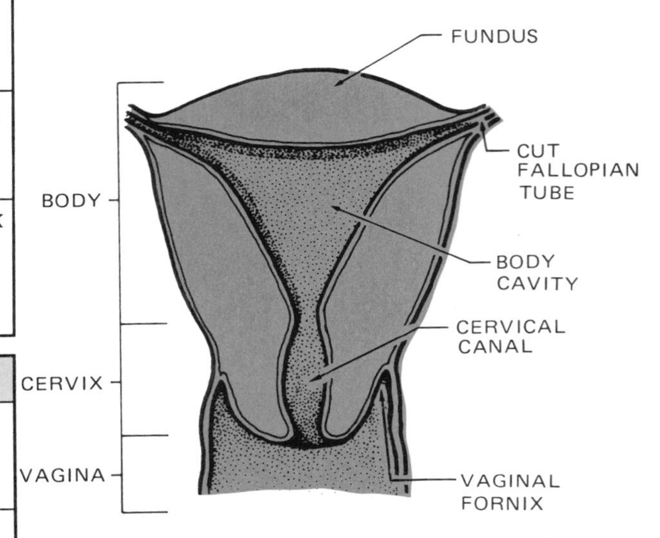

Figure 14-4 The uterus and surrounding tissues.

The Vagina

The vagina (vah-JYE-nah) is a muscular tube lined with mucosa that extends from the cervix to the outside of the body. (The combining forms *COLP/O* and *VAGIN/O* both mean vagina.)

The **vaginal fornix (FOR-nicks)** is the space within the vagina that surrounds the cervix. (Plural **fornices.**)

The **hymen (HIGH-men)** is a membranous fold of tissue that partly or completely covers the external vaginal orifice. (An **orifice** is an entrance into, or an outlet from, a body cavity or canal.)

The External Female Genitalia

The term **genitalia (jen-ih-TAY-lee-ah)** means reproductive organs. The external genitalia are those reproductive organs located outside of the body cavity.

The female external genitalia are located below the **mons pubis** (monz **PYOU**-bis) which is the rounded fleshy prominence over the pubic symphysis.

The female external genitalia are also known as the **vulva (VUL-vah)** or the **pudendum (pyou-DEN-dum).** (The combining form *VULV/O* means vulva.)

The Labia

The **labia majora** and **labia minora** protect the external genitalia and the urethral meatus. (The **urethral meatus** is the external opening of the urethra.)

The Clitoris

The clitoris (**KLIT**-oh-ris) is an organ of sensitive, erectile tissue located anterior to the vaginal orifice and in front of the urethral meatus.

Bartholin's glands

Bartholin's glands are two small, rounded glands on either side of the vaginal opening which produce a mucus secretion that lubricates the vagina.

The Perineum

The perineum (per-ih-**NEE**-um) is the region between the vaginal orifice and the anus. (The combining form *PERINE/O* means perineum.)

The Mammary Glands

The mammary glands, also known as **breasts,** are milk-producing glands that develop in response to hormones from the ovaries during puberty. (The combining form *MAMM/O* means breast and *MAST/O* means breast or nipple.)

Each breast is fixed to the overlying skin and the underlying pectoral muscles by suspensory ligaments. The **nipple,** also known as the **mammary papilla,** is surrounded by the **areola** (ah-**REE**-oh-lah), which is the dark-pigmented area.

The breasts consist of **mammary glands,** which are also known as **lactiferous glands** (lack-**TIF**-er-us), that produce milk.

The **lactiferous duct** carries milk to the nipple. (The combining forms *LACT/I* and *LACT/O* mean milk.)

OVULATION

Normally each month one ovum matures, ruptures from its graafian follicle and through the surface of the ovary. This process is called **ovulation (oh**-view-**LAY**-shun), and it is during this time that the female is fertile.

After the ovum has been released, the ruptured graafian follicle enlarges, takes on a yellow fatty substance and becomes the **corpus luteum (KOR**-pus **LOO**-tee-um). (The combining form *LUTE/O* means yellow.)

The corpus luteum then secretes the hormone progesterone, which maintains the growth of the uterine lining in preparation for the fertilized egg.

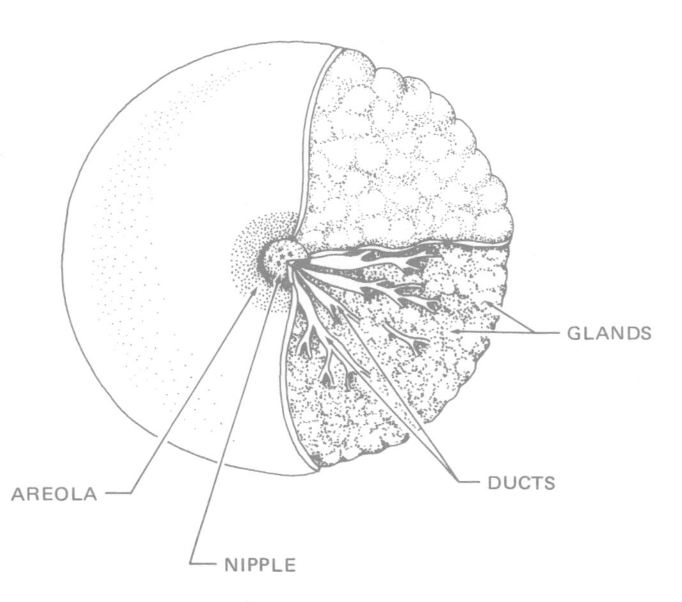

Figure 14-5 Structures of a breast.

After the ovum is released from the ovary it is caught up by the fimbriae of the fallopian tube. Peristaltic action and the small hairs that line the fallopian tube move the ovum toward the uterus.

It usually takes the ovum about five days to pass through the fallopian tube. If sperm are present, fertilization takes place within the fallopian tube.

If the ovum is not fertilized it dies, the corpus luteum degenerates, progesterone production stops and the endometrium sloughs off as the menstrual flow.

THE MENSTRUAL CYCLE

Menstruation (men-stroo-**AY**-shun), also known as **menses (MEN**-seez), is the normal periodic discharge of the superficial layers of the endometrium of the uterus along with some blood. (The combining forms *MEN/O, MENSTRU/O* and *MENSTRUAT/O* mean menstruation or taking place monthly.)

The flow is called **menorrhea** (**men**-oh-**REE**-ah); and **menarche** (meh-**NAR**-key) is the beginning of the menstrual function that occurs at the onset of puberty.

Puberty is the stage of life when the secondary sex characteristics begin to develop and the individual becomes capable of reproducing.

Menopause (**MEN**-oh-pawz), also known as the **climacteric** (klye-**MACK**-ter-ick), is the normal cessation (stopping) of the monthly flow. It usually occurs after the age of forty-five.

The Time Periods of the Menstrual Cycle

The average menstrual cycle consists of 28 days, grouped into four time periods:

Days 1-5 (Menstrual Period)
These are the days during which bloody fluid containing disintegrated endometrial cells, glandular secretions, and blood cells are discharged through the vagina.
Days 6-13 (Postmenstrual Period)
After the menstrual period is ended, the lining of the uterus begins to repair itself as the hormone estrogen is released by the maturing graafian follicle in the ovaries. This is also the period of the growth of the ovum in the graafian follicle.
Days 13-14 (Ovulatory Period)
On about the 14th day of the cycle, ovulation occurs and the egg leaves the ovary to travel slowly down the fallopian tube.
Days 15-28 (Premenstrual Period)
If fertilization does not occur, the levels of progesterone and estrogen fall and this leads to the breakdown of the uterine endometrium and the beginning of a new menstrual cycle (days 1-5).

FERTILIZATION

The union of ovum and sperm is called fertilization. **Conception** is the beginning of a new individual that results from fertilization.

During **coitus** (**KOH**-ih-tus), also known as **copulation** (**kop**-you-**LAY**-shun) or **sexual intercourse,** the male **ejaculates** approximately 100 million sperm cells into the female's vagina. (The combining form *EJACULAT/O* means to throw or hurl out.)

The sperm travel upward through the vagina, into the uterus and on into the fallopian tube, and it is here that fertilization takes place.

PREGNANCY

After fertilization occurs in the fallopian tube, the fertilized egg, called a **zygote** (**ZYE**-goht), travels to the uterus. The corpus luteum in the ovary continues to produce progesterone and estrogen, which continue preparation of the uterine lining.

Implantation is the attachment and embedding of the zygote within the endothelial lining of the uterus.

From this time, and up to the third month of pregnancy, the developing child is called an **embryo** (**EM**-bree-oh).

From the third month of pregnancy to the time of birth the unborn child is referred to as a **fetus** (**FEE**-tus). (The combining forms *FET/I* and *FET/O* mean fetus or unborn child in the womb.)

The Placenta

The placenta (plah-**SEN**-tah), also known as the **afterbirth,** allows the exchange of nutrients, oxygen and waste products between the mother and child without ever allowing maternal blood and fetal blood to mix.

The **umbilical cord** (um-**BIL**-ih-kal) is the structure that connects the fetus to the placenta. (The combining form *UMBILIC/O* means navel and the navel is formed where the umbilical cord was attached to the fetus.)

The outer layer of the placenta, the one that is attached to the uterine wall, is derived from maternal endometrium (the lining of the uterus).

The **chorion** (**KOH**-ree-on), which is the outermost membrane that surrounds the developing embryo, forms the inner layer of the placenta.

From the third month of pregnancy onward the placenta produces its own hormone, **human chorionic gonadotropin** (**koh**-ree-**ON**-ick **gon**-ah-doh-**TROH**-pin). This hormone stimulates the ovary to continue producing progesterone and estrogen which are essential to maintaining the pregnancy.

The Amnion

The amnion (**AM**-nee-on) is a membrane that covers the fetal side of the placenta. It forms the **amniotic cavity** and protects the fetus by holding it suspended in the **amniotic fluid** (**am**-nee-**OT**-ick).

Gestation

Gestation (jes-**TAY**-shun), which lasts about nine calendar months, is the period of development of the child in the mother's uterus. (The combining forms *GEST/O* and *GESTAT/O* mean to carry young or offspring.)

The term **pregnancy,** which is often used interchangeably with gestation, actually means the condition of having a developing child in the uterus. (The combining form *PREGN/O* means pregnant.)

Pregnancy may be described in terms of the number of weeks of gestation (40 altogether) or it may be divided into three **trimesters** of three months each.

Quickening is the first movements of the fetus felt in the uterus. This usually occurs during the 16th to 20th week of pregnancy.

A **nulligravida** (**null**-ih-**GRAV**-ih-dah) is a woman who has never been pregnant. (The prefix *NULLI-* means none and the combining form *GRAVID/O* means pregnant.)

A **nullipara** (nuh-**LIP**-ah-rah) is a woman who has never borne offspring. (The combining form *PAR/O* means labor or act of bearing.)

A **primigravida** (**pre**-mih-**GRAV**-ih-dah) is a woman during her first pregnancy and a **primipara** (prye-**MIP**-ah-rah) is a woman who has borne one child. (The prefix *PRIMI-* means first.)

Multiparous (mul-**TIP**-ah-rus) means having given birth two or more times.

Childbirth

Parturition (**par**-tyou-**RISH**-un), also known as **labor** and **childbirth,** is the act of giving birth to an offspring. (The combining form *PART/O* means labor and childbirth.)

Labor occurs in three stages. The first stage begins with contractions of the uterus and gradual **dilatation** of the cervix.

Dilatation (dil-ah-**TAY**-shun), also known as **dilation** (dye-**LAY**-shun), is the increase in diameter of a body opening.

Effacement (eh-**FAYS**-ment) is the thinning and shortening of the cervix that occurs during labor.

During this stage the **operculum** (oh-**PER**-kyou-lum), which is the plug of mucus that fills the cervical canal during pregnancy, is dislodged. (The combining form *OPERCUL/O* means cover or lid.)

The second stage is the delivery of the infant. The **amniotic sac,** also known as the **bag of waters,** ruptures. Also, the uterine contractions become stronger and more frequent until the child is expelled.

Presentation is the term used to describe the portion of the fetus that can be touched by the examining finger during labor.

Normally the head presents first, and the stage at which the head can be seen at the vaginal orifice is called **crowning.**

The third stage is the expulsion of the placenta as the **afterbirth.** The term **delivery** means the expulsion of the infant and afterbirth.

Multiple Births

If more than one egg is passing down the fallopian tube when sperm are present, multiple fertilizations are possible.

Fraternal twins result from the fertilization of separate ova by separate sperm cells.

Identical twins are formed from the fertilization of a single egg cell by a single sperm. As the fertilized egg cell divides, it somehow separates into two parts and each part produces a separate embryo.

Postpartum

Postpartum, also be spelled **post partum,** means after childbirth or delivery.

The term **natal** refers to birth. A **neonate** is a newborn infant during the first four weeks after birth, and **neonatal** means pertaining to a newborn infant.

The terms **prenatal** and **antenatal** refer to events and development that occur before birth. **Postnatal** means occurring after birth.

Meconium (meh-**KOH**-nee-um) is a material that collects in the intestine of a fetus and forms the first stools of a newborn.

For the mother, **puerperium (pyou-er-PEE**-ree-um) is the period of three to six weeks after childbirth until the uterus returns to its normal size.

Uterine involution is the return of the uterus, after childbirth, to its normal size and former condition.

Lochia (LOH-kee-ah) is the vaginal discharge that takes place during the first week or two after childbirth. It consisting of blood, tissue and mucus.

Colostrum (kuh-**LOS**-trum) is the fluid secreted by the breasts during pregnancy and the first days postpartum. It consists, in part, of immunologically active substances.

Lactation (lack-**TAY**-shun) is the process of forming and secreting milk from the breasts as nourishment for the infant.

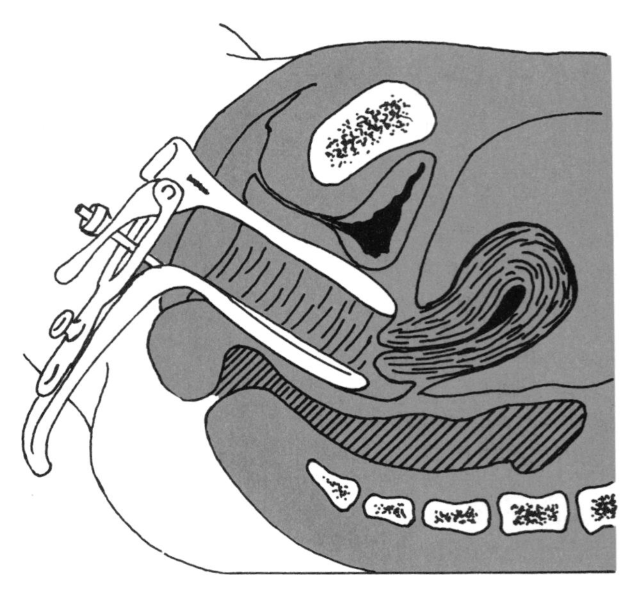

Figure 14-6 A speculum in position for an examination of the vagina and cervix.

DIAGNOSTIC PROCEDURES RELATED TO THE REPRODUCTIVE SYSTEMS

- A **speculum (SPECK**-you-lum) is an instrument resembling a duck's bill that is used to dilate the opening of a canal or cavity, such as the vagina, in order to facilitate inspection of its interior.

- A **Papanicolaou test (pap**-ah-**nick**-oh-**LAY**-ooh), also known as a **pap smear,** is an exfoliative test for the detection and diagnosis of conditions of the cervix and surrounding tissues.

- **Colposcopy** (kol-**POS**-koh-pee) is the examination of the tissues of the cervix and vagina using a **colposcope.**

- **Laparoscopy (lap**-ah-**ROS**-koh-pee) is the visual examination of the interior of the abdomen using a **laparoscope.** (The combining form *LAPAR/O* means abdomen.)

Diagnostic Procedures Related to Pregnancy

- **Amniocentesis** (**am**-nee-oh-sen-**TEE**-sis) is a surgical procedure in which a needle is passed through the abdominal and uterine walls to obtain a specimen of amniotic fluid to evaluate fetal health and diagnose certain congenital disorders.
- **Diagnostic ultrasound** is the use of high-frequency sound waves for the purpose of evaluating fetal development.
- An **electronic fetal monitor** is a device that allows observation of the fetal heart rate and the maternal uterine contractions.
- **Pelvimetry** is the measurement of the dimensions of the pelvis to determine its capacity to allow passage of the fetus through the birth canal.

PATHOLOGY RELATED TO THE MALE REPRODUCTIVE SYSTEM

General Pathology

- **Azoospermia** (ay-**zoh**-oh-**SPER**-me-ah) is the absence of sperm in the semen.
- **Oligospermia** (**ol**-ih-goh-**SPER**-me-ah), also known as a **low sperm count,** is a deficient amount of sperm in the semen.
- **Impotence** (**IM**-poh-tens) is the inability of the male to copulate.
- **Sterility** is the inability to reproduce or have children. (This term is applied to both the male and the female.)
- **Feminism,** also known as **effemination,** is the production of secondary female physical characteristics in a male.
- **Gynecomastia** (**jin**-eh-koh-**MAS**-tee-ah) is the condition of the excessive mammary development in the male. (The combining form *GYNEC/O* means female.)

Pathology of the Testes and Related Structures

- **Testitis** (tes-**TYE**-tis), also known as **orchitis** (or-**KEY**-tis), is an inflammation of a testis.
- **Anorchism** (an-**OR**-kizm) is the congenital absence of one or both testicles.
- **Cryptorchidism** (krip-**TOR**-kih-dizm), also known as an **undescended testis,** is a developmental defect in which one testis fails to descend into the scrotum.
- **Epididymitis** (**ep**-ih-did-ih-**MY**-tis) is an inflammation of the epididymis.
- A **hydrocele** (**HIGH**-droh-seel) is a hernia of fluid in the testes or the tubes leading from the testes.
- A **seminoma** (**see**-mih-**NO**-mah) is a malignant neoplasm of the testis.

Pathology Related to the Prostate Gland

- **Prostatitis** (**pros**-tah-**TYE**-tis) is an inflammation of the prostate gland.
- **Benign prostatic hypertrophy,** also known as **prostatomegaly** (**pros**-tah-toh-**MEG**-ah-lee), is an overgrowth of the glandular tissue of the prostate.

Pathology of the Penis

- **Phimosis** (fye-**MOH**-sis) is a narrowing of the opening of the foreskin so that it cannot be retracted (pulled back) to expose the glans penis.
- **Balanitis** (**bal**-ah-**NIGH**-tis) is an inflammation of the glans penis and is usually associated with phimosis.

PATHOLOGY RELATED TO THE FEMALE REPRODUCTIVE SYSTEM

General Pathology

- **Pelvic inflammatory disease** is any inflammation, especially one caused by bacterial infection, of the female reproductive organ.
- **Endometriosis (en-**doh-**me-**tree-**OH-** sis) is a condition in which tissue resembling uterine endometrium occurs abnormally in various locations in the pelvic cavity.
- **Toxic shock syndrome** is a severe staphylococcus infection. It is most common in menstruating women; however, it does occur in other patients.

Pathology of the Ovaries and Fallopian Tubes

- **Oophoritis (oh-**of-oh-**RYE-**tis) is an inflammation of an ovary.
- An **ovarian cyst** is a collection of fluid or solid material within a sac in the ovary.
- **Pyosalpinx (pye-**oh-**SAL-**pinks) is an accumulation of pus in the fallopian tube.
- **Salpingitis (sal-**pin-**JYE-**tis) is an inflammation of a fallopian tube. (This term also means an inflammation of the eustachian tube.)

Pathology of the Uterus

- **Anteversion (an-**tee-**VER-**zhun) is an abnormal tipping, tilting or turning forward of the entire uterus, including the cervix.
- **Prolapse of uterus** is a falling or sinking down of the uterus until it protrudes through the vaginal orifice.
- **Retroversion (ret-**roh-**VER-**zhun) is abnormal tipping of the entire uterus backward, with the cervix pointing forward towards the pubic symphysis.
- A **leiomyoma (lye-**oh-my-**OH-**mah), also known as a **fibroid,** is a benign tumor derived from the smooth muscle of the uterus.
- **Pyometritis (pye-**oh-meh-**TRY-**tis) is a purulent inflammation of the uterus. (The combining form *PY/O* means pus, and **purulent** means containing pus.)
- **Cervicitis (ser-**vih-**SIGH-**tis) is an inflammation of the uterine cervix.
- **Endocervicitis (en-**doh-**ser-**vih-**SIGH-**tis) is an inflammation of the mucous membrane lining of the cervix.

Pathology of the Vagina

- **Vaginitis (vaj-**ih-**NIGH-**tis), also known as **colpitis** (kol-**PYE-**tis), is an inflammation of the vagina.
- **Trichomonas vaginitis (trick-**oh-**MOH-**nas) is an inflammation of the vagina caused by a parasitic protozoan.
- **Leukorrhea (loo-**koh-**REE-**ah) is a profuse whitish mucous discharge from the uterus and vagina. (The combining form *LEUK/O* means white.)
- **Moniliasis** (mon-ih-**LYE-**ah-sis) is an infection of the skin or mucous membrane caused by a yeast-like fungus. It is usually localized in the mouth or the vagina.

Pathology of the External Genitalia

- **Pruritus vulvae** (proo-**RYE-**tus **VUL-**vee) is a condition of severe itching of the external female genitalia.

Pathology of the Breasts

- A **galactocele** (gah-**LACK-**toh-seel), also known as a **galactoma (gal-**ack-**TOH-**mah), is a cystic enlargement of the mammary gland containing milk. (The combining form *GALACT/O* means milk.)

- **Mastitis** (mas-**TYE**-tis) is an inflammation of the breast that is usually associated with lactation but may occur for other reasons.
- **Fibrocystic breast disease** is the presence of single or multiple cysts in the breasts. These cysts are usually benign but may become malignant.

Pathology of the Menstrual Cycle

- **Amenorrhea** (ah-**men**-oh-**REE**-ah) is an absence of the monthly flow of menstruation.
- **Dysmenorrhea** (**dis**-men-oh-**REE**-ah) is a difficult or painful monthly flow.
- **Oligomenorrhea** (**ol**-ih-goh-**men**-oh-**REE**-ah) means a scanty monthly flow. (The combining form *OLIG/O* means scanty.)
- **Menorrhagia** (**men**-oh-**RAY**-jee-ah) is excessive menstrual flow. (The suffix *-RRHAGIA* means bursting or breaking forth.)

SEXUALLY TRANSMITTED DISEASES

- **Sexually transmitted diseases,** also called **social diseases** and **venereal diseases** (VD), are common communicable diseases that are acquired during sexual intercourse or other genital contact.
- **Acquired immune deficiency syndrome** (AIDS) is a contagious and fatal disorder that can be transmitted through sexual intercourse with an infected partner.
- **Chlamydia** (klah-**MID**-ee-ah) is a sexually transmitted disease that is frequently the initial cause of pelvic inflammatory disease.
- **Genital herpes,** also known as **herpes genitalis** is a highly contagious venereal disease caused by the herpes simplex viruses (HVS) types 1 and 2.
- **Gonorrhea** (**gon**-oh-**REE**-ah) is a highly contagious venereal disease caused by the bacteria *Neisseria gonorrhoeae.*
- **Syphilis** (**SIF**-ih-lis) is a highly contagious venereal disease caused by the spirochete *Treponema pallidum.*

  The characteristic sore of the first stage of syphilis is called a **chancre** (**SHANG**-ker).

PATHOLOGY RELATED TO PREGNANCY AND CHILDBIRTH

- An **ectopic pregnancy** (eck-**TOP**-ick), also known as an **extrauterine pregnancy,** is a pregnancy that takes place outside of the uterus.
- A **tubal pregnancy** is an ectopic pregnancy that occurs within the fallopian tube.
- An **abortion** is the interruption or termination of pregnancy before the fetus is considered viable.

  Viable means capable of living outside the uterus. (The combining form *ABORT/O* means miscarriage or the premature expulsion of a nonviable fetus.)

  A **spontaneous abortion,** also known as a **miscarriage,** occurs without outside action.

  An **induced abortion** is deliberately caused by human action.
- **Rubella** (roo-**BEL**-ah), also known as **German measles** or **three-day measles,** is a viral infection characterized by fever and a diffuse, fine, red rash. If the mother has rubella during the early stages of pregnancy, this may cause congenital abnormality in the infant.
- **Hyperemesis gravidarum** (**high**-per-**EM**-eh-sis **grah**-vih-**DAH**-rum) is excessive or persistent vomiting during pregnancy.
- **Preeclampsia** (**pree**-ee-**KLAMP**-see-ah), also known as **toxemia of pregnancy,** is character-

ized by the onset of acute hypertension after the twenty-fourth week of gestation.

- **Eclampsia** (eh-**KLAMP**-see-ah) is the most serious form of toxemia of pregnancy and is characterized by grand mal convulsion, coma, hypertension, proteinuria and edema.

- **Gestational diabetes mellitus** is a form of diabetes characterized by a deficiency of insulin occurring during pregnancy and which disappears after delivery.

- **Abruptio placentae** (ab-**RUP**-she-oh plah-**SEN**-tee) is an abnormal condition in which the placenta separates from the uterine wall prematurely before the birth of the fetus.

- **Placenta previa** (plah-**SEN**-tah **PREE**-vee-ah) is the abnormal implantation of the placenta in the lower portion of the uterus.

- **Breech presentation** is when the buttocks or feet are presented first.

- A **premature infant** is any neonate born before the 37th week of gestation.

- **Stillbirth** is the birth of a fetus that died before or during delivery.

- A **congenital anomaly** is a malformation, such as the absence of a limb or the presence of an extra toe, that is present at birth.

  An **anomaly** (ah-**NOM**-ah-lee) is a deviation from what is regarded as normal.

The Rh Factor

When the mother's blood is Rh negative (lacking the Rh factor) and the father's is Rh positive (containing the Rh factor), the baby may inherit the Rh positive factor from the father.

In this situation, the baby gives the Rh factor to the mother. Her body develops anti-Rh antibodies and gives them to the baby. These antibodies can destroy the baby's red blood cells.

Blood tests of the parents can identify this potential problem and, if it exists, a vaccine is administered to the mother to prevent any further difficulty.

Genetic Disorders

- An **inherited disorder,** also known as a **genetic disorder,** is any disease or condition that is genetically determined. (There are more than 2000 known inherited disorders.)

- **Cystic fibrosis** is an inherited disorder of the exocrine glands. One of the primary characteristics is abnormally thick secretions of mucus.

- **Down's syndrome,** also known as **trisomy 21,** is a genetic syndrome characterized by varying degrees of mental retardation and multiple defects.

- **Tay-Sachs disease** is an inherited neurodegenerative disease marked by progressive physical and mental retardation and early death.

PROCEDURES RELATED TO THE REPRODUCTIVE SYSTEMS

General Procedures

- **Contraception** is the prevention of pregnancy. A **contraceptive** is the measure taken, or device used, to lessen the likelihood of conception and pregnancy.

- **Sterilization** is any procedure rendering an individual (male or female) incapable of reproduction.

Procedures Related to the Male Reproductive System

- **Circumcision** (ser-kum-**SIZH**-un) is the surgical removal of the foreskin of the penis and is usually performed a few days after birth.

- **Orchidectomy** (**or**-kih-**DECK**-toh-me), also known as **orchectomy**, **orchiectomy** (**or**-kee-**ECK**-toh-me) and **testectomy** is the surgical removal of a testis.
- **Castration** (kas-**TRAY**-shun) also known as **bilateral orchidectomy,** is the removal of both testes.
- A **vasectomy** (vah-**SECK**-toh-me) is a male sterilization procedure that involves cutting or tying off the vas deferens.
- **Prostatectomy** (**pros**-tah-**TECK**-toh-me) is the surgical removal of all or part of the prostate gland.
- A **transurethral prostatectomy,** also called a **transurethral resection,** is the removal of all or part of the prostrate through the urethra.

Procedures Related to the Female Reproductive System

- **Oophorectomy** (**oh**-of-oh-**RECK**-toh-me), also known as **ovariectomy**, (**oh**-vay-ree-**ECK**-toh-me) is the surgical removal of an ovary.
- **Salpingectomy** (**sal**-pin-**JECK**-toh-me) is the surgical removal of a fallopian tube.
- **Tubal ligation** is a surgical procedure in which the fallopian tubes are ligated and a section is removed for purposes of sterilization. (**Ligate** means to bind or tie.)
- A **hysterectomy** (**his**-teh-**RECK**-toh-me) is the surgical removal of the uterus.
- **Dilation and curettage** (D & C), also known **dilatation and curettage,** as is a procedure in which the cervix is dilated (enlarged) and the endometrium of the uterus is scraped with the curette.

  Curettage (**kyou**-reh-**TAHZH**) is the removal of material from the surface by scraping with an instrument called a **curette.**

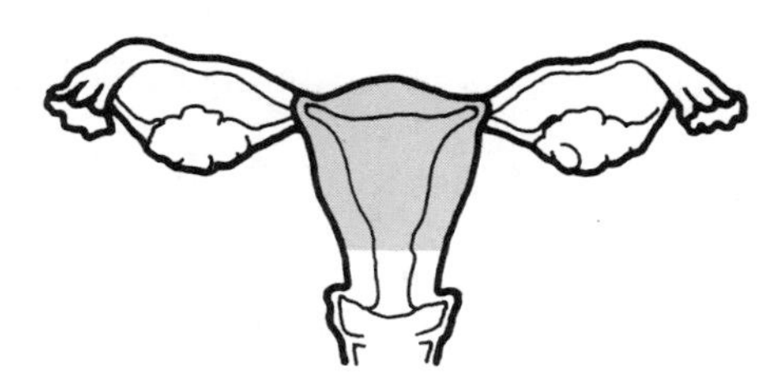

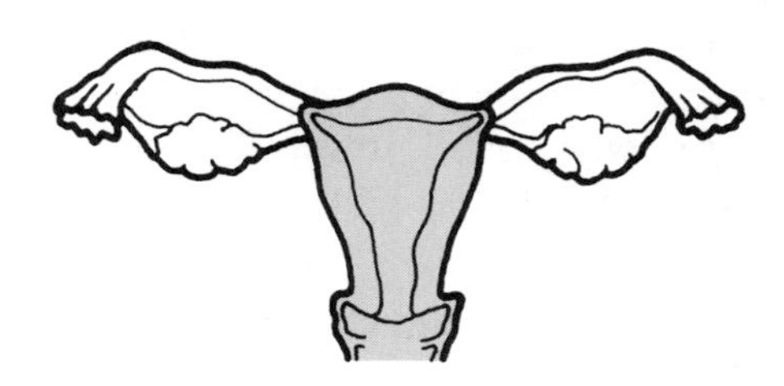

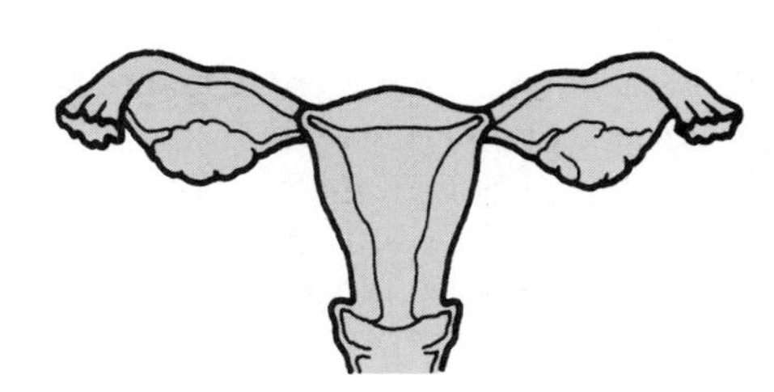

Figure 14-7 Types of hysterectomy.

- **Conization** (**kon**-ih-**ZAY**-shun) is the removal of a cone of tissue or the partial removal of the cervix.
- **Hymenectomy** (**high**-men-**ECK**-toh-me) is the surgical removal of the hymen.
- A **lumpectomy** is the surgical removal of a lump from the breast.
- **Mastectomy** is the surgical removal of all or part of the breast.

- **Mammoplasty** (**MAM**-oh-**plas**-tee) is the surgical repair or restructuring of the breast.

Procedures Related to Childbirth

- **Genetic counseling** is the process of determining the risk of occurrence of a genetic disorder.
- A **cesarean section** is the delivery of the child through an incision in the maternal abdominal and uterine wall.
- An **episiotomy** (eh-**piz**-ee-**OT**-oh-me) is a surgical incision of the vulva in order to facilitate delivery and prevent laceration of the tissues. (A **laceration** is a jagged tear of the tissue.)
- **Apgar score** is an evaluation of an infant's physical condition, usually performed one minute after, and again five minutes after birth.

IMPORTANT TERMS: THE REPRODUCTIVE SYSTEMS

This list will help you identify and review the major terms from this chapter.

When you work with the audio tape for this chapter, listen to the word, repeat it and then place a ✓ next to it on the list below.

- ☐ **Abruptio placentae** (ab-**RUP**-she-oh plah-**SEN**-tee)
- ☐ **Amenorrhea** (ah-**men**-oh-**REE**-ah)
- ☐ **Amniocentesis** (**am**-nee-oh-sen-**TEE**-sis)
- ☐ **Amnion** (**AM**-nee-on)
- ☐ **Amniotic** (**am**-nee-**OT**-ick)
- ☐ **Anomaly** (ah-**NOM**-ah-lee)
- ☐ **Anorchism** (an-**OR**-kizm)
- ☐ **Anteversion** (**an**-tee-**VER**-zhun)
- ☐ **Areola** (ah-**REE**-oh-lah)
- ☐ **Azoospermia** (ay-**zoh**-oh-**SPER**-me-ah)
- ☐ **Balanitis** (**bal**-ah-**NIGH**-tis)
- ☐ **Bulbourethral** (**bul**-boh-you-**REE**-thral)
- ☐ **Castration** (kas-**TRAY**-shun)
- ☐ **Cervicitis** (**ser**-vih-**SIGH**-tis)
- ☐ **Cervix** (**SER**-vicks)
- ☐ **Chlamydia** (klah-**MID**-ee-ah)
- ☐ **Chorionic gonadotropin** (**koh**-ree-**ON**-ick **gon**-ah-doh-**TROH**-pin)
- ☐ **Chorion** (**KOH**-ree-on)
- ☐ **Circumcision** (**ser**-kum-**SIZH**-un)
- ☐ **Climacteric** (klye-**MACK**-ter-ick)
- ☐ **Clitoris** (**KLIT**-oh-ris)
- ☐ **Coitus** (**KOH**-ih-tus)
- ☐ **Colostrum** (kuh-**LOS**-trum)
- ☐ **Colpitis** (kol-**PYE**-tis)
- ☐ **Colposcopy** (kol-**POS**-koh-pee)
- ☐ **Conization** (**kon**-ih-**ZAY**-shun)
- ☐ **Copulation** (**kop**-you-**LAY**-shun)
- ☐ **Corpus luteum** (**KOR**-pus **LOO**-tee-um)
- ☐ **Cryptorchidism** (krip-**TOR**-kih-dizm)
- ☐ **Curettage** (**kyou**-reh-**TAHZH**)
- ☐ **Dilatation** (dil-ah-**TAY**-shun)
- ☐ **Dilation** (dye-**LAY**-shun)
- ☐ **Dysmenorrhea** (**dis**-men-oh-**REE**-ah)
- ☐ **Eclampsia** (eh-**KLAMP**-see-ah)
- ☐ **Ectopic** (eck-**TOP**-ick)
- ☐ **Effacement** (eh-**FAYS**-ment)
- ☐ **Embryo** (**EM**-bree-oh)

- ☐ **Endocervicitis (en-**doh-**ser-**vih-**SIGH-**tis)
- ☐ **Endometriosis (en-**doh-**me-**tree-**OH-**sis)
- ☐ **Epididymitis (ep-**ih-did-ih-**MY-**tis)
- ☐ **Epididymis (ep-**ih-**DID-**ih-mis)
- ☐ **Episiotomy** (eh-**piz-**ee-**OT-**oh-me)
- ☐ **Fallopian** (fal-**LOH-**pee-an)
- ☐ **Fetus (FEE-**tus)
- ☐ **Fimbriae (FIM-**bree-ee)
- ☐ **Fornix (FOR-**nicks)
- ☐ **Galactocele** (gah-**LACK-**toh-seel)
- ☐ **Galactoma (gal-**ack-**TOH-**mah)
- ☐ **Gamete (GAM-**eet)
- ☐ **Genitalia (jen-**ih-**TAY-**lee-ah)
- ☐ **Gestation** (jes-**TAY-**shun)
- ☐ **Glans penis** (glanz **PEE-**nis)
- ☐ **Gonorrhea (gon-**oh-**REE-**ah)
- ☐ **Graafian follicles (GRAF-**ee-an **FOL-**lick-kulz)
- ☐ **Gynecomastia (jin-**eh-koh-**MAS-**tee-ah)
- ☐ **Hydrocele (HIGH-**droh-seel)
- ☐ **Hymen (HIGH-**men)
- ☐ **Hymenectomy (high-**men-**ECK-**toh-me)
- ☐ **Hyperemesis gravidarum (high-**per-**EM-**eh-sis **grah-**vih-**DAH-**rum)
- ☐ **Hysterectomy (his-**teh-**RECK-**toh-me)
- ☐ **Impotence (IM-**poh-tens)
- ☐ **Infundibulum (in-**fun-**DIB-**you-lum)
- ☐ **Lactation** (lack-**TAY-**shun)
- ☐ **Lactiferous** (lack-**TIF-**er-us)
- ☐ **Laparoscopy (lap-**ah-**ROS-**koh-pee)
- ☐ **Leiomyoma** (lye-oh-my-**OH-**mah)
- ☐ **Leukorrhea (loo-**koh-**REE-**ah)
- ☐ **Lochia (LOH-**kee-ah)
- ☐ **Mammoplasty (MAM-**oh-**plas-**tee)
- ☐ **Mastitis** (mas-**TYE-**tis)
- ☐ **Meconium** (meh-**KOH-**nee-um)
- ☐ **Menarche** (meh-**NAR-**key)
- ☐ **Menopause (MEN-**oh-pawz)
- ☐ **Menorrhagia (men-**oh-**RAY-**jee-ah)
- ☐ **Menorrhea (men-**oh-**REE-**ah)
- ☐ **Menses (MEN-**seez)
- ☐ **Menstruation (men-**stroo-**AY-**shun)
- ☐ **Moniliasis** (mon-ih-**LYE-**ah-sis)
- ☐ **Mons pubis** (monz **PYOU-**bis)
- ☐ **Multiparous** (mul-**TIP-**ah-rus)
- ☐ **Nulligravida (null-**ih-**GRAV-**ih-dah)
- ☐ **Nullipara** (nuh-**LIP-**ah-rah)
- ☐ **Oligomenorrhea (ol-**ih-goh-**men-**oh-**REE-**ah)
- ☐ **Oligospermia (ol-**ih-goh-**SPER-**me-ah)
- ☐ **Oophorectomy (oh-**of-oh-**RECK-**toh-me)
- ☐ **Oophoritis (oh-**of-oh-**RYE-**tis)
- ☐ **Operculum** (oh-**PER-**kyou-lum)
- ☐ **Orchidectomy (or-**kih-**DECK-**toh-me)
- ☐ **Orchiectomy (or-**kee-**ECK-**toh-me)
- ☐ **Ova (OH-**vah)
- ☐ **Ovariectomy (oh-**vay-ree-**ECK-**toh-me)
- ☐ **Ovaries (OH-**vah-rees)

- ◻ **Ovulation** (**oh**-view-**LAY**-shun)
- ◻ **Papanicolaou** (**pap**-ah-**nick**-oh-**LAY**-ooh)
- ◻ **Parturition** (**par**-tyou-**RISH**-un)
- ◻ **Perineum** (per-ih-**NEE**-um)
- ◻ **Phimosis** (fye-**MOH**-sis)
- ◻ **Placenta** (plah-**SEN**-tah)
- ◻ **Placenta previa** (plah-**SEN**-tah **PREE**-vee-ah)
- ◻ **Preeclampsia** (**pree**-ee-**KLAMP**-see-ah)
- ◻ **Prepuce** (**PRE**-pyous)
- ◻ **Primigravida** (**pre**-mih-**GRAV**-ih-dah)
- ◻ **Primipara** (prye-**MIP**-ah-rah)
- ◻ **Prostatectomy** (**pros**-tah-**TECK**-toh-me)
- ◻ **Prostatomegaly** (**pros**-tah-toh-**MEG**-ah-lee)
- ◻ **Prostatitis** (**pros**-tah-**TYE**-tis)
- ◻ **Pruritus vulvae** (proo-**RYE**-tus **VUL**-vee)
- ◻ **Pudendum** (pyou-**DEN**-dum)
- ◻ **Puerperium** (**pyou**- er-**PEE**-ree-um)
- ◻ **Pyometritis** (**pye**-oh-meh-**TRY**-tis)
- ◻ **Pyosalpinx** (**pye**-oh-**SAL**-pinks)
- ◻ **Retroversion** (**ret**-roh-**VER**-zhun)
- ◻ **Rubella** (roo-**BEL**-ah)
- ◻ **Salpingectomy** (**sal**-pin-**JECK**-toh-me)
- ◻ **Salpingitis** (**sal**-pin-**JYE**-tis)
- ◻ **Scrotum** (**SKROH**-tum)
- ◻ **Semen** (**SEE**-men)
- ◻ **Seminal** (**SEM**-ih-nal)
- ◻ **Seminiferous** (**see**-mih-**NIF**-er-us)
- ◻ **Seminoma** (**see**-mih-**NO**-mah)
- ◻ **Spermatozoa** (**sper**-mah-toh-**ZOH**-ah)
- ◻ **Syphilis** (**SIF**-ih-lis)
- ◻ **Testitis** (tes-**TYE**-tis)
- ◻ **Trichomonas** (**trick**-oh-**MOH**-nas)
- ◻ **Umbilical** (um-**BIL**-ih-kal)
- ◻ **Uterus** (**YOU**-ter-us)
- ◻ **Vagina** (vah-**JYE**-nah)
- ◻ **Vaginitis** (**vaj**-ih-**NIGH**-tis)
- ◻ **Vas deferens** (vas **DEF**-er-enz)
- ◻ **Vasectomy** (vah-**SECK**-toh-me)
- ◻ **Vulva** (**VUL**-vah)
- ◻ **Zygote** (**ZYE**-goht)

EXERCISES

DEFINING WORD PARTS

Write the definition for each of these word parts.

1. *ABORT/O* ______________________________
2. *CERVIC/O* ______________________________
3. *COLP/O* ______________________________
4. *CORP/U* ______________________________
5. *DIDYM/O* ______________________________
6. *EJACULAT/O* ______________________________
7. *FET/I, FET/O* ______________________________
8. *FLEX/O* ______________________________
9. *FUND/O* ______________________________
10. *GALACT/O* ______________________________
11. *GEST/O, GESTAT/O* ______________________________
12. *GRAVID/O* ______________________________
13. *GYNEC/O* ______________________________
14. *HYSTER/O* ______________________________
15. *LACT/I, LACT/O* ______________________________
16. *LAPAR/O* ______________________________

17. *LEUK/O* ______________________________

18. *LUTE/O* ______________________________

19. *MAMM/O* ______________________________

20. *MEN/O* ______________________________

21. *MENSTRU/O, MENSTRUAT/O* ______________________________

22. *METR/O, METRI/O* ______________________________

23. *NULLI-* ______________________________

24. *OLIG/O* ______________________________

25. *OO/O, OV/I, OV/O* ______________________________

26. *OOPHOR/O* ______________________________

27. *OPERCUL/O* ______________________________

28. *ORCH/O, ORCHI/O, ORCHID/O* ______________________________

29. *OVARI/O* ______________________________

30. *PAR/O* ______________________________

31. *PART/O* ______________________________

32. *PEN/I* ______________________________

33. *PERI-* ______________________________

34. *PERINE/O* ______________________________

35. *PREGN/O* ______________________________

36. *PRIAP/O* ______________________________

37. *PROSTAT/O* ______________________________

38. *PY/O* ______________________________

39. *SALPING/O* ______________________________

40. *SEMIN/I* ______________________________

41. *SPERM/O, SPERMAT/O* ______________________________

42. *UMBILIC/O* ______________________________

43. *UTER/O* ______________________________

44. *VAGIN/O* ______________________________

45. *VULV/O* ______________________________

DEFINITIONS

Circle the letter next to the correct answer.

1. The _______________ carries the sperm up into the pelvic region, around the bladder and then down toward the urethra.
   a) ejaculatory duct
   b) seminal vesicle
   c) sperminiferous tubule
   d) vas deferens

2. The inner layer of the uterus is called the _______________
   a) corpus.
   b) endometrium.
   c) myometrium.
   d) perimetrium.

3. In the female the _______________ is the area between the vaginal orifice and the anus.
   a) clitoris
   b) mons pubis
   c) perineum
   d) vulva

4. Semen consists of sperm plus the secretions of the _______________.
   a) Cowper's glands.
   b) prostate gland.
   c) seminal vesicles.
   d) a, b and c.

5. Immediately after conception, the fertilized egg is called a/an _______________
   a) embryo.
   b) fetus.
   c) gamete.
   d) zygote.

6. The _______________ are two small, rounded glands on either side of the vaginal opening which produce a mucous secretion that lubricates the vagina.
   a) Bartholin's glands
   b) bulbourethral glands
   c) Cowper's glands
   d) graafian follicles

7. The _______________ is the funnel-shaped opening into the fallopian tube.
   a) fimbria
   b) fundus
   c) infundibulum
   d) oviduct

8. The _______________ is the outermost membrane that surrounds the developing embryo and forms the inner layer of the placenta.
   a) amniotic sac
   b) chorion
   c) hymen
   d) operculum

9. The _______________ produce the hormone progesterone that is responsible for the preparation and maintenance of the uterus in pregnancy.
   a) graafian follicles
   b) ovaries
   c) seminal vesicles
   d) testes

10. The uterus is normally in a bent forward position called _______________
    a) anteflexion.
    b) anteversion.
    c) retroflexion.
    d) retroversion.

MISSING WORDS

Write the missing word on the line.

1. The _______________________ is the dark area surrounding the nipple.
2. The _______________________ cord connects the fetus to the placenta.
3. _______________________ is the stage in life when the secondary sex characteristics begin to develop.
4. A/an _______________________ is a woman during her first pregnancy.
5. _______________________ _______________________ disease is an inflammation, especially one caused by bacterial infection, of the female reproductive organs.
6. The characteristic sore of the first stage of _______________________ is called a chancre.
7. A/an _______________________, or extrauterine, pregnancy is one that takes place outside of the uterus.

8. Sexually transmitted diseases are also called social diseases and ______________________ diseases.

9. During delivery, a/an ______________________ presentation is when the buttocks or feet are presented first.

10. A/an ______________________ is the measure taken, or device used, to lessen the likelihood of conception and pregnancy.

11. ______________________ is the most serious form of toxemia of pregnancy.

12. A/an ______________________ ______________________ is the delivery of the child through an incision in the maternal abdominal and uterine wall.

13. ______________________, also known as bilateral orchidectomy, is the removal of both testes.

14. ______________________ means capable of living outside of the uterus.

15. If the mother has ______________________, also known as German measles, during the early stages of pregnancy this may cause congenital abnormality in the infant.

SPELLCHECK

Select the correct spelling and write it on the line.

1. In the male, the ______________________ gland circles the upper end of the urethra.
   prostate
   prostotate
   prostrate

2. The ______________________ is the muscular tube that extends from the cervix to the outside of the body.
   vagena
   vagina
   vegina

3. The ______________________ is located anterior to the vaginal orifice and in front of the urethral meatus.
   claterus
   cliteris
   clitoris

4. ______________________ is the normal periodic discharge from the uterus.
   Menstration
   Menstruation
   Menustration

5. The ______________________ is also known as the afterbirth.
   placenta
   plasenta
   plesenta

6. The first stage of labor begins with regular contractions of the uterus and the gradual ______________________ of the cervix.
   dielation
   dilatation
   diolatation

7. ______________________ is the normal stopping of the monthly flow, and it usually occurs after the age of 45.
   Menapause
   Menepause
   Menopause

8. ______________________ is the thinning and shortening of the cervix that occurs during labor.
   Affecement
   Effacement
   Effecement

9. ______________________ is the fluid secreted by the breasts during pregnancy and the first days postpartum.
   Colestrium
   Colostrium
   Colostrum

10. The ______________________ duct is one of the two final portions of the seminal vessels.
    ejackulatory
    ejaculatory
    ejaculotory

11. The female is fertile during ______________________.
    ovalation
    ovulation
    ovuletion

12. A ______________________ test is also known as a pap smear.
    Papanicolaou
    Papanencolaou
    Papincolaou

13. ______________________ is the process of forming and secreting milk from the breasts as nourishment for the infant.
    Lactation
    Lactetion
    Lactition

14. ______________________ is the ejaculatory fluid which contains sperm.
    Seamen
    Semen
    Semin

15. The ______________________ tubes are also known as oviducts or uterine tubes.
    fallopen
    fallopian
    fellopian

CASE STUDIES

Write the correct answer on the line.

1. Mary Smith developed ______________________ ______________________ which is caused by the herpes simplex viruses types 1 and 2.
2. Daniel Grossman was born with ______________________ which is an inherited disorder that is characterized by abnormally thick secretions of mucus.
3. Rita Orton saw her doctor because of ______________________ or the lack of menstruation.
4. During the delivery, Barbara Klein required a/an ______________________ to prevent laceration of the tissues.
5. Mr. Morgan underwent a/an ______________________ resection for the removal of part of the prostate gland.
6. Dr. Silverman explained to Jane O'Brien that the birth was complicated because of placenta ______________________ which is the abnormal implantation of the placenta in the lower portion of the uterus.
7. During her pregnancy Eleanor Jimenez was diagnosed as having ______________________ diabetes mellitus.
8. The Reicher infant was born with ______________________ syndrome, which is also known as trisomy 21.
9. As a means of sterilization, Harry Belcher had a/an ______________________ performed. During the procedure his doctor removed a portion of the vas deferens.
10. Within a few days of birth Harold Solomon underwent ______________________ to remove the foreskin of the penis.

11. Janet Dole has a/an ____________________ ____________________ which is a collection of fluid within a sac in the ovary.

12. During Kate Marshall's pregnancy ____________________ was performed to evaluate fetal health and to diagnose certain congenital disorders.

13. Mr. Romer was treated for benign ____________________ ____________________ which is also known as prostatomegaly.

14. Harriet Ingram was diagnosed as having a leiomyoma, also known as a/an ____________________, which is a benign tumor derived from the smooth muscle of the uterus.

15. Because of the prolonged bleeding problem, Jane Orton required ____________________ and ____________________ which is usually referred to as a D & C.

WORD BUILDING

Write the correct word or word part on the line.

1. Breast removal
   a) The combing form ____________________ means breast.
   b) The suffix ____________________ means surgical removal.
   c) The term ____________________ means the surgical removal of a breast.

2. Inflammation of the prostate
   a) The combining form ____________________ means prostate gland.
   b) The suffix ____________________ means inflammation.
   c) The term ____________________ means inflammation of the prostate gland.

3. White flow
   a) The combining form ____________________ means white.
   b) The suffix ____________________ means flow or discharge.
   c) The term ____________________ means a profuse whitish mucous discharge from the uterus and vagina.

LABELING EXERCISES

Identify the numbered items on this diagram.

1. ____________________
2. ____________________
3. ____________________
4. ____________________
5. ____________________

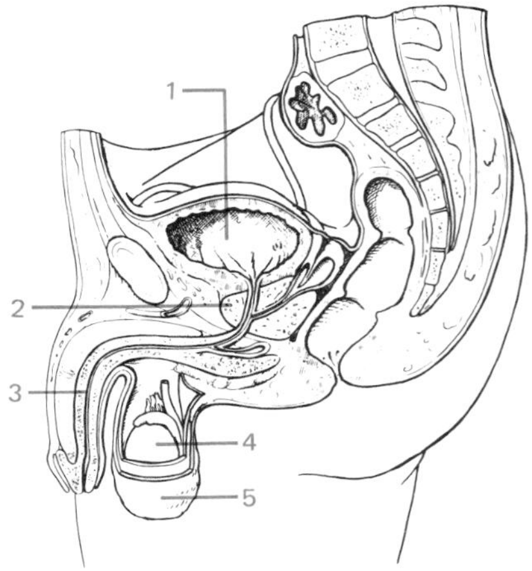

15

DIAGNOSTIC AND IMAGING PROCEDURES

LEARNING GOALS

In this chapter you will learn to:

- describe the basic diagnostic procedures.
- identify and describe the basic diagnostic positions.
- describe the major radiographic imaging techniques and differentiate between the action of x-rays and nuclear imaging.
- differentiate between projection and position and describe the basic radiographic projections.

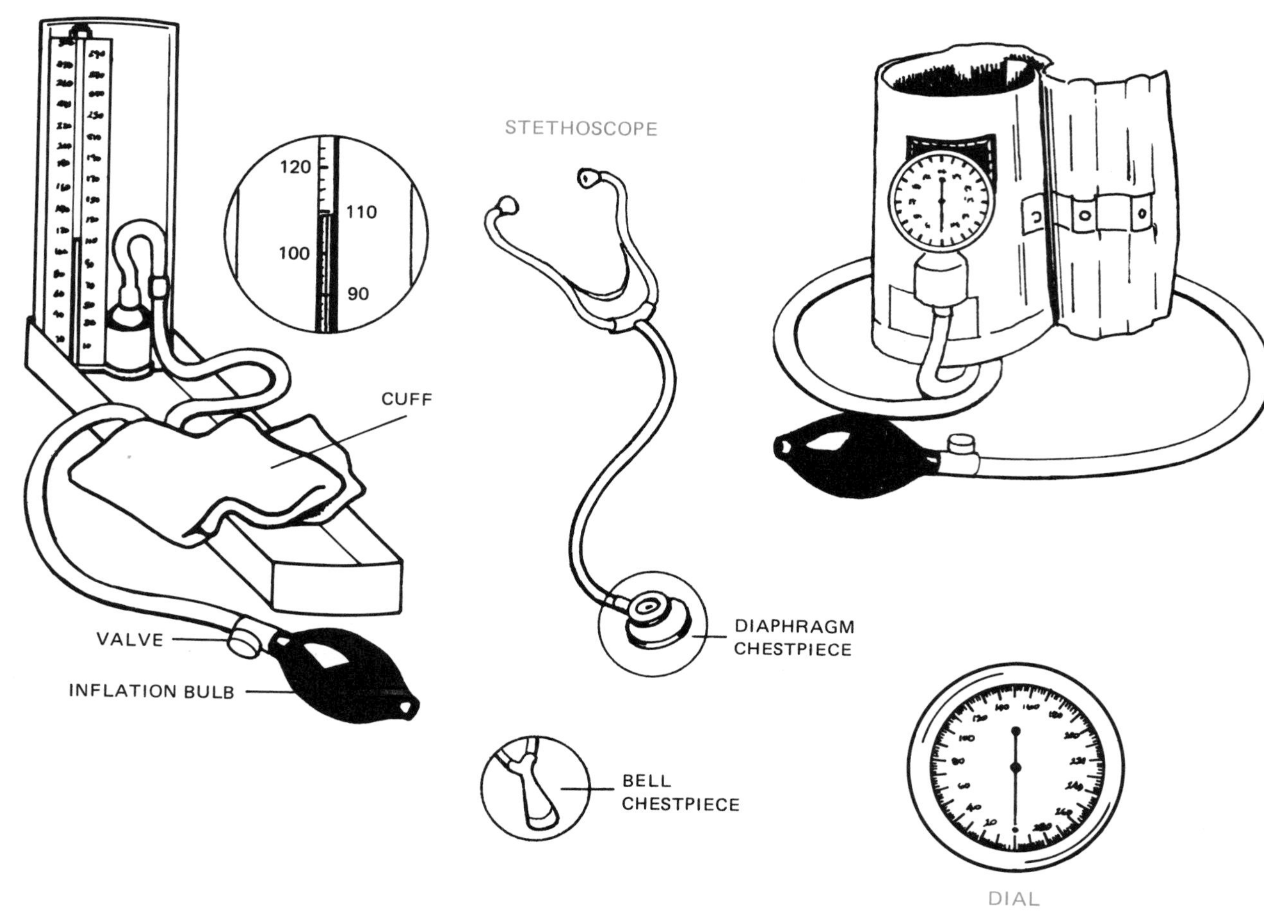

Figure 15-1 Stethoscope and sphygmomanometers.

BASIC DIAGNOSTIC PROCEDURES

Auscultation (aws-kul-**TAY**-shun) is listening through a **stethoscope** (**STETH**-oh-skope) for sounds within the body to determine the condition of the lungs, pleura, heart and abdomen.

Palpation (pal-**PAY**-shun) is an examination technique in which the examiner's hands are used to feel the texture, size, consistency and location of certain body parts. (Be careful not to confuse palpation with palpitation, which is discussed in Chapter 5.)

Percussion (per-**KUSH**-un) is an examination technique that uses sharp, short blows to the surface of the body with a finger or instrument.

Blood pressure is measured with a **sphygmomanometer** (**sfig**-moh-mah-**NOM**-eh-ter) and a **stethoscope.**

Endoscopy (en-**DOS**-koh-pee) is the visual examination of any cavity of the body by means of an **endoscope.** The instruments and procedures are named for the body parts involved.

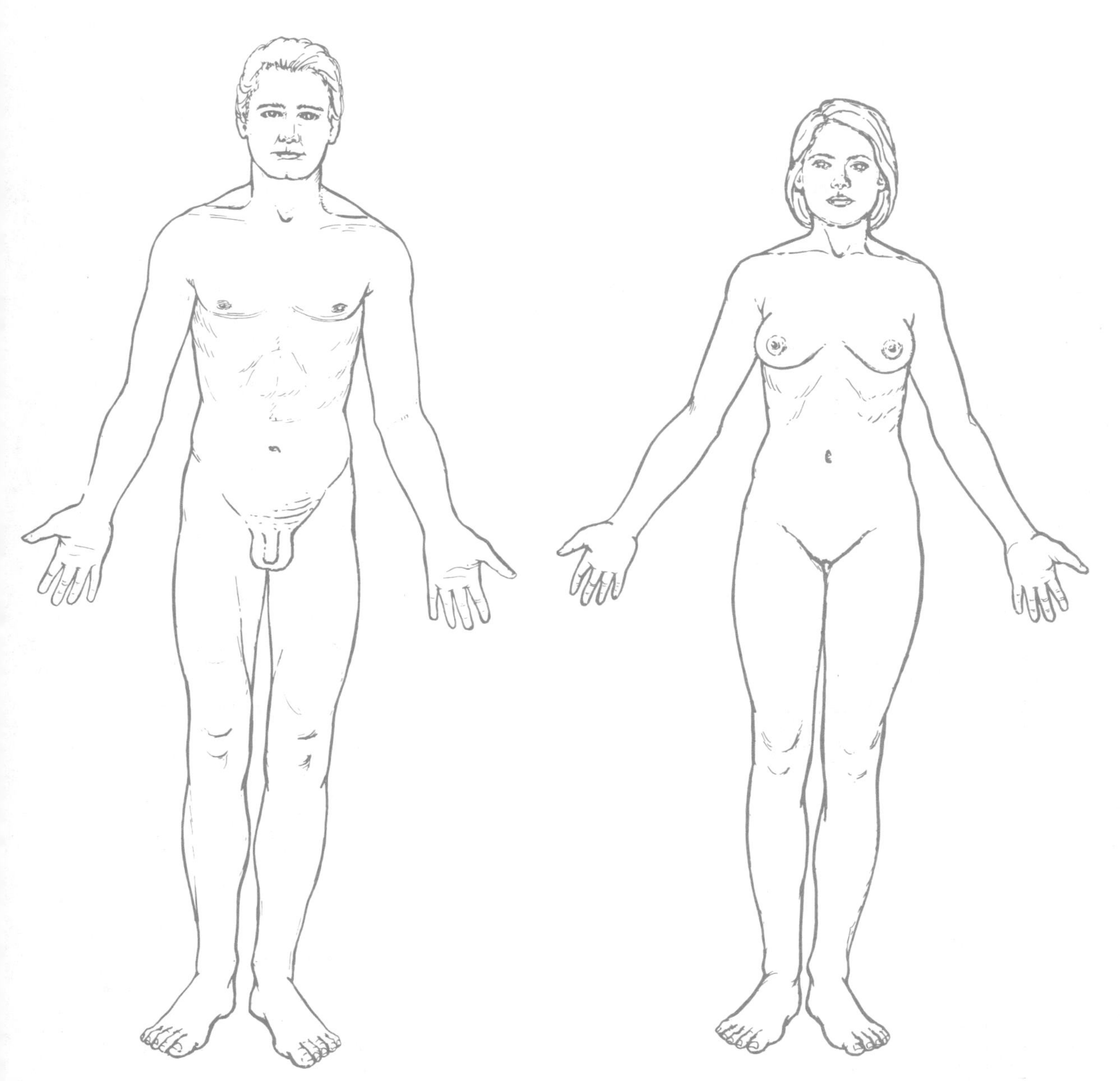

Figure 15-2 The anatomical position.

EXAMINATION POSITIONS

The Anatomical Position

The anatomical position is the position in which the patient is standing up.

In the anatomical position the body is erect, facing forward with the arms at the sides and the palms toward the front. Other positions are described in terms of how they vary from this position.

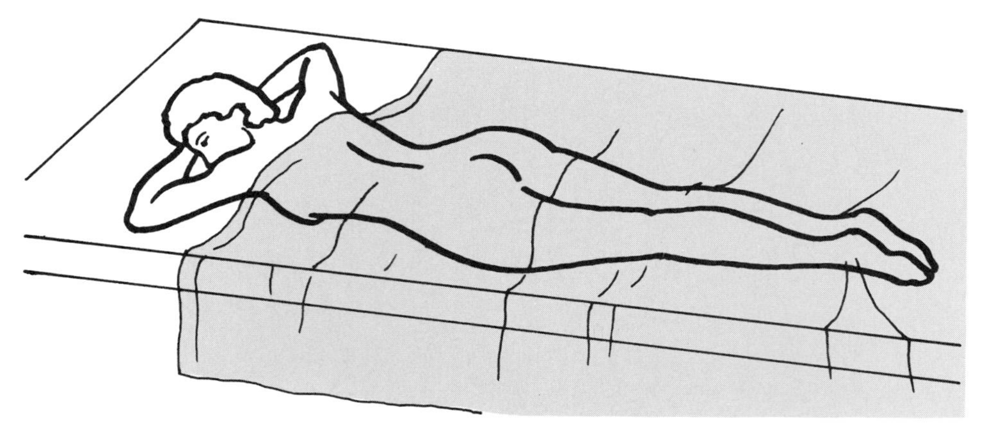

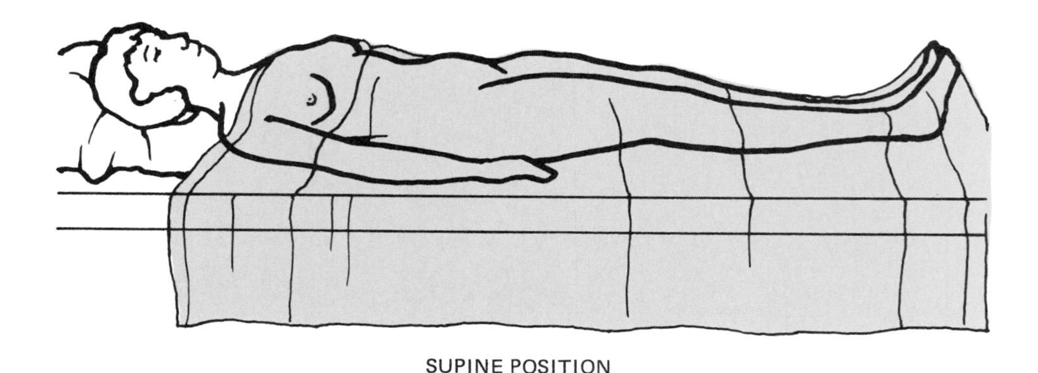

Figure 15-3 Patients in the prone and supine positions.

Recumbent Positions

The term recumbent (ree-**KUM**-bent) may be used to describe any position in which the patient is lying down.

The term **decubitus** (dee-**KYOU**-bih-tus) also means the act of lying down or the position assumed in lying down.

In radiography, the term **decubitus** is used to describe the position of the patient when he is lying down — either on his back, front or side.

The Prone Position

In a prone position the recumbent patient is lying on his or her belly — with the face down.

In this position, the arms may be placed under the head for comfort. This position is used for the examination of the back and buttocks.

The Supine Position

In a supine position (**SUE**-pine), also known as the **horizontal recumbent position,** the patient is lying on his or her back — with the face up. (The combining form *SUPIN/O* means lying on the back.)

This position is used for examination and treatment of the anterior surface of the body and for x-rays.

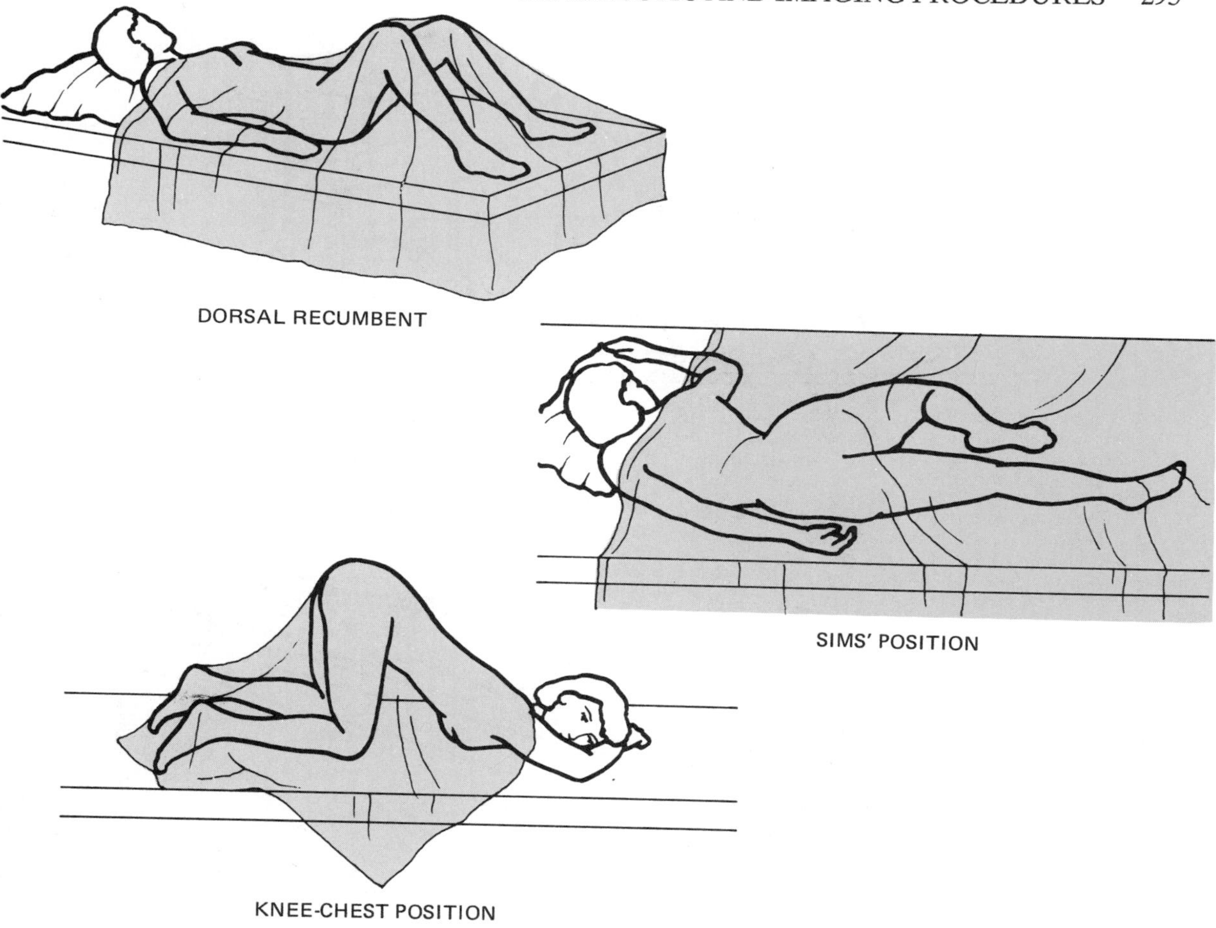

Figure 15-4 Patients in the dorsal recumbent, Sims', and knee-chest positions

The Dorsal Recumbent Position

In the dorsal recumbent position the patient is supine with his or her knees bent. This position is used for the examination of the abdominal area and may be used for vaginal or rectal examinations.

The Sims' Position

In the Sims' position the patient is on the left side of the chest, with the right knee and right thigh drawn up. The left arm is placed along the back. The Sims' position is used in the examination and treatment of the rectal area.

The Knee-Chest Position

In the knee-chest position the patient is face down so that the hips are flexed (bent) with his or her knees and chest resting on the table. This position is used for rectal examinations.

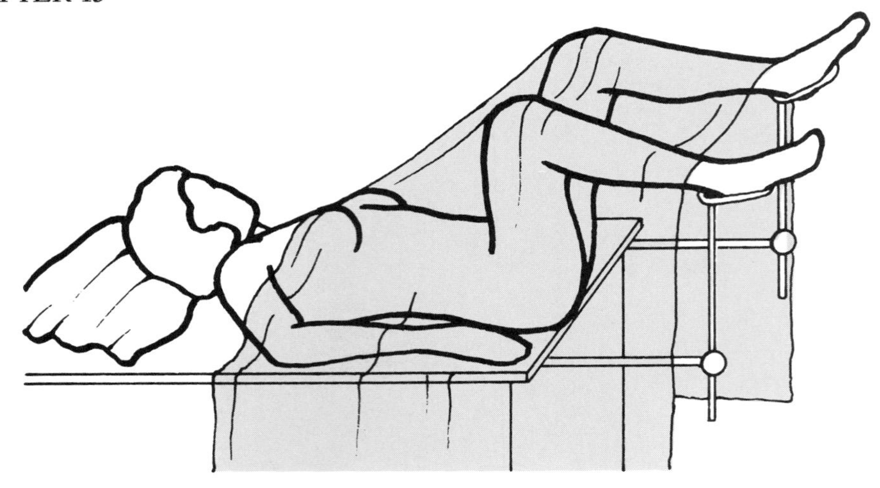

LITHOTOMY POSITION

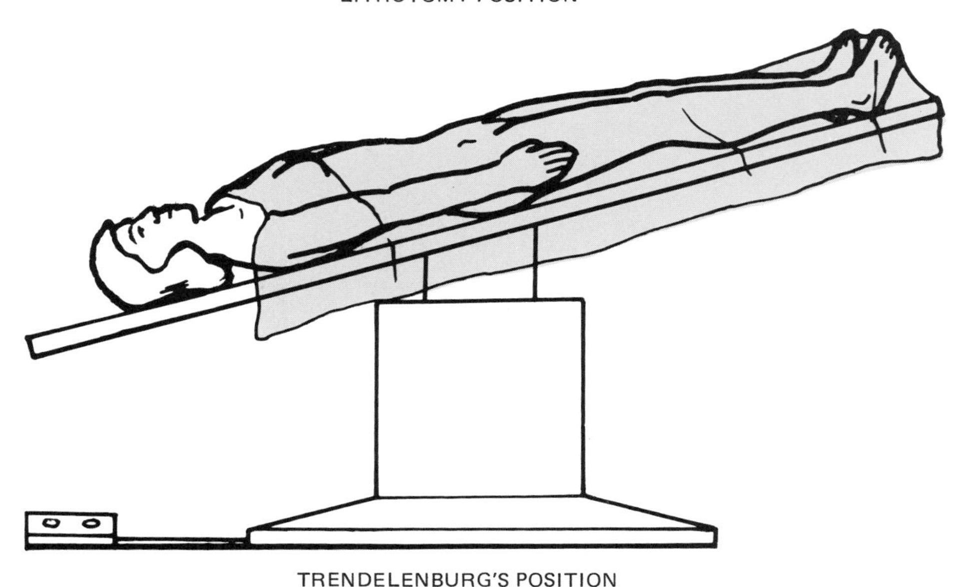

Figure 15-5 Patients in the lithotomy and Trendelenburg's positions.

The Lithotomy Position

In the lithotomy position (lih-**THOT**-oh-me) the patient is supine with the feet and legs raised and supported in stirrups. This position is used for vaginal and rectal examinations.

The Trendelenburg's Position

In the Trendelenburg's position the patient is supine with the feet elevated. The knees may be bent. This position is used for some radiographic examinations and is also used for the treatment of shock.

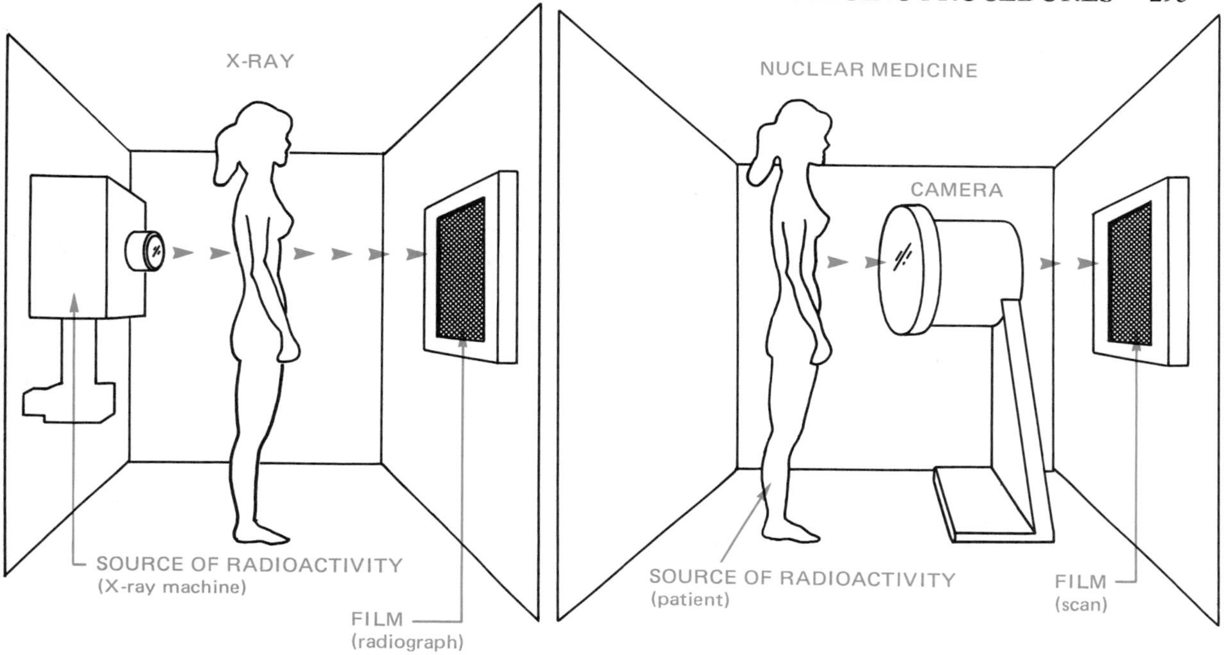

Figure 15-6 In radiography, the source of radioactivity is the x-ray machine. In nuclear medicine the source of radioactivity comes from within the patient.

RADIOGRAPHY

Radiography, also known as **x-ray,** is the creation of an image of hard tissue internal structures of the body by exposure of sensitized film through the use of radiation. The resulting film is known as a **radiograph, radiogram** or an **x-ray.**

X-rays are a form of radiation that are invisible high-energy electromagnetic waves produced by an x-ray machine. **Ionization** is the ability of these x-rays to change the substances through which they pass.

Ionization is beneficial in producing radiographs and in treating cancer. However, excessive exposure to this type of radiation is dangerous and may cause death.

NUCLEAR MEDICINE

Nuclear medicine, also known as **radionuclide imaging (ray-** dee-oh-**NEW-**klyd), is that branch of radiology utilizing radioactive elements and compounds for both diagnosis and treatment.

In conventional x-rays, radiation passes through the body from an outside source. But nuclear medicine involves detecting radiation from a radioactive chemical placed within the body, or mixed with a sample of blood or urine for laboratory analysis.

Nuclear Scans

Nuclear scans, also referred to simply as **scans**, provide images that give information about function as well as the structure of an organ or system. Scans can even visualize some organs that cannot be seen on conventional x-rays.

A patient undergoing a scan is given a **radiopharmaceutical,** which is a drug or chemical that contains a radionuclide designed to concentrate in a particular part of the body.

Radiopharmaceuticals are usually administered by injection but may be administered by mouth or inhalation.

A special instrument is used to detect the radiation given off by the drug and convert it to an image that can be photographed or displayed on a television screen. The instrument most often used is a **gamma camera.** The images obtained are called **scans** or **scintigrams.**

- A **bone scan** helps to detect fractures, tumors and inflammation, and to determine whether bone growth is normal.
- A **brain scan** is often used together with an image of the brain produced by tomography to detect brain tumors or problems in blood flow within, or to and from, the brain.
- A **liver scan** is useful in diagnosing cirrhosis and hepatitis, as well as in detecting tumors, cysts, or an abscess of the liver.
- A **lung scan** is most often done to detect blood clots that have traveled through the bloodstream to the lungs.
- A **thyroid scan** utilizes radioactive iodine because iodine accumulates in the thyroid and the rate of uptake is an indicator of thyroid function.

Radioimmunoassay

Radioimmunoassay (**ray**-dee-oh-**im**-you-no-**AS**-ay), also known as **radioassay,** is a laboratory technique in which a radioactively labeled substance is mixed with a blood specimen.

This test is used to determine the concentration of an antigen, antibody, or other proteins in the blood serum.

Immunofluorescence (im-you-no-**floo**-oh-**RES**-ens) is a method of tagging antibodies with a fluorescent dye to detect or localize antigen-antibody combinations. (The combining form *FLUOR/O* means luminous.)

Radiation Therapy

Radiation therapy, also known as **radiotherapy,** is the treatment of neoplastic disease through the use of x-rays or gamma rays.

Teletherapy is radiation therapy administered by a machine that is positioned at some distance from the patient. For example, a teletherapy unit rotates around the patient. (The combining form *TELE/O* means distant or far. The combining form *THERAP/O* means therapy.)

Brachytherapy (brack-ee-**THER**-ah-pee) is the use of radioactive materials in the treatment of malignant neoplasms by placing the radioactive sources in contact with or implanted into the tissues to be treated. (The prefix *BRACHY-* means short.)

OTHER IMAGING TECHNIQUES

Tomography

Tomography (toh-**MOG**-rah-fee), also known as **laminagraphy (lam**-ih-**NAG**-rah-fee), is any imaging method that produces images of cross-sections of the body.

Computerized axial tomography, also known as **computed tomography** (CT) and **computer aided tomography** (CAT), is an imaging method by which a computer is used to reconstruct two-dimensional cross-section images of body structures into a three-dimensional image.

Positron emission tomography, also known as PET, uses radioactive tracers (radiopharmaceuticals) to produce enhanced images of selected body areas. PET is used predominantly to measure cellular, organ, or system function.

Magnetic Resonance Imaging

Magnetic resonance imaging, also known as **nuclear magnetic resonance,** uses a combination of radio waves and a strong magnetic field to produce images of the soft tissues (tissues other than bones).

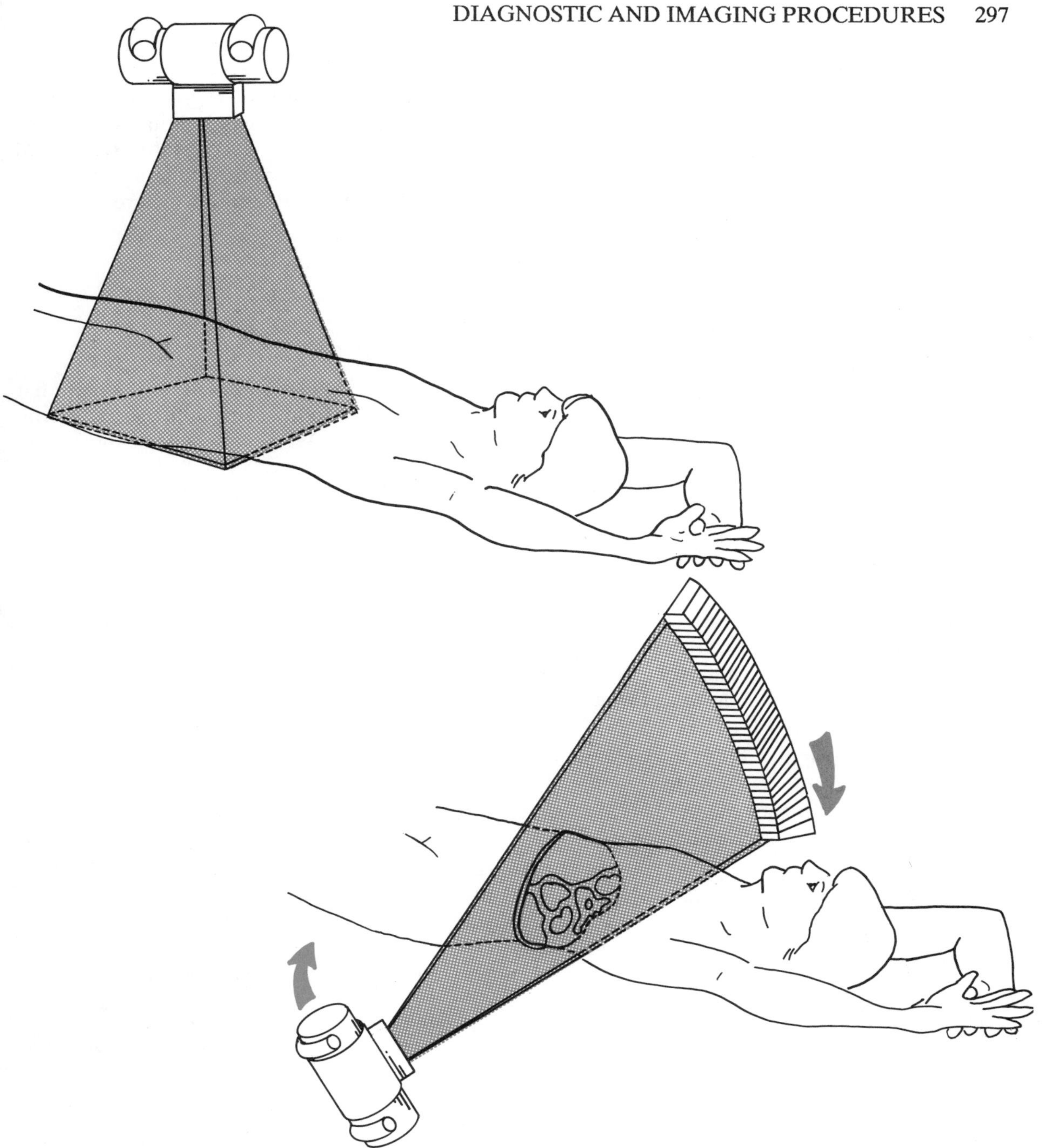

Figure 15-7 Conventional x-rays superimpose anatomy. Tomography provides cross-sectional images.

Ultrasound

Ultrasound, also known as **ultrasonography,** (**ul**-trah-son-**OG**-rah-fee) is the imaging of deep structures of the body by recording the echoes of pulses of sound waves above the range of human hearing. The resulting record is called an **ultrasonogram** or a **sonogram.**

Thermography

Thermography (ther-**MOG**-rah-fee) is a technique utilizing an infrared camera to photographically portray the body's surface temperature. The resulting record is a **thermogram.** (The combining form *THERM/O* means heat.)

Radiographic Contrast Medium

A contrast medium is a substance used to facilitate radiographic imaging of internal structures that otherwise are hard to see on x-ray films.

Radiopaque (**ray**-dee-oh-**PAYK**) means that the substance does not permit x-rays to pass through it. A radiopaque contrast medium, such as barium sulfate, appears on the x-ray as white or light gray.

Radiolucent (ray-dee-oh-**LOO**-sent) means that the substance permits x-rays to pass through it. A radiolucent contrast medium, such as air, appears on the x-ray as black or dark gray.

Fluoroscopy

Fluoroscopy (**floo**-or-**OS**-koh-pee) is an examination using a fluoroscope that involves the use of x-rays projected on a fluorescent screen. Fluoroscopy can be used to visualize body parts in motion.

Cineradiography

Cineradiography (**sin**-eh-**ray**-dee-**OG**-rah-fee) is the filming with a movie or video camera of the images that appear on a fluorescent screen.

Xeroradiography

Xeroradiography (**zee**-roh-ray-dee-**OG**-rah-fee) is an x-ray process in which images are produced by exposing an electrostatically charged photoreceptor plate (rather than using a traditional x-ray film). The resulting picture is printed on paper.

RADIOGRAPHIC POSITIONING AND PROJECTIONS

Projections

The term **projection** describes the path that the x-ray beam follows through the body from entrance to exit. When the name of the projection combines two terms into a single word, the term listed first is the one that the x-ray penetrates first.

For example, in an anteroposterior projection the x-rays travel through the body from anterior (front) toward the posterior (back) and expose the film which is located behind the patient.

Positioning

The term **positioning** describes the specified body position and the part of the body closest to the film. For example, in a left lateral position the left side of the body is placed nearest the film.

The basic projections described in the next section may be used for most body parts. These projections may be exposed with the patient in a standing or recumbent position.

Basic Radiographic Projections

- An **anteroposterior projection** (A.P.) has the patient positioned with her back parallel to the film. The x-ray beam travels from anterior (front) to posterior (back).
- A **posteroanterior projection** (P.A.) has the patient positioned facing the film and parallel to it. The x-ray beam travels through the body from posterior to anterior.

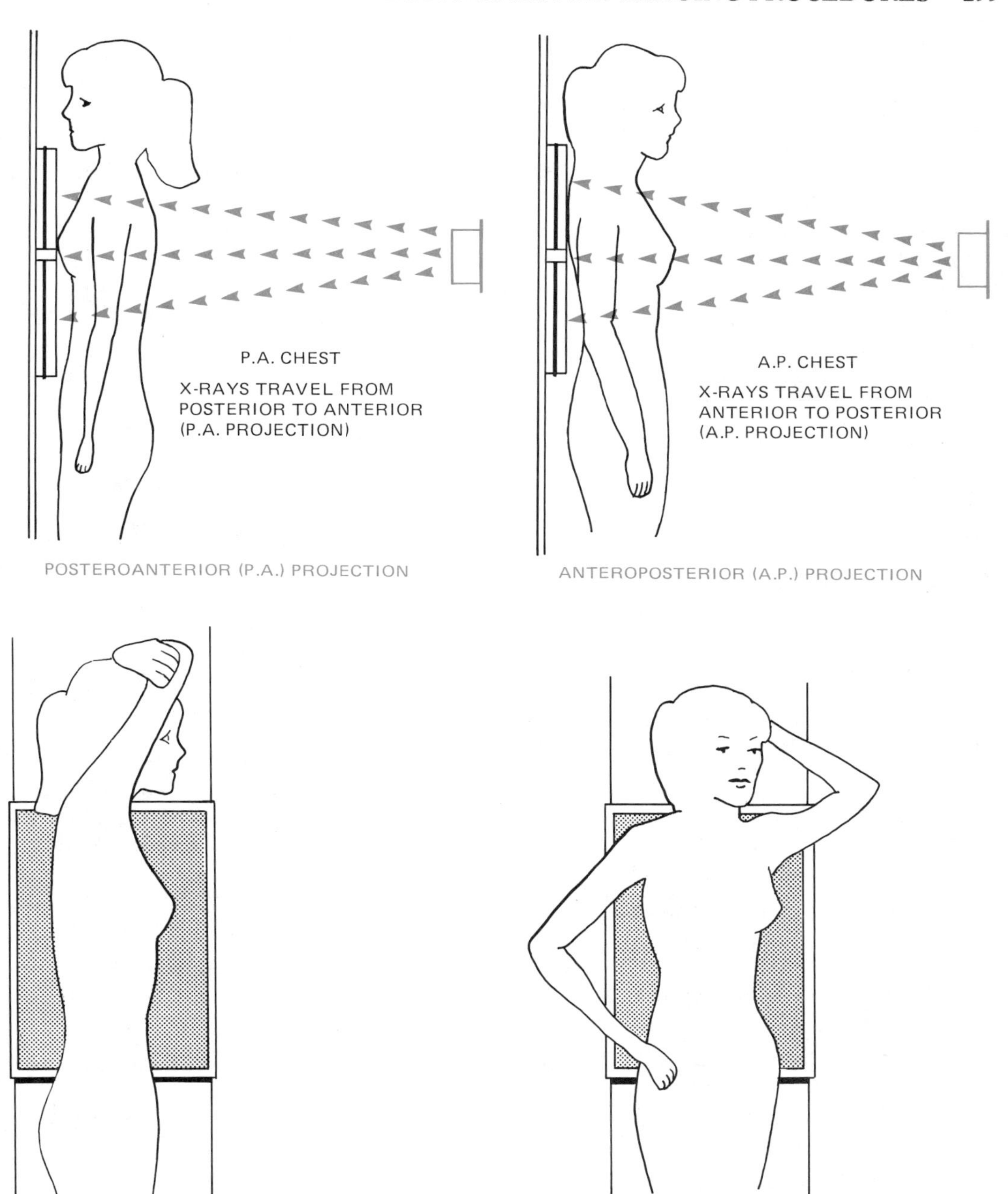

Figure 15-8 Radiographic projections.

- A **lateral projection** (Lat.), also known as a **side view,** has the patient positioned at right angles to the film. This view is named for the side of the body nearest the film.
- An **oblique projection** (Obli.) has the patient positioned so that his body is slanted sideways to the film. This is halfway between a parallel and a right angle position. This view is named for the side of the body nearest the film. (**Oblique** means slanted sideways.)
- For a **left posterior oblique** (L.P.O.) projection the patient is positioned so that her back is toward the film. She is then turned at a slight angle so that the left portion of her back is nearest the film.
- For a **right posterior oblique projection** (R.P.O.) the patient is positioned so that her back is toward the film. She is then turned at a slight angle so that the right portion of her back is nearest the film.
- For a **left anterior oblique projection** (L.A.O.) the patient is positioned facing the film and turned slightly so that the left side of her body is nearest the film.
- For a **right anterior oblique projection** (R.A.O.) the patient is positioned facing the film and turned slightly so that the right side of her body is nearest the film.

IMPORTANT TERMS: DIAGNOSTIC AND IMAGING PROCEDURES

This list will help you identify and review the major terms from this chapter.

When you work with the audio tape for this chapter, listen to the word, repeat it and then place a ✓ next to it on the list below.

- ☐ **Auscultation** (**aws**-kul-**TAY**-shun)
- ☐ **Brachytherapy** (**brack**-ee-**THER**-ah-pee)
- ☐ **Cineradiography** (**sin**-eh-**ray**-dee-**OG**-rah-fee)
- ☐ **Decubitus** (dee-**KYOU**-bih-tus)
- ☐ **Endoscopy** (en-**DOS**-koh-pee)
- ☐ **Fluoroscopy** (**floo**-or-**OS**-koh-pee)
- ☐ **Immunofluorescence** (**im**-you-no-**floo**-oh-**RES**-ens)
- ☐ **Laminagraphy** (**lam**-ih-**NAG**-rah-fee)
- ☐ **Lithotomy** (lih-**THOT**-oh-me)
- ☐ **Palpation** (pal-**PAY**-shun)
- ☐ **Percussion** (per-**KUSH**-un)
- ☐ **Radioimmunoassay** (**ray**-dee-oh-**im**-you-no-**AS**-ay)
- ☐ **Radiolucent** (ray-dee-oh-**LOO**-sent)
- ☐ **Radionuclide** (**ray**-dee-oh-**NEW**-klyd)
- ☐ **Radiopaque** (**ray**-dee-oh-**PAYK**)
- ☐ **Recumbent** (ree-**KUM**-bent)
- ☐ **Sphygmomanometer** (**sfig**-moh-mah-**NOM**-eh-ter)
- ☐ **Stethoscope** (**STETH**-oh-skope)
- ☐ **Supine** (**SUE**-pine)
- ☐ **Thermography** (ther-**MOG**-rah-fee)
- ☐ **Tomography** (toh-**MOG**-rah-fee)
- ☐ **Xeroradiography** (**zee**-roh-ray-dee-**OG**-rah-fee)

EXERCISES

DEFINING WORD PARTS

Write the definition for each of these word parts.

1. *BRACHY-* ______________________________
2. *FLUOR/O* ______________________________
3. *SUPIN/O* ______________________________
4. *TELE/O* ______________________________
5. *THERM/O* ______________________________

DEFINITIONS

Circle the letter next to the correct answer.

1. In the ______________ position, the patient is supine with the feet and legs raised and supported in stirrups.
   a) lithotomy
   b) recumbent
   c) Sims'
   d) Trendelenburg's

2. In a/an ______________ examination, the source of radiation comes from the machine.
   a) immunofluorescence
   b) nuclear medicine
   c) ultrasound
   d) x-ray

3. _______________ is an x-ray process in which images are produced by exposing an electrostatically charged photoreceptor plate.
   a) Cineradiography
   b) Fluoroscopy
   c) Thermography
   d) Xeroradiography

4. _______________ is any imaging method that produces images of cross-sections of the body.
   a) Laminagraphy
   b) Teletherapy
   c) Tomography
   d) a and c.

5. The term _______________ may be used to describe any position in which the patient is lying down.
   a) anatomical
   b) decubitus
   c) recumbent
   d) b and c.

MISSING WORDS

Write the missing word on the line.

1. The term ______________________ describes the path that the x-ray beam follows through the body from entrance to exit.
2. A ______________________ results from the use of a camera to photographically portray the body's surface temperature.
3. A/an ______________________ projection has the patient positioned so that his body is slanted sideways to the film.
4. A ______________________ substance does not permit x-rays to pass through it.
5. A patient undergoing a nuclear scan is given a/an ______________________ which is a drug or chemical that contains a radionuclide designed to concentrate in a particular part of the body.
6. ______________________ is the ability of x-rays to change the substances through which they pass.
7. ______________________ ______________________ ______________________, also known as PET, uses radioactive tracers to produce enhanced images of selected body areas.
8. ______________________ is the filming with a movie or video camera of the images that appear on a fluorescent screen.

SPELLCHECK

Select the correct spelling and write it on the line.

1. A ______________________ is used to measure blood pressure.
   sfignometer
   sphygmomanometer
   sphygnomanometer

2. A ______________________ is used to listen for sounds within the body.
   stethascope
   stethescope
   stethoscope

3. ______________________ is also known as x-ray.
   Radeography
   Radiography
   Radography

4. ______________________ is also known as radioassay.
   Radioemmunoassay
   Radioimmunassay
   Radioimmunoassay

5. A ______________________ results from the use of sound waves above the range of human hearing.
   sonagram
   sonegram
   sonogram

6. In an ______________________ projection the patient is positioned so that his body is slanted sideways to the film.
   olbeque
   oblique
   oblioque

7. The term ______________________ means any position in which the patient is lying down.
   recombant
   recumbant
   recumbent

8. In a ______________________ position, the patient is lying on his or her back with the face up.
   sopine
   supiane
   supine

9. In the ______________________ position the patient's feet are elevated.
   Trandelenburg's
   Trendelenburg's
   Trendelinburg's

10. An ______________________ projection has the patient positioned with her back parallel to the film. The x-ray beam travels from front to back.
    antereoposterior
    anterioposterior
    anteroposterior

CASE STUDIES

Write the correct answer on the line.

1. Mr. Johnson underwent ______________________ in which the radioactive source was implanted into the tissues to be treated.

2. In order to produce images of the soft tissues, Homer Potter's doctor used ______________________ ______________________ ______________________ which uses a combination of radio waves and a strong magnetic field.

3. For the rectal examination, the patient was placed in the ______________________ position with his face down, his hips flexed and his knees and chest resting on the table.

4. During her examination of the patient, Dr. LaPinta used ______________________ to feel the texture, size, consistency and location of certain body parts.

5. For the ______________________ projection, Jack Wriggly was positioned facing the film and parallel to it.

6. Maria Martinez was placed in the ______________________ ______________________ position, lying on her back with her knees bent.

7. For the ______________________ projection, Alicia Walters was positioned at right angles to the film.

8. During the examination, Dr. Ulrich used ______________________ which involves the use of sharp, short blows to the surface of the body with a finger or instrument.

9. Dr. Oshone used ______________________ to visualize the body parts in motion.

10. For a left ______________________ ______________________ projection Mrs. Brown was positioned so that she was facing the film and turned slightly so that the left side of her body was nearest the film.

WORD BUILDING

Write the correct word or word part on the line.

1. From front to back
   a) The combining form ______________________ means front.
   b) The combining form ______________________ means back.
   c) The term ______________________ describes a front to back projection.
2. From back to front
   a) The combining form ______________________ means back.
   b) The combining form ______________________ means front.
   c) The term ______________________ describes a back to front projection.
3. Radiation therapy
   a) The prefix ______________________ means short.
   b) The combining form ______________________ means therapy.
   c) The term ______________________ means radiation therapy in which the radioactive material is placed in contact with, or implanted in, the tissues to be treated.
4. More radiation therapy
   a) The combining form ______________________ means distant or far.
   b) The combining form ______________________ means therapy.
   c) The term ______________________ means radiation therapy administered by a machine that is positioned at some distance from the patient.
5. Body surface temperature
   a) The combining form ______________________ means heat.
   b) The suffix ______________________ means the process of recording a picture or record.
   c) The term ______________________ means to use a special camera to photographically portray the body's surface temperature.

CHALLENGE WORD BUILDING

Write the correct word or word part on the line. (These word parts are not included in this chapter. However, they are covered in other chapters and also may be found in Appendix A.)

1. Endoscopy of the bronchi
   a) The combining form ______________________ means bronchial tube or windpipe.
   b) The suffix ______________________ means visual examination.
   c) The term ______________________ means visual examination of the bronchi.

2. Endoscopy of the larynx
   a) The combining form ______________________ means larynx.
   b) The suffix ______________________ means visual examination.
   c) The term ______________________ means visual examination of the larynx.

3. Endoscopy of the large intestine
   a) The combining form ______________________ sigmoid colon.
   b) The suffix ______________________ means visual examination.
   c) The terms ______________________ means visual examination of the sigmoid colon.

4. Endoscopy of the stomach
   a) The combining form ______________________ means stomach.
   b) The suffix ______________________ means visual examination.
   c) The term ______________________ means visual examination of the stomach.

5. Endoscopy of the rectum
   a) The combining form ______________________ means anus and rectum.
   b) The suffix ______________________ means visual examination.
   c) The term ______________________ means visual examination of the anus and rectum.

6. Endoscopy of the esophagus
   a) The combining form ______________________ means esophagus.
   b) The suffix ______________________ means visual examination.
   c) The term ______________________ means visual examination of the esophagus.

7. Endoscopy of a joint
   a) The combining form ______________________ means joint.
   b) The suffix ______________________ means visual examination.
   c) The term ______________________ means visual examination of a joint.

LABELING EXERCISES

Identify the numbered items on the diagrams and this and on the following page.

1. ______________________

2. ______________________

3. ______________________

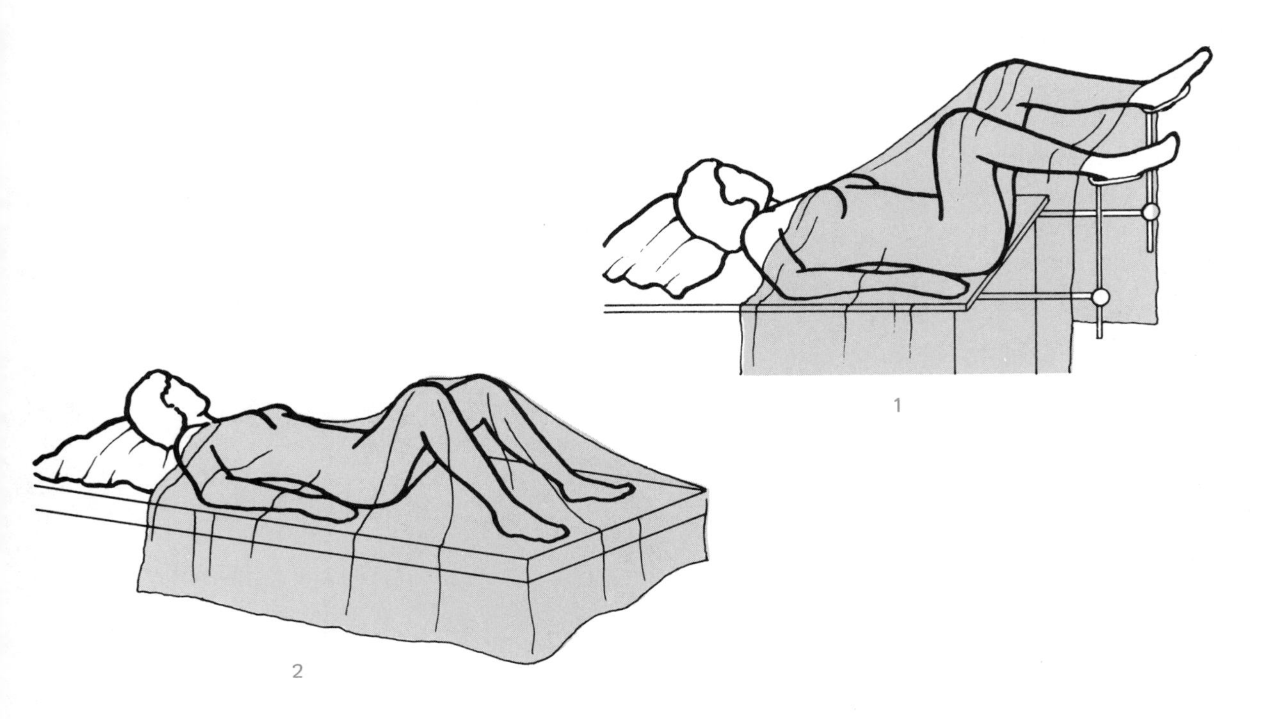

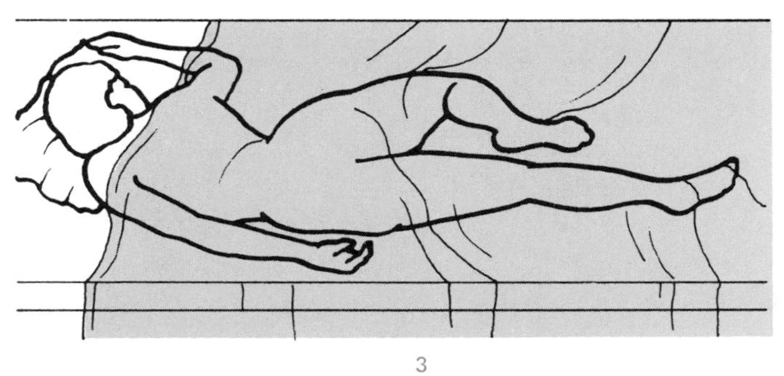

LABELING EXERCISES (continued)

4. ______________________

5. ______________________

6. ______________________

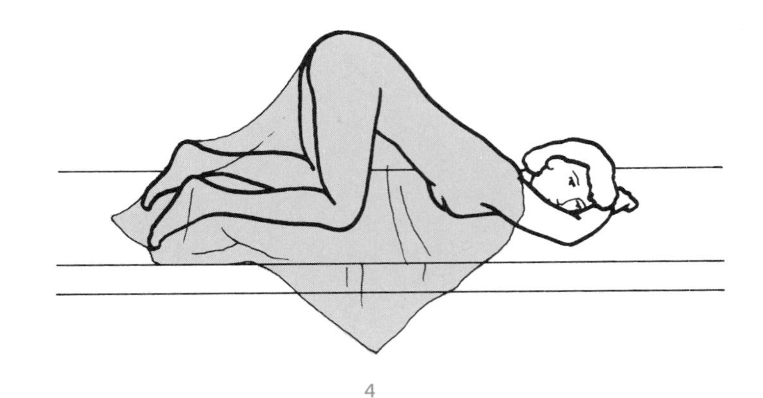

4

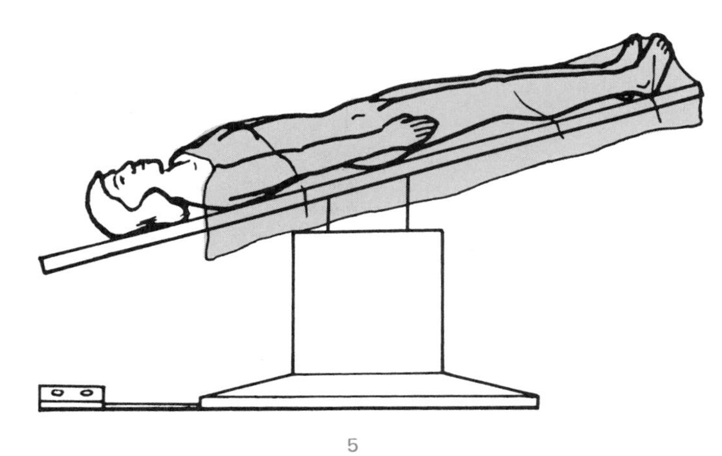

5

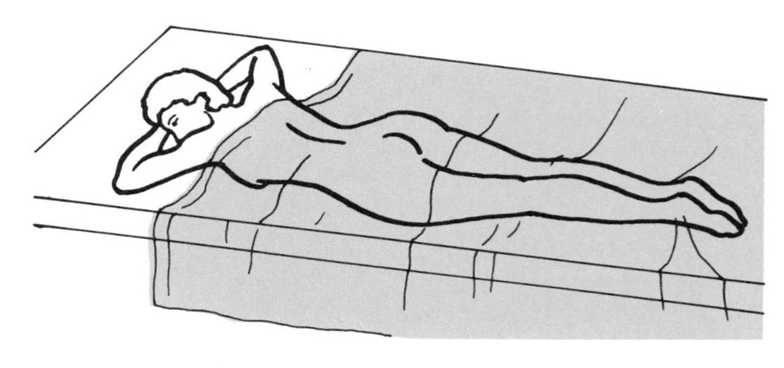

6

16

MENTAL DISORDERS AND PHARMACOLOGY

LEARNING GOALS

In this chapter you will learn to:

- differentiate between neurotic disorders and psychoses.
- recognize and define the terms used to describe the major types of mental disorders.
- define pharmacology and the basic terms related to it.
- identify the routes of drug administration and describe three types of injections.
- recognize and define the terms associated with anesthesia, analgesics and commonly used groups of drugs.

MENTAL DISORDERS

Psychology is the study of behavior and of the functions and processes of the mind. (The combining form *PSYCH/O* means mind.

Psychosomatic disorders (**sigh**-koh-soh-**MAT**-ick) are a variety of physical symptoms of mental origin that do not involve tissue damage. (The prefix *SOMA-* means body.)

Neurotic Disorders

A **neurosis** (new-**ROH**-sis), also known as a **neurotic disorder,** is a mental disorder without any demonstrable organic basis. The individual may have considerable insight and usually has good contact with reality. Although behavior may be greatly affected, it usually remains within socially acceptable limits. (Plural, **neuroses.**)

An **anxiety state** is a feeling of apprehension, tension or uneasiness that stems from the anticipation of danger, the source of which is largely unknown or unrecognized.

Hypochondriasis (**high**-poh-kon-**DRY**-ah-sis) is a neurotic disorder in which the conspicuous feature is excessive concern with one's health.

Neurasthenia (**new**-ras-**THEE**-nee-ah) is a neurotic disorder characterized by fatigue, irritability, headache, depression, insomnia, difficulty in concentrating and lack of capacity for enjoyment.

Psychosis

A psychosis (sigh-**KOH**-sis) is any major mental disorder in which impairment of mental function has developed to a degree that it seriously interferes with insight, the ability to meet the ordinary demands of life, or the ability to maintain adequate contact with reality. (Plural, **psychoses.**)

Affective psychoses are mental disorders in which there are recurrent severe disturbances of mood accompanied by other symptoms such as delusions.

Affect is the outward manifestation of a person's mood. **Apathy** is an absence or suppression of emotion, feeling, concern or passion. (One meaning of the suffix *-PATHY* is feeling or emotion.)

A **delusion** (dee-**LOO**-zhun) is a false personal belief that is maintained in spite of obvious proof or evidence to the contrary.

A **manic-depressive psychosis** is characterized by periods of severe depression mixed with manic phases.

Depression is a mood disturbance characterized by feelings of sadness, discouragement and despair. This is an abnormal condition when the feelings are exaggerated and do not appear to be associated with life events.

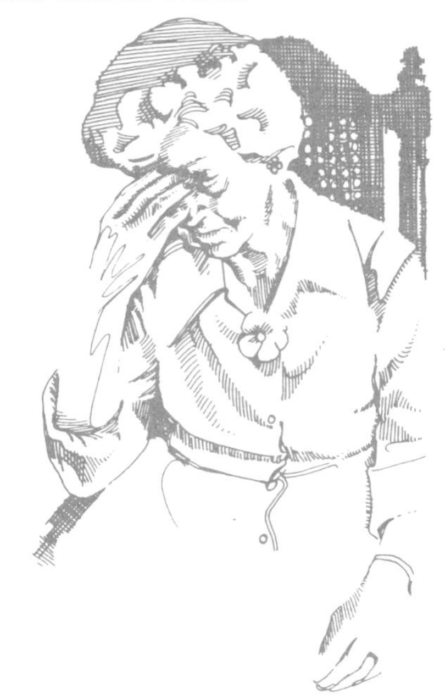

Figure 16-1 Depression affects people of all ages.

Mania is characterized by an expansive emotional state, over-talkativeness and increased motor activity. (The combining form *MAN/I* means rage.)

Paranoia (**par**-ah-**NOI**-ah) is a psychosis, acute or chronic, characterized by delusions of being influenced, persecuted or treated in some special way.

Schizophrenia (**skiz**-oh-**FREE**-nee-ah) is a group of psychoses in which there is a fundamental disturbance of personality. There is also a characteristic distortion of thinking which may include a sense of being controlled by alien forces, bizarre delusions and disturbed perception.

The combining form *SCHIZ/O* means divided, split or cleft. Although schizophrenia is sometimes called **split personality,** this is not an accurate description of the disorder.

Personality Disorders

A personality disorder is any of a large group of mental disorders characterized by rigid, inflexible and maladaptive behavior patterns that impair a person's ability to function in society.

An **antisocial type** is a personality disorder characterized by repeated behavioral patterns that lack moral and ethical standards and bring a person into continuous conflict with society.

A **compulsive type** is a personality disorder characterized by feelings of personal insecurity, doubt and incompleteness leading to excessive conscientiousness, stubbornness, and caution.

A **passive-aggressive type** is a personality disorder characterized by aggressive behavior manifested in passive ways, such as obstructionism, procrastination and intentional inefficiency. (The combining form *AGGRESS/O* means attack.)

Phobias

A phobia (**FOH**-bee-ah) is a neurotic state characterized by an abnormally intense dread of certain objects or specific situations that would not normally have that effect. (The combining form *PHOB/O* means fear.)

Acrophobia (**ack**-roh-**FOH**-bee-ah) is an excessive fear of being in high places. (The combining form *ACR/O* means top.)

Agoraphobia (**ag**-oh-rah-**FOH**-bee-ah) is the overwhelming fear of being in crowded places and incapacitating anxiety on traveling away from the safety of home. (The combining form *AGOR/A* means marketplace.)

Alcoholism

Alcoholism is an extreme dependence on excessive amounts of alcohol associated with a cumulative pattern of deviant behavior.

Delirium tremens (dee-**LIR**-ee-um **TREE**-mens) is an acute and sometimes fatal psychotic reaction in alcoholics. It is characterized by clouded consciousness, disorientation, fear, delusion and hallucinations.

Delirium is a mental state in which one experiences confusion and decreased awareness of surroundings. (The combining form *DELIRI/O* means wandering in the mind.)

A **hallucination** (hah-**loo**-sih-**NAY**-shun) is a sense perception (sight, touch, sound, smell or taste) that has no basis in external stimulation. (The combining form *HALLUCIN/O* means to wander in the mind.)

Other Disorders

- **Anorexia nervosa** (**an**-oh-**RECK**-see-ah ner-**VOH**-sah) is a disorder in which the main features are persistent, active refusal to eat and a marked loss of weight.
- **Autism** (**AW**-tizm) is a syndrome mainly affecting children in which responses to auditory and sometimes to visual stimuli are abnormal. The combining form *AUT/O* means self, and children with this syndrome often seem withdrawn into themselves.
- **Bulimia** (byou-**LIM**-ee-ah) is an episodic pattern of binge eating that is usually followed by purging through the use of vomiting or laxatives.

- **Dementia** (dee-**MEN**-she-ah) is a decrease in intellectual functioning of sufficient severity to interfere with occupational or social performance, or both.

- **Dyslexia** (dis-**LECK**-see-ah) is a disorder in which the main feature is a serious impairment of reading skills that cannot be explained in terms of general intellectual retardation or of inadequate schooling.

- **Fetishism** (**FET**-ish-izm) is a disorder in which nonliving objects are utilized as a preferred or exclusive method of stimulating erotic arousal.

- **Hyperkinetic syndrome of childhood** is a group of disorders in which the essential features are short attention span, distractibility and being overactive.

  Hyperkinetic (**high**-per-kih-**NET**-ick) means increased motor activity. (One meaning of the prefix *HYPER-* is increased or excessive.)

- **Involutional melancholia** (**in**-voh-**LOO**-shun-al **mel**-an-**KOH**-lee-ah) is a severe depression occuring in middle age or later.

  One meaning of **involution** refers to progressive degeneration occurring naturally with advancing age.

- **Kleptomania** (**klep**-toh-**MAY**-nee-ah) is a disorder characterized by a recurrent failure to resist impulses to steal objects not for immediate use or their monetary value. (The combining form *KLEPT/O* means to steal.)

- **Malingering** (mah-**LING**-ger-ing) is a disorder in which the predominant feature is the presentation of fake or grossly exaggerated physical or psychiatric illness apparently under voluntary control.

- **Masochism** (**MASS**-oh-kizm) is a disorder in which having physical or psychological pain inflicted gives sexual gratification to the recipient.

- **Megalomania** (**meg**-ah-loh-**MAY**-nee-ah) is an unreasonable conviction of one's own extreme greatness, goodness or power. (The combining form *MEGAL/O* means great or large.)

- **Narcissism** (**NAR**-sih-sizm) is an abnormal interest in oneself and is characterized by a preoccupation with self-love.

- **Pica** (**PYE**-kah) is a perverted appetite of nonorganic origin in which there is persistent eating of non-nutritional substances such as clay.

- **Pyromania** (**pye**-roh-**MAY**-nee-ah) is a disorder characterized by a recurrent failure to resist impulses to set fires. (The combining form *PYR/O* means fire.)

- **Sadism** (**SAY**-dizm) is a disorder of obtaining sexual gratification through the infliction of pain or humiliation on others.

- **Sadomasochism** (**say**-doh-**MASS**-oh-kizm) is a state characterized by both sadistic and masochistic tendencies.

- **Transsexualism** (trans-**SECKS**-you-ah-lizm) is a disturbance of gender identity accompanied by the desire to change one's sex.

- **Transvestism** (trans-**VES**-tizm) is a sexual deviation in which there is recurrent and persistent dressing in clothes of the opposite sex.

- **Voyeurism** (**VOI**-yer-izm) is a sexual deviation in which the individual seeks gratification from looking at sexual objects or acts.

Psychoanalysis

Psychoanalysis is a system of treating mental disorders by gathering from the patient his past emotional experience and the facts of his mental life, in order to discover the mechanism by which a pathological mental state has been produced.

In psychoanalysis, the **psyche** (**SIGH**-kee) consists of the total components of the id, ego and superego. (**Psyche** means the mind of an individual.)

The **id** is defined as that part of the psyche, functioning in the unconscious, that is the source of instinctive energy, impulses and drives.

The **ego** is defined as that part of the psyche that experiences and maintains conscious contact with reality.

The **superego** is defined as that part of the psyche, functioning mostly in the unconscious, that develops when the standards of the parents and of society are incorporated into the ego.

PHARMACOLOGY

Pharmacology is the study of the nature, uses and effects of drugs. A **pharmacist** is a specialist who is licensed in formulating and dispensing medications. (The combining form *PHARMAC/O* means drug.)

A **prescription** is an order for medication, therapy or a therapeutic device given (usually in writing) by a properly authorized person to a person properly authorized to dispense or perform the order.

A **prescription drug** is a medication that may be purchased only with a prescription from an appropriately licensed professional. For example, a drug prescribed by a physician or dentist.

An **over-the-counter drug** is a medication that may be purchased without a written prescription.

A **brand name** drug is sold under the name given the drug by the manufacturer. A brand name is always spelled with a capital letter.

A **generic drug** is one that is usually named for its chemical structure and is not protected by a brand name or trademark.

Drug Action and Interaction

A **contraindication** is a factor in the patient's condition that makes the use of a drug dangerous or ill-advised.

A **palliative** (**PAL**-ee-ay-tiv) is a substance that serves to ease pain or the severity of a disease but does not cure it.

A **placebo** (plah-**SEE**-boh) is a substance containing no active ingredients that is given for its suggestive effects or to please a person.

A **drug interaction** occurs when the effect of one drug is modified (changed) when it is administered at the same time as another drug.

Potentiation, also known as **synergism** (**SIN**-er-jizm), is a drug interaction that occurs when the effect of one drug is potentiated (increased) by another drug.

An **adverse reaction,** also known as a **side effect,** is a drug response that accompanies the principal response for which the drug was taken.

An **idiosyncratic reaction** (id-ee-oh-sin-**KRAT**-ick) is an unexpected reaction to a drug. (The combining form *IDI/O* means peculiar to the individual or organ.)

Addiction is compulsive, uncontrollable dependence on a substance, habit or practice to the degree that stopping causes severe emotional, mental or physiological reactions.

Routes of Drug Administration

Inhalation administration refers to vapor and gases that are taken in through the nose or mouth and absorbed into the bloodstream through the lungs. For example, the gases used for general anesthesia are administered by inhalation.

Topical administration refers to the drugs, such as lotions and ointments, that are applied to the skin for local action.

Transdermal administration, usually with a patch, is the application of a drug that is absorbed through the skin and into systemic circulation.

With **sublingual administration** the medication is placed under the tongue and allowed to dissolve slowly in the mouth. (The combining form *LINGU/O* means tongue.)

Oral administration refers to drugs that are taken by mouth and are designed to be absorbed into the system from the stomach or small intestine. These drugs may be in the forms such as liquids, pills or capsules.

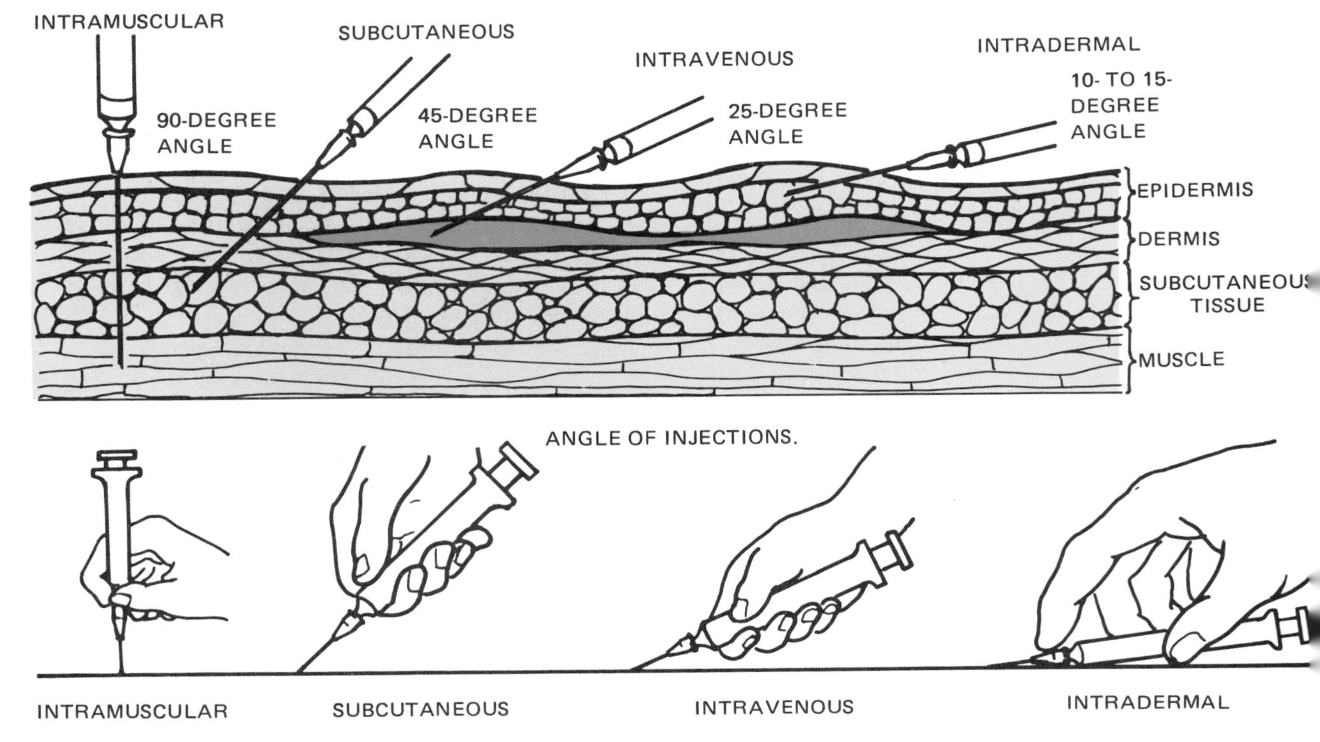

Figure 16-2 Types of parenteral injections.

An **enteric coating** is a special coating applied to tablets or capsules that prevents release and absorption of their contents until they reach the small intestine. (The combining form *ENTER/O* means small intestine.)

Rectal administration is the insertion of medication in the rectum by use of either **suppositories** or liquid solutions.

Parenteral Administration

Parenteral (pah-**REN**-ter-al) administration is the administration of medication by injection through a hypodermic syringe.

An **intradermal injection** is given within the structure of the outer layers of the skin.

A **subcutaneous injection** is given just beneath the skin.

An **intramuscular injection** is given within the substance of a muscle.

An **intravenous injection** is given directly into a vein. An alternative is to administer the drug through an IV (intravenous) line that is already in place in the patient's vein.

Anesthesia

Anesthesia is the absence of normal sensation, especially sensitivity to pain. Anesthesia is induced by an **anesthetic** and may be topical, local, regional or general. (The suffix *-ESTHESIA* means sensation or feeling.)

A **topical anesthesia** is usually applied as a liquid, ointment or spray form and numbs the surface of the skin.

Local anesthesia, also known as **infiltration anesthesia,** is localized or **regional anesthesia** produced by injection of an anesthetic immediately adjacent to the area where loss of sensation is desired.

A **nerve block** is a type of regional anesthesia in which the anesthetic agent is injected close to the nerves whose conduction is to be temporarily interrupted.

Epidural anesthesia is the process of achieving regional anesthesia of the pelvic, abdominal, genital, or other area by the injection of a local anesthetic into the epidural space of the spinal cord.

General anesthesia involves the total loss of body sensation and consciousness as induced by various anesthetic agents, given primarily by inhalation or intravenous injection.

Analgesics

An **analgesic (an-al-JEE-zick)** is a drug that relieves pain without affecting consciousness.

Nonnarcotic analgesics, which are used for mild to moderate pain, act at the site of the pain and do not produce dependence.

Narcotic analgesics, which are used for severe pain, act on the central nervous system and may cause dependence or addiction.

A **narcotic,** also known as an **opiate,** is a substance that produces insensibility or stupor and is generally derived from opium or produced synthetically.

Morphine, Demerol, and **codeine** are all narcotics used to control severe pain. They are highly addictive.

Brompton's mixture is an analgesic solution containing a variety of narcotic drugs that is used to control pain in terminally ill patients.

Sedatives and Hypnotics

A **sedative** is a drug that depresses the central nervous system and produces diminished responsiveness without producing sleep.

A **hypnotic** is a drug that depresses the central nervous system and usually produces sleep. (The combining form *HYPN/O* means sleep.)

Be careful not to confuse a hypnotic with hypnosis. They really are very different! **Hypnosis** is a state of narrowly focused attention and increased suggestibility that may be used for pain control, to speed psychological change and for relaxation.

A **barbiturate** (bar-**BIT**-you-rayt) is a class of drugs whose major action is a calming or depressed effect on the central nervous system.

Amobarbital (am-oh-BAR-bih-tal) is a barbiturate that is used as a sedative and hypnotic.

Phenobarbital (fee-no-BAR-bih-tal) is a barbiturate that is used as a sedative and to control convulsions.

Drugs to Treat Infections

An **antiseptic** is a substance that kills or inhibits the growth of microorganisms. The term is commonly used to describe preparations, such as an iodine tincture, that are applied to the skin.

A **disinfectant** is an agent that is used to destroy pathogenic microorganisms. The term is commonly used to describe substances, such as 70% isopropyl alcohol, applied to inanimate objects such as equipment and clothing.

Germicide is the general term used to describe agents capable of destroying microorganisms. More specific names are given drugs within the category. For example, a bactericide is a type of germicide.

A **bactericide** (back-**TEER**-ih-sighd) is a substance that causes the death of bacteria. These include primarily the antibiotic groups of **penicillins** and **cephalosporins.** (The combining form *BACTERI/O* means bacteria. The suffix *-CIDE* means causing death.)

Antibiotics are drugs made from naturally occurring and synthetic substances that are used to combat bacterial infection.

A **bacteriostatic** (back-**tee**-ree-oh-**STAT**-ick) is an agent that inhibits, slows or retards the growth of bacteria. These include primarily the antibiotic groups of **tetracyclines, sulfonamides,** and **erythromycin.** (The suffix *-STATIC* means stopping, controlling, slowing.)

An **antifungal (an-**tih-**FUNG**-gal) drug, such as nystatin, is used to treat fungal infections.

An **antiviral** (**an**-tih-**VYE**-ral) is a drug, such as acyclovir, used to treat viral infections or to provide temporary immunity.

Drugs to Treat Blood Pressure and Heart Function

A **vasoconstrictor** (**vas**-oh-kon-**STRICK**-tor) is a drug which constricts (narrows) the blood vessels.

A **vasodilator** (**vas**-oh-dye-**LAYT**-or) is a drug which dilates (expands) the blood vessels.

An **antihypertensive** (**an**-tih-**high**-per-**TEN**-siv) is a drug that is used to lower blood pressure.

An **antiarrhythmic** (**an**-tih-ah-**RITH**-mick) is a drug used to control irregularities of the heartbeat.

A **beta-blocker** is a drug that is used as an antihypertensive and antiarrhythmic.

An **anticoagulant** (**an**-tih-koh-**AG**-you-lant), also known as a **thrombolytic** (**throm**-boh-**LIT**-ick), slows blood clotting (coagulation) and prevents new clots from forming.

Prostaglandin (**pros**-tah-**GLAN**-din) is used to stimulate contractions of the uterus and other smooth muscles. It also has the ability to lower blood pressure and to regulate several other body functions.

Drugs Used to Treat Cancer

An **antineoplastic** (**an**-tih-nee-oh-**PLAS**-tick) is a drug that blocks the growth of neoplasms and is used to treat cancer.

An **immunosuppressant** (**im**-you-no-soo-**PRES**-ant) is a drug that prevents or reduces the body's normal reactions to invasion by disease or by foreign tissues.

A **cytotoxic drug** (**sigh**-toh-**TOK**-sick) is one that kills or damages cells. It is used as an antineoplastic and as an immunosuppressant.

Drugs to Treat Mental Disorders

Tranquilizers, also known as **antianxiety drugs,** are used to suppress anxiety and to relax muscles.

An **antidepressant** is a drug that prevents or relieves depression.

An **antipsychotic** (**an**-tih-sigh-**KOT**-ick) is a drug used to treat symptoms of severe psychiatric disorders.

Psychotropic drugs (**sigh**-koh-**TROP**-pick) are agents used to treat emotional and mental disorders.

Drugs to Control Spasms and Convulsions

An **antispasmodic,** also known as an **anticholinergic drug,** acts to control spasmodic activity of the smooth muscles. (The combining form *SPASMOD/O* means sudden contraction tightening or cramping.)

Atropine (**AT**-roh-peen) is a drug that is used primarily as an antispasmodic for smooth muscles such as the intestine.

An **anticonvulsant** (**an**-tih-kon-**VUL**-sant) is a drug that prevents seizures and convulsions.

Other Types of Drugs

- An **antidote** (**an**-tih-doht) is a drug or other substance that opposes the action of a poison.
- An **antihistamine** (**an**-tih-**HIS**-tah-meen) is a drug used to counteract the effects of histamine (which is released in allergic reactions).
- An **anti-inflammatory** is a drug used to counteract or suppress inflammation.
- A **corticosteroid drug** is a hormonal preparation used primarily as an anti-inflammatory and as an immunosuppressant.
- A **diuretic** (**dye**-you-**RET**-ick) is a medication that increases urine secretion.
- An **emetic** (eh-**MET**-ick) is a substance that produces vomiting.

Gamma globulin, also known as **immune globulin,** is an agent obtained from human plasma that may be used for immunization against diseases such as measles.

IMPORTANT TERMS: THE MIND AND DRUGS

This list will help you identify and review the major terms from this chapter.

When you work with the audio tape for this chapter, listen to the word, repeat it and then place a ✓ next to it on the list below.

- ☐ **Acrophobia** (**ack**-roh-**FOH**-bee-ah)
- ☐ **Agoraphobia** (**ag**-oh-rah-**FOH**-bee-ah)
- ☐ **Amobarbital** (**am**-oh-**BAR**-bih-tal)
- ☐ **Analgesic** (**an**-al-**JEE**-zick)
- ☐ **Anorexia nervosa** (**an**-oh-**RECK**-see-ah ner-**VOH**-sah)
- ☐ **Antiarrhythmic** (**an**-tih-ah-**RITH**-mick)
- ☐ **Anticoagulant** (**an**-tih-koh-**AG**-you-lant)
- ☐ **Anticonvulsant** (**an**-tih-kon-**VUL**-sant)
- ☐ **Antidote** (**an**-tih-doht)
- ☐ **Antifungal** (**an**-tih-**FUNG**-gal)
- ☐ **Antihistamine** (**an**-tih-**HIS**-tah-meen)
- ☐ **Antihypertensive** (**an**-tih-**high**- per-**TEN**-siv)
- ☐ **Antineoplastic** (**an**-tih-nee-oh-**PLAS**-tick)
- ☐ **Antipsychotic** (**an**-tih-sigh-**KOT**-ick)
- ☐ **Antiviral** (**an**-tih-**VYE**-ral)
- ☐ **Atropine** (**AT**-roh-peen)
- ☐ **Autism** (**AW**-tizm)
- ☐ **Bacteriostatic** (back-**tee**-ree-oh-**STAT**-ick)
- ☐ **Bactericide** (back-**TEER**-ih-sighd)
- ☐ **Barbiturate** (bar-**BIT**-you-rayt)
- ☐ **Bulimia** (byou-**LIM**-ee-ah)
- ☐ **Cytotoxic** (**sigh**-toh-**TOK**-sick)
- ☐ **Delirium tremens** (dee-**LIR**-ee-um **TREE**-mens)
- ☐ **Delusion** (dee-**LOO**-zhun)
- ☐ **Dementia** (dee-**MEN**-she-ah)
- ☐ **Diuretic** (**dye**-you-**RET**-ick)
- ☐ **Dyslexia** (dis-**LECK**-see-ah)
- ☐ **Fetishism** (**FET**-ish-izm)
- ☐ **Hallucination** (hah-**loo**-sih-**NAY**-shun)
- ☐ **Hyperkinetic** (**high**-per-kih-**NET**-ick)
- ☐ **Hypochondriasis** (**high**-poh-kon-**DRY**-ah-sis)
- ☐ **Idiosyncratic** (**id**-ee-oh-sin-**KRAT**-ick)
- ☐ **Immunosuppressant** (**im**-you-no-soo-**PRES**-ant)
- ☐ **Involutional melancholia** (**in**-voh-**LOO**-shun-al **mel**-an-**KOH**-lee-ah)
- ☐ **Kleptomania** (**klep**-toh-**MAY**-nee-ah)
- ☐ **Malingering** (mah-**LING**-ger-ing)
- ☐ **Masochism** (**MASS**-oh-kizm)
- ☐ **Megalomania** (**meg**-ah-loh-**MAY**-nee-ah)
- ☐ **Narcissism** (**NAR**-sih-sizm)
- ☐ **Neurasthenia** (**new**-ras-**THEE**-nee-ah)
- ☐ **Neurosis** (new-**ROH**-sis)
- ☐ **Palliative** (**PAL**-ee-ay-tiv)
- ☐ **Paranoia** (**par**-ah-**NOI**-ah)
- ☐ **Parenteral** (pah-**REN**-ter-al)
- ☐ **Phenobarbital** (**fee**-no-**BAR**-bih-tal)

- □ **Phobia** (**FOH**-bee-ah)
- □ **Pica** (**PYE**-kah)
- □ **Placebo** (plah-**SEE**-boh)
- □ **Prostaglandin** (**pros**-tah-**GLAN**-din)
- □ **Psyche** (**SIGH**-kee)
- □ **Psychosis** (sigh-**KOH**-sis)
- □ **Psychosomatic** (**sigh**-koh-soh-**MAT**-ick)
- □ **Psychotropic** (**sigh**-koh-**TROP**-pick)
- □ **Pyromania** (**pye**-roh-**MAY**-nee-ah)
- □ **Sadism** (**SAY**-dizm)
- □ **Sadomasochism** (**say**-doh-**MASS**-oh-kizm)
- □ **Schizophrenia** (**skiz**-oh-**FREE**-nee-ah)
- □ **Synergism** (**SIN**-er-jizm)
- □ **Thrombolytic** (**throm**-boh-**LIT**-ick)
- □ **Transsexualism** (trans-**SECKS**-you-ah-lizm)
- □ **Transvestism** (trans-**VES**-tizm)
- □ **Vasoconstrictor** (**vas**-oh-kon-**STRICK**-tor)
- □ **Vasodilator** (**vas**-oh-dye-**LAYT**-or)
- □ **Voyeurism** (**VOI**-yer-izm)

EXERCISES

DEFINING WORD PARTS

Write the definition for each of these word parts.

1. *ACR/O* ________________
2. *AGGRESS/O* ________________
3. *AGOR/A* ________________
4. *AUT/O* ________________
5. *BACTERI/O* ________________
6. *-CIDE* ________________
7. *DELIRI/O* ________________
8. *ENTER/O* ________________
9. *-ESTHESIA* ________________
10. *HALLUCIN/O* ________________
11. *HYPN/O* ________________
12. *IDI/O* ________________
13. *KLEPT/O* ________________
14. *LINGU/O* ________________
15. *MAN/I* ________________
16. *MEGAL/O* ________________

17. *-PATHY* ______________________________

18. *PHARMAC/O* ______________________________

19. *PHOB/O* ______________________________

20. *PSYCH/O* ______________________________

21. *PYR/O* ______________________________

22. *SCHIZ/O* ______________________________

23. *SOMA-* ______________________________

24. *SPASMOD/O* ______________________________

25. *-STATIC* ______________________________

DEFINITIONS

Circle the letter next to the correct answer.

1. A ______________ drug is one that is usually named for its chemical structure and is not protected by a trademark.
   a) brand name
   b) generic
   c) prescription
   d) a and c.

2. A/an ______________ is a drug that depresses the central nervous system and produces diminished responsiveness without producing sleep.
   a) analgesic
   b) hypnotic
   c) palliative
   d) sedative

3. ______________ is a disorder in which the predominant feature is the presentation of fake or grossly exaggerated physical or psychiatric illness apparently under voluntary control.
   a) Dementia
   b) Malingering
   c) Masochism
   d) Narcissism

4. Parenteral administration is the administration of medication ______________
   a) by injection
   b) orally
   c) rectally
   d) sublingually

5. _______________ is sense perception that has no basis in external stimulation.
   a) Delirium
   b) Delusion
   c) Hallucination
   d) Voyeurism

6. The _______________ is the part of the psyche that experiences and maintains conscious contact with reality.
   a) ego
   b) id
   c) subconscious
   d) superego

7. A/an _______________ is an agent used to destroy pathogenic microorganisms on objects such as equipment and clothing.
   a) antiseptic
   b) bacteriostatic
   c) disinfectant
   d) a and b.

8. A/an _______________ drug is one that kills or damages cells. It is used as an immunosuppressant.
   a) antineoplastic
   b) antiviral
   c) corticosteroid
   d) cytotoxic

9. _______________ disorders are a variety of physical symptoms of mental origin that do not involve tissue damage.
   a) Affective psychoses
   b) Hyperkinetic
   c) Megalomania
   d) Psychosomatic

10. _______________ drugs are agents used to treat emotional and mental disorders.
    a) Antihypertensive
    b) Barbiturate
    c) Psychotropic
    d) Sedative

MISSING WORDS

Write the missing word on the line.

1. A/an _______________________, also known as an anticholinergic drug, acts to control spasmodic activity of the smooth muscles.
2. _______________________ is characterized by an expansive emotional state, over-talkativeness and increased motor activity.
3. A/an _______________________ is a drug that expands the blood vessels.
4. A/an _______________________ state is a feeling of apprehension, tension or uneasiness that stems from the anticipation of danger, the source of which is largely unknown or unrecognized.
5. _______________________ anesthesia is regional anesthesia of the pelvic, abdominal, genital or other area by the injection of a local anesthetic into the space around the spinal cord.
6. _______________________ is an absence or suppression of emotion, feeling, concern or passion.
7. A/an _______________________ is a drug used as an antihypertensive and antiarrhythmic.
8. _______________________ is a drug used primarily as an antispasmodic for smooth muscles such as the intestine.
9. A/a _______________________ injection is administered within the structures of the outer layers of skin.
10. A/an _______________________ reaction is an unexpected reaction to a drug.

SPELLCHECK

Select the correct spelling and write it on the line.

1. An _______________________ is a drug used to combat bacterial infections.
   antabiotic
   antebiotic
   antibiotic
2. _______________________ is a drug used as a sedative and to control convulsions.
   Pfenobarbital
   Phenabarbital
   Phenobarbital
3. _______________________ is a mental state in which one experiences confusion and decreased awareness of surroundings.
   Delerium
   Delirium
   Dilerium

4. An ______________________ is a drug that relieves pain without affecting consciousness.
   Analgesic
   Anelgesic
   Anilgesic

5. A ______________________ is a class of drugs whose major action is a calming or depressed effect on the central nervous system.
   barbeturate
   barbiturate
   barbituate

6. ______________________ is a group of psychoses in which there is a fundamental disturbance of personality.
   Schizaphrenia
   Schezophrenia
   Schizophrenia

7. ______________________, also known as antianxiety drugs, are used to suppress anxiety and to relax muscles.
   Trankquillizers
   Tranquilizers
   Tranquillizers

8. A ______________________ is a medication that increases urine secretion.
   diaretic
   diuretic
   dioretic

9. In ______________________, the psyche consists of the total components of the id, ego, and superego.
   psychioanalysis
   psychoanalysis
   psychoanalyzis

10. An ______________________ is a drug used to counteract the effects of allergic reactions.
   antahistamine
   antehistamine
   antihistamine

11. ______________________ is a narcotic used to control severe pain. It is highly addictive.
   Codene
   Codeine
   Codine

12. A ______________________ is an order for medication, therapy or a therapeutic given by a properly authorized person to a person properly authorized to dispense or perform the order.
perscription
perscreption
prescription

13. ______________________ is a narcotic used to control severe pain. It is highly addictive.
Demarol
Demerol
Demirol

14. An ______________________ is a drug that prevents or reduces the body's normal reactions to invasion by disease or by foreign tissues.
immunosuppresant
immunosupressant
immunosuppressant

15. A ______________________ is a false personal belief that is maintained in spite of obvious proof or evidence to the contrary.
dalusion
delusion
deluzion

CASE STUDIES

Write the correct answer on the line.

1. John Doe had an uncontrollable dependence on a drug. Because of his ______________________ stopping involved severe emotional, mental and physiological reactions.
2. Angela Espinoza's pregnancy was the condition, or ______________________, that made the use of the drug dangerous and ill-advised.
3. Jane Hilldigger was deathly afraid of heights. Jane's fear is called ______________________.
4. Mr. Unger purchased the _________-_____-___________ drug without a written prescription.
5. Robby Baldwin has ______________________ syndrome of childhood. He has a short attention span, is easily distracted and overactive.
6. The doctor changed Mrs. Totten's medication after she had a/an ______________________ reaction, or side effect, caused by the drug previously prescribed.
7. Dr. Diaz prescribed a drug with a/an ______________________ coating which prevents the release and absorption of the drug until it reaches the small intestine.

8. Two-year-old Jimmy Donaldson drank a poisonous substance that his mother kept stored under the kitchen sink. The doctor in the emergency room administered a/an ______________________ to counteract the effects of the poison.

9. A/an ______________________ drug was prescribed to treat Mr. Crawford's fungus infection.

10. Ron Pryor suffers from ______________________ which is characterized by a severe impairment of reading skills.

11. Ruth Franklin suffers from ______________________ which is a disorder characterized by an episodic pattern of binge eating that is usually followed by purging through the use of vomiting or laxatives.

12. During labor, Carmella's doctor administered ______________________ to stimulate the contractions of the uterus.

13. Mr. Oliver was so severely depressed that he was unable to function. His doctor prescribed a/an ______________________ drug to relieve the depression.

14. Marvin Stauffer suffers from a severe psychiatric disorder. A/an ______________________ is used to treat his symptoms.

15. Ingrid Klein suffers from ______________________ which is characterized by a recurrent failure to resist impulses to steal objects not for immediate use or their monetary value.

WORD BUILDING

Write the correct word or word part on the line.

1. Setting fires
   a) The combining form ______________________ means fire.
   b) The combining form ______________________ means rage or madness.
   c) The term ______________________ means a disorder characterized by a recurrent failure to resist impulses to set fires.

2. Without feeling
   a) The prefix ______________________ means without.
   b) The suffix ______________________ means feeling or sensation.
   c) The term ______________________ means the absence of sensitivity to pain.

3. Fear of crowded places
   a) The combining form ______________________ means marketplace.
   b) The combining form ______________________ means fear.
   c) The term ______________________ means an overwhelming fear of being in crowded places.

4. Killing bacteria
   a) The combining form ______________________ means bacteria
   b) The suffix ______________________ means causing death.
   c) The term ______________________ means a substance that causes the death of bacteria.

5. Slowing bacteria
   a) The combining form ______________________ means bacteria
   b) The suffix ______________________ means causing controlling or slowing.
   c) The term ______________________ means a substance that retards and slows the growth of bacteria.

LABELING EXERCISES

Identify the types of injections shown on the diagram.

1. ______________________
2. ______________________
3. ______________________
4. ______________________

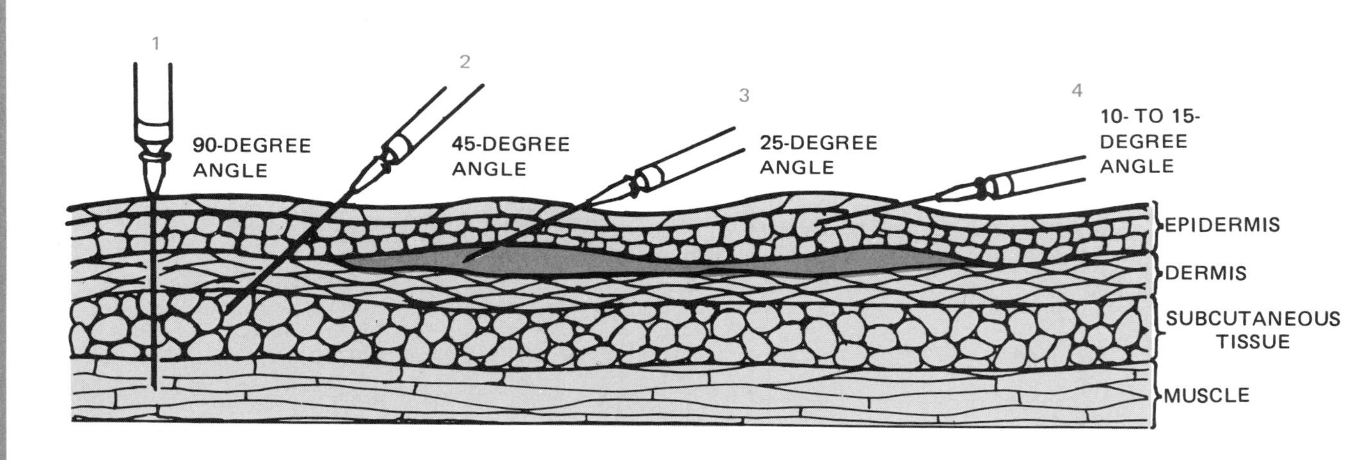

Appendix A: Prefixes, Combining Forms and Suffixes

-A-	
a-	away from, negative, no, not, without
ab-	away from
abdomin/o	abdomen
-able	capable of, able to
abort/o	premature expulsion of a nonviable fetus
abrad/o, abras/o	rub or scrape off
abrupt/o	broken away from
abs-	away from
abscess/o	going away, collection of pus
absorpt/o	suck up, suck in
ac-	toward, to
-ac	pertaining to
acanth/o	spiny, thorny
acetabul/o	acetabulum (hip socket)
-acious	characterized by
acne/o	point or peak
acou/o, acous/o	hearing, sense of hearing
acquir/o	get, obtain
-acusia, -acusis, acust/o	hearing, sense of hearing
acr/o	extremities, top, point
acromi/o	acromion, point of shoulder blade
acu/o	sharp, severe, sudden

continued ...

acuit/o, acut/o	sharp, sharpness
ad-, -ad	toward, to, in direction of
aden/o	gland
adenoid/o	adenoids
adhes/o	stick to, cling to
adip/o	fat
adnex/o	bound to
adren/o, adrenal/o	adrenal glands
-aemia	blood
aer/o	air, gas
aesthe-, -aesthesia, aesthet/o	sensation, sense of perception
af-	toward, to
affect/o	exert influence on
ag-	toward, to
agglutin/o	clumping, stick together
aggress/o	attack, step forward
-ago	attack, diseased state or condition
agor/a	marketplace
-agra	excessive pain, seizure, attack of severe pain
-aise	comfort, ease
al-	like, similar
-al	pertaining to
alb/i, alb/o, albin/o	white
albumin/o	albumin, protein

continued ...

alg/e, alg/o	pain
algesi/o *-algesia*	suffering, pain, the sense of pain, sensitivity to pain
-algesic	painful
algi-, -algia	suffering, pain
align/o	bring into line or correct position
aliment/o	to nourish
all/o, all-	other, different
allucin/o	wander in the mind
alopec/o	mangy, baldness
alveol/o	alveolus, air sac, small sac
amb-, ambi-	both, on both sides
ambly/o	dim, dull
ambul/o, *ambulat/o*	to walk
ametr/o	out of proportion
-amine	nitrogen compound
amni/o	amnion, fetal membrane
amph-	around, on both sides, doubly
amput/o, *amputat/o*	cut away, cut off a part of the body
amyl/o	starch
an-	no, not, without
an-, ana-	up, apart, backward, excessive
andr/o	male
aneurysm/o	aneurysm
angi/o, *angi-, angio-*	relating to blood or lymph vessels
angin/o	choking, strangling

continued ...

anis/o	unequal
an/o	anus, ring
ankyl/o	crooked, bent, stiff, looped
anomal/o	irregularity
ante-	before, forward
anter/o	front
anthrac/o	coal dust
anti-	against, counter
anxi/o, *anxiet/o*	uneasy, anxious, distressed
aort/o	aorta
ap-	toward, to
-apheresis	removal
aphth/o	a small ulcer or eruption
apic/o	apex
aplast/o	defective development, lack of development
apo-	from, opposed, detached
aponeur/o	aponeurosis
apoplect/o	a stroke
append/o, *appendic/o*	appendix
aqu/i, aqu/o, *aque/o*	water
-ar	pertaining to
arc/o	bow, arc or arch
-arche	beginning
arachn/o	spider web, spider
areat/o	occurring in patches or circumscribed areas
areol/o	little open space
arrect/o	upright, lifted up, raised

continued ...

arteri/o	artery
arthr/o, articul/o	joint
-ary	pertaining to
as-	toward, to
-ase	enzyme
asphyxi/o	absence of a pulse
aspir/o, aspirat/o	to breathe in
asthen- -asthenia	weakness, lack of strength
-asthmat/o	a gasping, choking
at-	toward, to
atel/o	incomplete
ather/o	plaque, fatty substance
athet/o	uncontrolled
-atonic	lack of tone
atop/o	strange, out of place
atres/i	without an opening
atri/o	atrium
attenuat/o	diluted, weakened
aud-, audi/o, audit/o	ear, hearing, the sense of hearing
aur/i, aur/o	ear, hearing
auscult/o	listen
aut/o	self
axill/o	armpit
ax/o	axis, main stem
azot/o	urea, nitrogen

-B-	
bacill/o	little stick or rod

continued ...

bacteri/o	bacteria, rod or staff
balan/o	glans penis
bar/o	pressure, weight
bas/o	base, opposite of acid
bi-, -bin, bis-	twice, double, two
bi/o, bio-	pertaining to life
bifid/o	split, cleft into two parts
bifurcat/o	divide or fork into two branches
bil/i	bile, gall
bilirubin/o	bilirubin
-blast	embyronic, immature
blephar/o	eyelid
borborygm/o	rumbling sound
brachi/o	arm
brachy-	short
brady-	slow
brev/i, brev/o	short
bronch/i, bronch/o	bronchial tube, windpipe, bronchus
bronchi/o	bronchial tube
bronchiol/o	bronchiole, bronchiolus
brux/o	grind
bucc/o, bucca-	cheek
burs/o	bursa, sac of fluid near joint

-C-	
cac-, cac/o, caco-	evil, bad, diseased, weak
cadaver/o	dead body, corpse
calc/o	calcium

continued ...

calcane/o	calcaneus, heel bone
calc/i	calcium, lime, the heel
calcul/o	stone, little stone
cali/o, calic/o	cup, calyx
call/i, callos/o	hard, hardened and thickened
calor/i	heat
canalicul/o	little canal or duct
canth/o	corner of the eye
capill/o	hair
capit/o	head
capn/o, -capnia	smoke, carbon dioxide
capsul/o	little box
carb/o	carbon
carbuncul/o	carbunculus
carcin/o	cancerous
cardi/o	heart
cari/o	rottenness, decay
carot/o	stupor, sleep
carp/o	carpus, wrist bone
cartilag/o, cartilagin/o	gristle, cartilage
caruncul/o	bit of flesh
cat-, cata-, cath-	down, lower, under, downward
catabol/o	a breaking down
cathart/o	cleansing, purging
cathet/o	send down, insert
caud/o	tail, lower part of body

continued ...

caus/o, caust/o	burn, burning
cauter/o, caut/o	heat, burn
cav/i, cav/o	hollow, cave
cavern/o	containing hollow spaces
cec/o	cecum, blind gut
-cele	tumor, cyst, hernia
celi/o	belly, abdomen
cement/o	a rough stone, cementum
cent-	hundred
-centesis	surgical puncture to remove fluid
cephal/o, cephal-, -ceps	relating to a head, head
cera-	wax
cerebell/o	cerebellum
cerebr/o	brain, cerebrum
cerumin/o	cerumen
cervic/o	neck, cervix
chalas/o, -chalasis	relaxation, loosening
chalaz/o	a hailstone
cheil/o	lip
cheir/o, cheir-	hand
chem/i, chem/o, chemic/o	drug, chemical
chir/o, chiro-	hand
chlorhydr/o	hydrochloric acid
chol/e	bile, gall
cholangi/o	bile duct

continued ...

cholecyst/o	gall bladder
choledoch/o	common bile duct
cholesterol/o	cholesterol
chondr/o, chondri/o	cartilage
chord/o	cord, the spinal cord
chori/o	chorion, membrane
choroid/o	choroid layer of eye
chrom/o, chromat/o	color
chym/o	to pour, juice
cib/o	meal
cicatric/o	scar
-cidal	pertaining to death
-cide	causing death
cili/o	microscopic hair-like projections, eyelashes
cine/o	movement
circ/i	ring or circle
circulat/o	go around in a circle
circum-	around, about
circumcis/o	cutting around
circumscrib/o	confined, limited in space
cirrh/o	tawny, orange-yellow
cis/o	cut
-clasis, -clast	break
claudicat/o	limping
claustr/o	barrier
clav/i	key
clavicul/o, cleid/o	clavicle, collar bone

continued ...

climacter/o	crisis, rung of a ladder
clitor/o, clitorid/o	clitoris, a small hill
clon/o	violent action
clus/o	shut or close
-clysis	irrigation, washing
co-	together, with
coagul/o, coagulat/o	congeal, curdle, fix together
coarct/o, coarctat/o	press together, narrow
cocc/i, cocc/o, -coccus	berry-shaped bacterium, spherical bacterium
coccyg/o	coccyx, tailbone
cochle/o	snail, snail shell, spiral
coher/o, cohes/o	cling or stick together
coit/o	a coming together
col/o	colon, large intestine
coll/a	glue
coll/i	neck
colon/o	colon, large intestine
colp/o	vagina
column/o	pillar
com-	together, with
comat/o	deep sleep
comminut/o	break into pieces
communic/o	share, to make common
compatibil/o	sympathize with
con-	together, with
concav/o	hollow

continued ...

concentr/o	condense, intensify, remove excess water
concept/o	receive or take to oneself, become pregnant
conch/o	shell
concuss/o	shaken together, violently agitated
condyl/o	knuckle, knob
confus/o	disorder, confusion
conjunctiv/o	conjunctiva, joined together, connected
consci/o	aware, awareness
consolid/o, consolidat/o	become firm or solid
constipat/o	pressed together, crowded together
constrict/o	draw tightly together
contact/o	touched, infected
contagi/o	touching of something, unclean, infection
contaminat/o	pollute, render unclean by contact
contine/o, continent/o	keep in, contain, hold back, restrain
contra-	against, counter, opposite
contracept/o	prevention of conception
contus/o	bruise
convalesc/o	become strong, recover
convex/o	arched, vaulted
convolut/o	coiled, twisted
convuls/o	pull together
copi/o	plentiful, abundant
copulat/o	joining together, linking

continued ...

cor/o	pupil
cord/o	cord, spinal cord
cordi/o	heart
core/o	pupil
cori/o	skin, leather
corne/o	cornea
coron/o	crown, coronary
corp/u, corpor/o	body
corpuscul/o	little body
cort-	covering
cortic/o	cortex, outer region
cost/o	rib
cox/o	hip, hip joint
crani/o	skull
-crasia	a mixture or blending
crepit/o, crepitat/o	crackling, rattling
crin/o, -crine	secrete, separate
cris/o, critic/o	turning point
-crit	separate
cry/o	cold
crypt/o	hidden
cubit/o	elbow
cuboid/o	cube-like
culd/o	cul-de-sac, blind pouch
cult/o	cultivate, plow, till
-cusis	hearing
cusp/i	point, pointed flap
cut-, cutane/o	skin

continued ...

cyan/o	blue
cycl/o	ciliary body of eye, cycle
cyes/i, cyes/o, -cyesis	pregnancy
cyst-, -cyst	bag, bladder
cyst/o	urinary bladder, cyst, sac of fluid
cyt/o, -cyte	cell
-cytic	pertaining to a cell
-cytosis	condition of cells

-D-	
dacry/o, dacry-	tear, tear duct, lacrimal duct
dacryocyst/o	tear sac, lacrimal sac
dactyl/o, dactyl-	fingers, toes
dart/o	skinned, flayed
de-	from, not, down, lack of
debrid/e	open a wound
deca-, deci-	ten, tenth
decidu/o	falling off, shedding
decubit/o	lying down
defec/o, defecat/o	clear, free from waste
defer/o	carrying down or out
degenerat/o	gradual impairment, breakdown, diminished function
deglutit/o	swallow
dehisc/o	burst open, split
deliri/o	wandering in the mind, silly, crazy

continued ...

delt/o	greek letter delta or d, triangular shape
delus/o	mock, cheat, delude
-dema	swelling (fluid)
demi-	half
dem/o	people, population
dendr/o	tree, resembling a tree, branching
dent-, dent/i, dent/o	tooth, relating to the teeth
depilat/o	hair removal
depress/o	press down lower, pressed or sunk down
derm/o, dermat/o, derma-	skin
-desis	bind, tie together, surgical fixation of bone or joint
deteriorat/o	worsening or gradual impairment
dextr/o	right side
di-	double, apart from, two
dia-	through, between, apart, complete
diaphor/o	sweat
diaphragmat/o	diaphragm, wall across
diastol/o	standing apart, expansion
didym/o	testes, twins, double
diffus/o	pour out, spread apart
digest/o	divide, distribute
digit/o	finger or toe
dilat/o, dilatat/o	spread out, expand

continued ...

dilut/o	dissolve, separate
diphther/o	membrane
dipl/o, dipla-	double
dips/o, -dipsia	thirst
dis-	negative, apart, absence of
dislocat/o	displacement
dissect/o	cutting apart
disseminat/o	widely scattered
dist/o	far
distend/o, distent/o	stretch apart, expand
diur/o, diuret/o	tending to increase urine output
divert/i	turning aside, bypath
domin/o	controlling, ruling
don/o	give
dors/i, dors/o	back of body
drom/o, -drome	run, running, to run
duct/o	to lead, carry
-duct	opening
duoden/i, duoden/o	duodenum
dur/o	dura mater
-dynia	pain
dys-	difficult, painful, bad

-E-	
e-	out of, from
-eal	pertaining to
ec-	out, outside
ecchym/o	pouring out of juice

continued ...

ech/o	sound
eclamps/o, eclampt/o	flashing or shining forth
-ectasia, -ectasis	stretching, dilation, enlargement
ecto-	out, outside,
-ectomy	surgical removal, cutting out, excision
eczemat/o	boil over, eruption
edem-, edemat/o	swelling, fluid, tumor
edentul/o	toothless
ef-	out
effect/o	bring about a response, activate
effus/o	pouring out
ejaculat/o	throw or hurl out
elasm/o	plate
eliminat/o	expel from the body
em-	in
emaciat/o	lean, wasted by disease
embol/o	something inserted or thrown in
embras/o	a sloped or beveled opening
embry/o	fertilized ovum, embryo
-emesis	vomiting
emet/o	vomit
-emia	blood, blood condition
emmetr/o	in proper measure
emolli/o	make soft, soften
en-	in, into, within

continued ...

encephal/o	brain
end/o, endo-	within, in, inside
endocrin/o	secrete within
enem/o	end in, inject
enter/o	small intestine
ento-	within
enzym/o	leaven
eosin/o	red, rosy, dawn-colored
epi-	upon, above, on, upper
epidemi/o	among the people, an epidemic
epididym/o	epididymis
epiglott/o	epiglottis
episi/o	vulva
epithel/i, epitheli/o	epithelium
equin/o	pertaining to a horse
erect/o	upright
erg/o	work
erot/o	sexual love
eruct/o, eructat/o	belch forth
erupt/o	break out, burst forth
erythem/o, erythemat/o	flushed, redness
erythr/o	red
es-	out of, outside, away from
-esis	state or condition, abnormal condition
eso-	inward
esophag/o	esophagus

continued ...

-esthesia, esthesi/o	sensation, feeling
esthet/o	feeling, nervous sensation, sense of perception
estr/o	female
ethm/o	sieve
eti/o	cause
eu-	well, good
evacu/o, evacuat/o	empty out
eviscer/o, eviscerat/o	disembowelment, protrusion of viscera
ex-	out of, outside, away from
exacerbat/o	irritate, aggravate
excis/o	cutting out
excori/o, excoriat/o	abrade or scratch
excret/o	separate, discharge
excruciat/o	intense pain, agony
exhal/o, exhalat/o	breathe out
-exia, -exis	condition
exo-	out of, outside, away from
exocrin/o	secrete out of
expector/o, expectorat/o	cough up, drive out of the chest
expir/o, expirat/o	breathe out
exstroph/o	turned or twisted out
extern/o	outside, outer
extra-	on the outside, beyond, outside

continued ...

extrem/o, extremit/o	outermost, extremity
extrins/o	from the outside, contained outside
exud/o, exudat/o	to sweat out

-F-	
faci-	facies, face
faci/o	the face, form
-facient	making, producing
fasci/o	fascia, fibrous band
fascicul/o	little bundle
fatal/o	pertaining to fate, death
fauc/i	narrow pass, throat
febr/i	fever
fec/i, fec/o	dregs, sediment
femor/o	femur, thigh bone
fenestr/o	window
fer/o	bear, carry
-ferent	carrying
-ferous	bearing, carrying, producing
fertil/o	fruitful, productive
fet/i, fet/o	the fetus, the unborn child in the womb
fibr/o	fiber
fibrill/o	muscular twitching
fibrin/o	fibrin, fibers, threads of a clot
fibros/o	fibrous connective tissue
fibul/o	fibula

continued ...

-fic, fic/o	making, producing, forming
filtr/o, filtrat/o	to strain through
fimbri/o	fringe
fiss/o, fissur/o	crack, split, cleft
fistul/o	tube or pipe
flamme/o	flame colored
flat/o	breaking wind, rectal gas
flex/o	bend
flu/o	flow
fluor/o	luminous
foc/o	point, focus
foll/i	bag, sac
follicul/o	follicle, small sac
foramin/o	opening
fore-	before, in front of
-form, form/o	form, figure, shape
fornic/o	arch, vault, brothel
foss/o	ditch, shallow depression
fove/o	pit
fract/o	break, broken
fren/o	bridle, any device that limits movement
frigid/o	cold
front/o	forehead, brow
-fuge	to drive away
funct/o, function/o	perform, function
fund/o	bottom, base, ground
fung/i	fungus

continued ...

furc/o	forking, branching
furuncul/o	furunculus, a boil, an infection
-fusion	pour

-G-	
galact/o	milk
gamet/o	wife or husband, sperm or egg
gangli/o, ganglion/o	ganglion
gangren/o	eating sore, gangrene
gastr/o	stomach, belly
gastrocnemi/o	gastrocnemius, calf muscle
gemin/o	twin, double
gen/o, genit/o	producing, produced by, birth, origin, race
-gene	production, origin, formation
-genesis, -genic	producing, forming
genit/o	related to birth or the reproductive organs
-genous	producing
ger/i	old age
germin/o	bud, sprout, germ
geront/o	old age
gest/o, gestat/o	bear, carry young or offspring
gigant/o	giant, very large
gingiv/o	gum
glauc/o	gray
glen/o	socket or pit

continued ...

gli/o	glue
-globin, -globulin	protein
globul/o	little ball
glomerul/o	glomerulus
gloss/o, glosso-	tongue, relating to the tongue
glott/i, glott/o	back of the tongue
gluc/o	glucose, sugar
glute/o	buttocks
glyc/o	glucose, sugar
glycer/o	sweet
glycogen/o	glycogen, animal starch
gnath/o	jaw
-gog, -gogue	make flow
goitr/o	goiter, enlargement of the thyroid gland
gon/e, gon/o	seed
gonad/o	sex glands
goni/o	angle
gracil/o	slender
grad/i	move, go, step, walk
-grade	go
-gram	tracing, picture, record
granul/o	granule(s)
-graph	instrument for recording, picture
-graphy	process of recording a picture or record
grav/i	heavy, severe
gravid/o	pregnancy
-gravida	pregnant woman

continued ...

gynec/o	woman, female
gyr/o	turning, folding

-H-	
hal/o, halit/o	breath
halluc/o	great or large toe
hallucin/o	to wander in the mind
hem-	relating to the blood
hem/e	deep red iron-containing pigment
hem/o, hemat/o	blood, relating to the blood
hemangi/o	blood vessel
hemi-	half
hepa-, hepar- hepat/o	liver
hered/o, heredit/o	inherited, inheritance
herni/o	hernia
herpet/o	creeping
heter/o, hetero-	other, different
hiat/o	opening
hidr/o	sweat
hil/o	hilum or hilus, notch or opening from a body part
hirsut/o	hairy, rough
hist/o, histi/o	tissue
holo-	all
hom/o	same, like, alike
home/o	sameness, unchanging
horde/o	barley corn

continued ...

hormon/o	excite, rouse, urge on
humer/o	humerus
hydr/o, hydra-	relating to water
hygien/o	healthful
hymen/o	hymen, a membrane
hyper-	over, above, increased, excessive, beyond
hyph-	under
hypn/o	sleep
hyp/o, hypo-	under, decreased, deficient, below
hyster/o	uterus, womb

-I-	
-iac	pertaining to
-iasis	condition, pathological state, abnormal condition
-ible	able to be, capable of being
-ic	pertaining to
ichthy/o	dry, scaly
icter/o, ictero-	jaundice
idio-, idi/o	peculiar to the individual or organ, one, distinct
-iferous	bearing, carrying, producing
-ific	making, producing
-iform	shaped or formed like, resembling
-igo	attack, diseased condition
-ile	capable of (being), able to, pertaining to
ile/o	ileum, small intestine

continued ...

ili/o	ilium, hip bone
illusi/o	deception
immun/o	immune, protected, safe
impact/o	pushed against, wedged against, packed
impress/o	pressing into
impuls/o	pressure or pushing force, drive, urging on
in-	in, into, not, without
incis/o	cutting into
incubat/o	incubation, hatching
indurat/o	hardened
infarct/o	filled in, stuffed
infect/o	tainted, infected
infer/o	below, beneath
infest/o	attack, assail, molest
inflammat/o	flame within, set on fire
infra-	beneath, below, inferior to
infundibul/o	funnel
ingest/o	carry or pour in
inguin/o	groin
inhal/o, inhalat/o	breathe in
inject/o	to force or throw in
innominat/o	unnamed, nameless
inocul/o	implant, ingraft, introduce
insipid/o	tasteless
inspir/o, inspirat/o	breathe in
insul/o	island
intact/o	untouched, whole

continued ...

inter-	between, among
intermitt/o	not continuous
intern/o	within, inner
interstiti/o	the space between things
intestin/o	intestine
intim/o	innermost
intoxic/o	put poison in
intra-	within, into, inside
intrins/o	contained within
intro-	within, into, inside
introit/o	entrance or passage
intussuscept/o	take up or receive within
involut/o	rolled up, curled inward
ion/o	ion, wander
ir/i, ir/o, irid/o, irit/o	rainbow, iris of eye
is/o	same, equal
isch/o	hold back
ischi/o	ischium
-ism	state of
iso-	equal
-istis, -itis	inflammation
-ium	structure, tissue

-J-	
jejun/o	jejunum
jugul/o	throat
juxta-	near, nearby

-K-	
kal/i	potassium
kary/o, karyo-	nucleus, nut
kata-, kath-	down
kel/o	growth, tumor
kera-	horn, hardness
kerat/o	horny, hard, cornea
ket/o, keton/o	ketones
kinesi/o	movement
-kinesis	motion
klept/o	to steal
kraur/o	dry
kyph/o	bent, hump

-L-	
labi/o	lip
labyrinth/o	maze, labyrinth, the inner ear
lacer/o, lacerat/o	torn, mangled
lacrim/o	tear, tear duct, lacrimal duct
lact/i, lact/o	milk
lactat/o	secrete milk
lamin/o	lamina
lapar/o	loin, flank, abdomen
laps/o	slip, fall, slide, gradual movement, especially downward
laryng/o	larynx, voice box
lat/i, lat/o	broad

continued ...

later/o	side
lav/o, lavat/o	wash, bathe
lax/o, laxat/o	loosen, relax
leiomy/o	smooth muscle
lemm/o	husk, peel, bark
lent/i	the lens of the eye
lenticul/o	shaped like a lens, pertaining to a lens
-lepsy	seizure
lept/o	thin, slender
lepto-	small, soft
letharg/o	drowsiness, oblivion
leuco-, leuk/o	white
lev/o, levat/o	raise, lift up
libid/o, libidin/o	sexual drive, desire, passion
ligament/o	ligament
ligat/o	a binding or tying off
lingu/o	tongue
lip/o	fat, lipid
-lite, lith/o, -lith	stone, calculus
-lithiasis	presence of stones
lob/i, lob/o	lobe, fairly well-defined part of an organ
loc/o	place
loch/i	childbirth, confinement
longev/o	long-lived, long life
lord/o	bent backward
lumb/o	lower back, loin

continued ...

lumin/o	light
lun/o	the moon
lunat/o	of the moon
lunul/o	crescent
lup/i, lup/o	wolf
lute/o	yellow
lymph/o	lymph, lymphatic tissue
lymphaden/o	lymph gland
lymphangi/o	lymph vessel
-lysis	setting free, break down, separation, destruction
-lyst	agent that causes lysis or loosening
-lytic	reduce, destroy

-M-	
macr/o, macro-	large, abnormal size or length, long
macul/o	spot
magn/o	great, large
major/o	larger
mal-	bad, poor, evil
malac/o, -malacia	abnormal softening
malign/o	bad, evil
malle/o	hammer
malleol/o	malleolus, little hammer
mamm/o	breast
man/i	rage, madness
man/i, man/o	the hand
mandibul/o	mandible, lower jaw
-mania	obsessive preoccupation

continued ...

manipul/o	handful, use of hands
manubri/o	handle
masset/o	chew
mast/o	breast, nipple
mastic/o, masticat/o	chew
mastoid/o	mastoid process
matern/o	maternal, of a mother
matur/o	ripe, ripened
maxill/o	maxilla, upper jaw
maxim/o	largest, greatest
meat/o	meatus, a passage
med-, medi/o	middle
mediastin/o	middle, in the middle
medic/o	medicine, physician, healing
medicat/o	medication, healing
medull/o	medulla, inner section, middle, soft, marrow
mega-, megal/o	large, great
-megalia, -megaly	large, great, extreme, enlargement
mei/o	less, meiosis
melan/o	black, dark
mellit/o	honey, honeyed
membran/o	membrane, thin skin
men/o	menses, menstruation, month, moon
mening/o, meningi/o	membranes, meninges
menisc/o	crescent

continued ...

mens-, mens/o	menses, menstruate, menstruation, monthly
menstru/o, menstruat/o	taking place monthly
ment/o	mind
mes-, meso-	middle
mesenter/o	mesentery, middle intestine
mesi/o	middle, median plane
meta-	beyond, over, between, change, transposition
metabol/o	a change
metacarp/o	metacarpals, hand bones
metatars/o	bones of the foot between the tarsus and toes
-meter	measure
meta-, metr/i, metr/o, metri/o	the uterus, womb
mi/o	smaller, less
micr/o, micro-	small
mictur/o, micturit/o	urinate
midsagitt/o	from front to back, at the middle
-mimetic	mimic, copy
mineral/o	mineral
minim/o	smallest, least
minor/o	smaller
mio-	less, smaller
mit/o	a thread
mitr/o	a miter having two points on top
mobil/o	capable of moving

continued ...

mon/o, mono-	one, single
monil/i	string of beads, genus of parasitic mold or fungi
morbid/o	disease, sickness
moribund/o	dying
morph/o	shape, form
mort/i, mort/o, mort/u	death, dead
mortal/i	pertaining to death, subject to death
mot/o, motil/o	motion, movement
mu/o	close, shut
muc/o, mucos/o	mucus
multi-	many, much
muscul/o	muscle
mut/a	genetic change
mut/o	unable to speak, dumb, inarticulate
my/o	muscle
myc/e, myc/o	fungus
mydri/o	wide
mydrias/i	dilation of the pupil
myel/o	spinal cord, bone marrow
myocardi/o	myocardium, heart muscle
myom/o	muscle tumor
myos/o	muscle
myring/o	tympanic membrane, eardrum
myx/o, myxa-	mucus, slime

-N-	
nar/i	nostril
narc/o	numbness, stupor
nas/i, nas/o	the nose
nat/i	birth
natr/o	sodium
nause/o	nausea, seasickness
ne/o, neo-	new, strange
necr/o	death
-necrosis	death of tissue
nect/o	bind, tie, connect
nephr/o, nephra-	kidney
nerv/o	nerve, nerve tissue
neu-, neur/i, neur/o	pertaining to the nerves, nerve, nervous tissue
neutr/o	neither, neutral
nev/o	birthmark, mole
niter-, nitro-	nitrogen
noct/i	night
nod/o	knot, swelling
nodul/o	little knot
nom/o	law, control
non-	no
nor-	chemical compound
norm/o	rule, order
nuch/o	the nape
nucle/o	nucleus
nucleol/o	little nucleus, nucleolus
nulli-	none
numer/o	number, count
nunci/o	messenger
nutri/o, nutrit/o	nourishment, food, nourish, feed
nyct/o, nyctal/o	night

-O-	
o-	egg, ovum
ob-	against
obes/o	extremely fat
obliqu/o	slanted, sideways
oblongat/o	oblong, elongated
obstetr/i, obstetr/o	midwife, one who stands to receive
occipit/o	back of the skull, occiput
occlud/o, occlus/o	shut, close up
occult/o	hidden, concealed
ocul/o, oculo-	eye
odont/o	tooth
olecran/o	olecranon, elbow
olfact/o	smell, sense of smell
olig/o	scanty, few
-olisthesis	slipping, dislocation
-ology	the science or study of
-oma	tumor, neoplasm
om/o, omo-	shoulder
oment/o	omentum, fat
omphal/o	the navel
onc/o	tumor
onych/o	fingernail or toenail

continued ...

oo/o	egg
oophor/o, oophoron-	ovary
opac/o, opacit/o	shaded, dark, impenetrable to light
oper/o, operat/o	perform, operate, work
opercul/o	cover or lid
ophthalm/o	eye, vision
-opia	vision
opisth/o	backward
-opsia, -opsis -opsy	vision, view of
opt/i, opt/o, optic/o	eye, vision
or/o	the mouth
orbit/o	circle, orbit, bony cavity or socket
orch/o, orchi/o, orchid/o	testis, testes
orect/i, orex/i	appetite
organ/o	organ
orgasm/o	swell, be excited
orth/o, ortho-	straight, normal, correct
os-	mouth, bone
-osis	an abnormal condition
osm/o, -osmia	smell, odor
osm/o	pushing, thrusting
oss/e, oss/i, oste/o	bone
-ostomosis, -ostomy	surgically creating a mouth or opening

continued ...

ot/o	ear, hearing
-otomy	cutting, surgical incision
-ous	pertaining to
ov/i, ov/o	egg, ovum
ovari/o	ovary
ox/i, ox/o, ox/y	oxygen
oxid/o	containing oxygen
oxy-	sharp, acid, quick, oxygen

-P-	
pachy-	thick
palat/o	palate, roof of mouth
pall/o, pallid/o	pale, lacking or drained of color
palliat/o	cloaked, hidden
palm/o	the palm
palpat/o	touch, feel, stroke
palpebr/o	eyelid
palpit/o	throbbing, quivering
pan-	all, entire, every
pancreat/o	pancreas
papill/i, papill/o	nipple-like
papul/o	pimple
par/o, para-	apart from, beside, near, abnormal
par/o	labor, act of bearing
-para	to bear, bring forth
paralys/o, paralyt/o	disable
parasit/o	near food, parasite
parathyroid/o	parathyroid glands

continued ...

pares/i	to disable
-paresis	slight paralysis
paret/o	to disable
pareuni/o	coitus
pariet/o	wall
parotid/o	parotid gland
-parous	having borne one or more children
paroxysm/o	sudden attack
part/o, -partum	birth, labor
parturit/o	childbirth, labor
patell/a, patell/o	patella, kneecap
path/o, pathia, -pathy	disease, suffering, feeling, emotion
-pathic	pertaining to, affected by disease
paus/o	cessation, stopping
pector/o	chest
pedi/a	child
ped/o	child, foot
pedicul/o	a louse
pelv/i, pelv/o	pelvic bone, pelvic cavity, hip
pen/i	penis
-penia	lack, deficiency, too few
peps/i, pept/o	digest, digestion
per-	excessive, through
percept/o	perceive, become aware
percuss/o	strike, tap, beat

continued ...

peri-	around, surrounding
perine/o	perineum
peristals/o, peristalt/o	constrict around
peritone/o	peritoneum
perme/o	to pass or go through
pernici/o	destructive, harmful
perone/o	fibular
perspir/o	perspiration
pertuss/i	intensive cough
petechi/o	skin spot
-pexy	surgical fixation, to put in place
phac/o	lens of eye
phag/o	eating, swallowing
-phage	one that eats, a cell that destroys
-phagia	eating, swallowing
phak/o	lens of eye
phalang/o	phalanges, finger and toe
phall/o	penis
pharmac/o	drug
pharyng/o	throat, pharynx
phas/o	speech
-phasia	speak
phe/o	dusky
pher/o	to bear or carry
-pheresis	removal
phil/o	to like, to love, attraction to

continued ...

-philia	attraction for, love of, increase in numbers
phim/o	muzzling, stopping up, constriction of an orifice
phleb/o	vein
phlegm/o	thick mucus
phob/o	fear
phon/o, -phonia	sound, voice
phor/o	carry, bear, movement
-phoresis	carrying, transmission
-phoria	to bear, carry, feeling, mental state
phot/o	light
phren/o	diaphragm, mind
-phylactic	protective, preventive
-phylaxis	protection
physi/o, physic/o	nature
-physis	to grow
-phyte	plant
pigment/o	paint, color, pigment
pil/i, pil/o	hair
pineal/o	pineal gland
pinn/i	external ear, auricle
pituit/o	pituitary
pituitar/o	mucous secretion
plac/o	flat plate or patch
placent/o	round flat cake, placenta
-plakia, plak/o	plate, thin flat layer or scale
plan/o	flat

continued ...

plant/i, plant/o	sole or bottom of foot
plas/i, plas/o	growth, development, formation, mold
-plasia	formation, development, growth
-plasm	to mold, formation
plasm/o	something molded or formed
plast/o	growth, development, mold
-plasty	surgical repair
-plegia	stroke, paralysis, palsy
-plegic	paralysis, one affected with paralysis
pleur/o	pleura, side of the body
plex/o	plexus, network
plic/o	fold or ridge
-pnea	breathing
-pneic	pertaining to breathing
pneu-	relating to the air or lungs
pneum/o, pneumon/o	lung, air
pod/o	foot
-poiesis	formation
poikil/o	varied, irregular
poli/o, polio-	gray matter of brain and spinal cord
pollic/o	thumb
poly-	many
polyp/o	polyp, small growth
pont/o	pons, a part of the brain
poplit/o	back of the knee

continued ...

por/o	pore, small opening
-porosis	passage, porous condition
port/i	gate, door
post-	after, behind
poster/o	back of body, behind
potent/o	powerful
pract/i, practic/o	practice, pursue an occupation
prandi/o, -prandial	meal, late breakfast, dinner
-praxia	action, condition concerning the performance of movements
-praxis	therapeutic treatment involving a specified method
pre-	before, in front of
precoc/i	early, premature
pregn/o	pregnant, full of
prematur/o	too early, untimely
preputi/o	foreskin, prepuce
presby/o	old age
press/o	press, draw
priap/o	penis
primi-	first
pro-	before, in behalf of
process/o	going forth
procident/o	fall down or forward
procreat/o	beget, reproduce
proct/o	anus and rectum
prodrom/o	running ahead, precursor
product/o	lead forward, yield, produce

continued ...

prolaps/o	fall downward, slide forward
prolifer/o	bear offspring, reproduce
pron/o, pronat/o	bent forward
prostat/o	prostate gland
prosth/o, prosthet/o	addition, appendage
prot/o, prote/o	first, original, protein
proxim/o	near
prurit/o	itch
pseud/o	false
psor/i, psor/o	itch
psych/o	mind
ptomat/o	a fall
-ptosis	drooping, sagging, prolapse, dropping down
-ptyal/o	spittle, spit, saliva
-ptysis	spitting
pub/o	pubis, part of hip bone
pubert/o	ripe age, adult
pudend/o	pudendum, shameful
puerper/i	childbearing, labor
pulm/o, pulmon/o	lung
pulpos/o	fleshy, pulpy
puls/o	beat, beating, striking
punct/o	sting, prick, puncture, little hole
pupill/o	pupil
pur/o	pus

continued ...

purpur/o	purple
pustul/o	infected pimple, blister
py/o	pus
pyel/o	renal pelvis, bowl of kidney
pylor/o	pylorus, gate keeper
pyr/o, pyret/o	fever, fire
pyramid/o	pyramid shaped

-Q-	
quadr/i, quadr/o	four

-R-	
rabi/o	rage, madness
rachi/o	spinal column, vertebrae
radi/o	radius, lateral lower arm bone
radiat/o	giving or passing off rays or radiant energy
radicul/o	root, nerve root
raph/o	seam, suture
-raphy	suturing, stitching
re-	back, again
recept/o	receive, receiver
recipi/o	receive, take to oneself
recticul/o	network
rect/o	rectum, straight
recuperat/o	recover, regain health
reduct/o	bring back together
refract/o	bend back, turn aside
regurgit/o, regurgitat/o	flood or gush back

continued ...

remiss/o	let go, relax, give up
ren/o	kidney
restor/o	rebuild, put back, restore
resuscit/o, resuscitat/o	revive
retent/o	hold back
retin/o	retina, net
retract/o	draw back or in
retr/o, retro-	behind, backward, back of
rhabdomy/o	striated muscle
-rhage, -rhagia	bursting forth
-rhaphy	suture
-rhea	flow, discharge
-rhexis	rupture
rheum/o, rheumat/o	a watery flow, subject to flow
rhin/o	nose
rhiz/o	root
rhonc/o	snore, snoring
rhythm/o	rhythm
rhytid/o	wrinkle
rigid/o	stiff
ris/o	laugh
roentgen/o	x-ray
rotat/o	rotate, revolve
-rrhage, -rrhagia	bursting forth
-rrhaphy	suture
-rrhea	flow, discharge
-rrhexis	rupture

continued ...

rug/o	wrinkle, fold

-S-	
sacc/i, sacc/o	sac
sacchar/o	sugar
sacr/o	sacrum
saliv/o	spittle, spit
salping/o	uterine (fallopian) tube, auditory (eustachian) tube
-salpinx	uterine (fallopian) tube
san/o	sound, healthy, sane
sangu/i, sanguin/o	blood
sanit/o	soundness, health
saphen/o	clear, apparent, manifest
sapr/o	dead or decaying
sarc/o, sarcomat/o	flesh (connective tissue), cancer of connective tissue
sarco-	flesh
-sarcoma	tumor, cancer
scalp/o	carve, scrape
scapul/o	scapula, shoulder blade
-schisis, schiz/o	split, cleft, divided
scirrh/o	hard
scler/o	sclera, white of eye, hard
-sclerosis	abnormal dryness, hardness, hardening
scoli/o	crooked, curved
-scope	instrument for visual examination
-scopic	pertaining to visual examination

continued ...

-scopy	see, visual examination
scot/o	darkness
scrib/o, script/o	write
scrot/o	bag or pouch
seb/o	sebum, wax, suet
secti/o	to cut
secret/o	produce and separate out
sect/o	cutting
segment/o	in pieces
sell/o	saddle
semi-	half
semin/i	seed, sperm, semen
sen/i	old
senesc/o	grow old
senil/o	old age
sens/i	feeling, sensation
sensitiv/o	sensitive (to), affected (by)
seps/o	infection
sept/o	infection, partition
ser/o	serum
seros/o	serous
sial/o	saliva, salivary glands
sialaden/o	salivary gland
sider/o	iron
sigm/o	sigma, the greek letter s
sigmoid/o	sigmoid colon
sin/o, sin/u	hollow, sinus, tube-like passage
sinistr/o	left, left side

continued ...

sinus/o	sinus
sit/u	place
skelet/o	skeleton
soci/o	companion, fellow being
solut/o, solv/o	loosened, dissolved
soma-, somat/o	body
somn/i, somn/o, -somnia	sleep
son/o	sound
sopor/o	sleep
spad/o	draw off, draw
spasm/o, -spasm spasmod/o	sudden involuntary, contraction, tightening or cramping
spec/i	look at, a kind or sort
specul/o	mirror
sperm/o, spermat/o	spermatozoa, sperm cells, seed
sphen/o	wedge, sphenoid bone
spher/o	round, sphere, ball
sphincter/o	tight binder or band
sphygm/o, -sphyxia	pulse
spin/o	spine, backbone
spir/o	breathe
spirill/o	little coil
spirochet/o	coiled microorganism
splen/o	spleen
spondyl/o	vertebra, vertebral column

continued ...

spontane/o	unexplained, of one's own accord
spor/o	seed, spore
sput/o	spittle, spit
squam/o	scale
-stalsis	contraction
staped/o, stapedi/o	the stapes, stirrup, middle ear bone
staphyl/o	cluster, bunch of grapes
stas/i, -stasis, stat/i, -static	stopping, controlling, slowing,
-statis	stopping, controlling
steat/o	fat, lipid, sebum
sten/o	narrowing, contracted
-stenosis	tightening, stricture
ster/o	solid structure
stere/o	solid, three-dimensional
steril/i	barren, sterile
stern/o	sternum, the breastbone
stert/o	snore, snoring
steth/o	chest
sthen/o, -sthenia	strength
stigmat/o	point, spot
stimul/o	goad, prick, incite
stol/o	send or place
stomat/o	mouth
-stomosis, -stomy	furnish with a mouth or outlet, new opening
strab/i	squint, squint-eyed
strat/i	layer
strept/o	twisted chain

continued ...

striat/o	stripe, furrow, groove
stric-	narrowing
strict/o	draw tightly together, bind or tie
strid/o	harsh sound
stup/e	benumbed, stunned
styl/o	pen, pointed instrument
sub-	under, less, below
subluxat/o	partial dislocation
sucr/o	sugar
sudor/i	sweat
suffoc/o, suffocat/o	choke, strangle
sulc/o	furrow, groove
super- super/o	above, excessive, higher than
superflu/o	overflowing, excessive
supin/o	lying on the back
supinat/o	bend backward, place on the back
suppress/o	press down
suppur/o, suppurat/o	to form pus
supra-	above, excessive
supraren/o	above or on the kidney, suprarenal gland
sutur/o	stitch, seam
sym-	with, together
symptomat/o	falling together, symptom
syn-	with, together
synaps/o, synapt/o	point of contact

continued ...

syncop/o	cut short, cut off
-syndesis	surgical fixation of vertebrae
syndesm/o	ligament
syndrom/o	running together
synovi/o	synovia, synovial membrane, lubricating fluid
syphil/i, syphil/o	syphilis
syring/o	tube
system/o, systemat/o	body system
systol/o	contraction

-T-	
tachy-	fast, rapid
tact/i	touch
talip/o	foot and ankle deformity
tars/o	ankle, instep, edge of the eyelid
tax/o	order, coordination
techn/o, techni/o	skill
tectori/o	covering, roof-like
tele/o	distant, far
tempor/o	the temple
tenac/i	holding fast, sticky
ten/o, tend/o	tendon, stretch out, extend, strain
tendin/o	tendon
tens/o	stretch out, extend, strain
terat/o	monster, malformed fetus
termin/o	the end, limit

continued ...

test/i, test/o	witness, testis, testicle,
testicul/o	testicle
tetan/o	rigid, tense
tetra-	four
thalam/o	thalamus, inner room
thalass/o	sea
thanas/o, thanat/o	death
the/o	put, place
thec/o	sheath
thel/o	nipple
therap/o, therapeut/o	treatment
therm/o	heat
thio-	sulfur
thorac/o	chest
-thorax	pleural cavity, chest
thromb/o	clot
thym/o	thymus gland
thyr/o, thyroid/o	shield, thyroid gland
tibi/o	tibia, shin bone
-tic	pertaining to
tine/o	gnawing worm, ringworm
tinnit/o	ringing, buzzing, tinkling
toc/o	birth, childbirth
-tocia, -tocin	labor, delivery, birth
tom/o	cut
-tome	instrument to cut
-tomy	cutting, incision
ton/o	tone, tension, stretching

continued ...

tone/o	stretch
tonsill/o	tonsil, throat
top/o	place, position, location
tors/o	twist, rotate
tort/i	twisted
tox/o, toxic/o	poison, poisonous
trabecul/o	little beam marked with cross bars or beams
trache/i, trache/o	trachea, windpipe
trachel-	neck
tract/o	draw, pull, path, bundle of nerve fibers
tranquil/o	quiet, calm, tranquil
trans-	across, through
transfus/o	pour across, transfer
transit/o	changing
transvers/o	across, crosswise
traumat/o	injury
trem/o	shaking, trembling
tremul/o	fine tremor or shaking
treponem/o	coiled, turning microbe
-tresia	opening
tri-	three
trich/o	hair
trigon/o	trigone
-tripsy	crushing stone
-trite	instrument for crushing
trochle/o	pulley
trop/o	turn, change

continued ...

troph/o, -trophic, -trophy	relating to nutrition, nourishment, development, growth
-tropia	turn
-tropic, -tropin	pertaining to a pituitary hormone
tub/i, tub/o	tube, pipe
tubercul/o	little knot, swelling
tunic/o	covering, cloak, sheath
turbinat/o	coiled, spiral-shaped
tuss/i	cough
tympan/o	tympanic membrane, eardrum

-U-	
ulcer/o	sore, ulcer
uln/o	ulna
ultra-	beyond, excess
umbilic/o	navel
un-	not
ungu/o	nail
uni-	one
ur/o	urine, urinary tract
-uresis	urination
ureter/o	ureter
urethr/o	urethra
urg/o	press, push
-uria	urination, urine
urin/o	urine or urinary organs
urtic/o	nettle, rash, hives
-us	thing
uter/i, uter/o	uterus, womb

continued ...

uve/o	vascular layer of eye, iris, choroid, ciliary body
uvul/o	uvula, little grape

-V-	
vaccin/i, vaccin/o	vaccine
vacu/o	empty
vag/o	wandering
vagin/o	vagina, sheath
valg/o	bent or twisted outward
valv/o, valvul/o	valve
var/o	bent or twisted inward
varic/o	swollen or dilated vein
vas/o	vessel, duct, vas deferens
vascul/o	little vessel
vaso-	vessel
vast/o	vast, great, extensive
vect/o	carry, convey
ven/o	vein
vener/o	coitus, sexual intercourse
venter-	the abdomen
ventilat/o	expose to air, fan
ventr/o	in front, belly side of body
ventricul/o	ventricle of brain or heart, small chamber
venul/o	venule, small vein
verg/o	twist, incline
verm/i	worm
verruc/o	wart
-version	to turn

continued ...

vers/o, vert/o	turn
vertebr/o	vertebra, backbone
vertig/o, vertigin/o	whirling round, turning around, revolution
vesic/o	urinary bladder
vesicul/o	seminal vesicle, blister, little bladder
vestibul/o	entrance, vestibule
vi/o	force
vill/i	shaggy hair, tuft of hair
vir/o	poison, virus
viril/o	masculine, manly
vis/o	seeing, sight
visc/o	sticky
viscer/o	viscera, internal organ
viscos/o	sticky
vit/a, vit/o	life
viti/o	blemish, defect
vitre/o	glassy, made of glass
voc/i	the voice
vol/o	the palm or sole
volv/o	roll, turn
vulgar/i	common
vulv/o	vulva, covering

-X-	
xanth/o	yellow
xen/o	strange, foreign
xer/o	dry
xiph/i, xiph/o	sword

-Z-	
zygomat/o	yoke, cheekbone
zygot/o	joined or yoked together

Appendix B: Abbreviations and Meanings

-A-	
A	accommodation; age; anterior
AAV	adenoassociated virus
Ab	antibody
ab	abortion
abd	abdomen
AB	abnormal
A/B	acid-base ratio
ABC	aspiration, biopsy, cytology
ABE	acute bacterial endocarditis
ABG	arterial blood gas
ABP	arterial blood pressure
AC	acromioclavicular; air conduction; alternating current
ac	acute
AC, ac	before meals
Acc	accommodation
ACD	acid-citrate-dextrose; anterior chest diameter
ACG	angiocardiography; apex cardiogram
ACH	adrenocortical hormone
ACP	acid phosphatase
ACTH	adrenocorticotropic hormone
ACVD	acute cardiovascular disease

continued ...

AD	abdominal diaphragmatic breathing; adenovirus; right ear
ADH	antidiuretic hormone
ADL	activities of daily living
ad lib	as desired
adm	admission
ADS	antibody deficiency syndrome
ADT	admission, discharge, transfer
AE	above elbow
AF	acid-fast; arterial fibrillation
AFB	acid-fast bacilli
AFIB	atrial fibrillation
AFP	alpha-fetoprotein
Ag	antigen
AG, A/G	albumin/globulin ratio
$AgNO_3$	silver nitrate
AH	abdominal hysterectomy
AHD	arteriosclerotic heart disease; autoimmune hemolytic disease
AHF	antihemophilic Factor VIII
AHG	antihemophilic globulin Factor VIII
AI	aortic insufficiency; atherogenic index
AID	acute infectious disease; artificial insemination donor

continued ...

AIDS	acquired immune deficiency syndrome
AIH	artificial insemination homologous
AIHA	autoimmune hemolytic anemia
aj	ankle jerk
AK	above knee
AKA	above-knee amputation
alb	albumin
ALG	antilymphocytic globulin
alk	alkaline
alk phos	alkaline phosphatase
ALL	acute lymphoblastic leukemia; acute lymphocytic leukemia
ALP	alkaline phosphatase
ALS	aldolase; amyotrophic lateral sclerosis; antilymphocytic serum
alt dieb	alternate days; every other day
alt hor	alternate hours
alt noct	alternate nights
AMA	against medical advice
amb	ambulate, ambulatory
AMI	acute myocardial infarction
AML	acute myeloblastic leukemia; acute myelocytic leukemia
amp	ampule
AMS	amylase
amt	amount

continued ...

ANA	antinuclear antibodies
ANF	antinuclear factor
ANLL	acute non-lymphocytic leukemia
ANS	autonomic nervous system
ant	anterior
AOD	adult-onset diabetes; arterial occlusive disease
A & P	anterior and posterior; auscultation and percussion
AP	angina pectoris; anteroposterior; anterior-posterior
aq	aqueous
ARC	AIDS-related complex
ARD	acute respiratory disease
ARF	acute respiratory failure
ARM	artificial rupture of membranes
AS	aortic stenosis; left ear
ASA	aspirin
ASAP	as soon as possible
ASCVD	arteriosclerotic cardiovascular disease
ASD	atrial septal defect
ASH	asymmetrical septal hypertrophy
ASHD	arteriosclerotic heart disease
ASIS	anterior superior iliac spine
ASO	arteriosclerosis obliterans
ASS	anterior superior spine

continued ...

AST	aspartate aminotransferase
as tol	as tolerated
ATP	adenosine triphosphate
Au	gold
AU	both ears
AUL	acute undifferentiated leukemia
ausc	auscultation
AV	atrioventricular; arteriovenous
ax	axillary
AZT	Aschheim-Zondek test

-B-	
B/A	backache
BA	bronchial asthma
BAC	blood alcohol concentration
BaE	barium enema
BAO	basal acid output
bas	basophils
BBB	bundle branch block
BBT	basal body temperature
BC	bone conduction
BCC	basal cell carcinoma
BE	below elbow; barium enema
BFP	biological false positive
BID, bid	twice a day
bil	bilateral
BIN, bin	twice a night
BK	below knee
BKA	below knee amputation
Bld	blood
BJ	Bence Jones
BM	bowel movement; bone marrow
BMR	basal metabolic rate
BMT	barium meal test
BNO	bladder neck obstruction
BNR	bladder neck resection
BOM	bilateral otitis media
B/P, BP	blood pressure
BPD	biparietal diameter
BPH	benign prostatic hyperplasia; benign prostatic hypertrophy
BR	bed rest
BRP	bathroom privileges
BS	blood sugar; bowel sounds; breath sounds
BSP	bromsulphalein
BT	bleeding time
BUN	blood urea nitrogen
BV	blood volume
Bx	biopsy

-C-	
C	Celsius; centigrade
c	with
Ca	calcium; cancer

continued ...

CA	cancer; carcinoma; chronological age
CAB	coronary artery bypass
CAD	coronary artery disease
cal	calorie
cap	capsule
CAPD	continuous ambulatory peritoneal dialysis
CAT	computerized axial tomography
cath	catheter; catheterize
CAVH	continuous arteriovenous hemofiltration
CBC	complete blood count
CBF	cerebral brain syndrome
CBI	continuous bladder irrigation
CBR	complete bed rest
CBS	chronic brain syndrome
CC	chief complaint; colony count; cardiac cycle; creatinine clearance
cc	cubic centimeter
CCA	circumflex coronary artery
CCCR	closed chest cardio-pulmonary resuscitation
CCF	cephalin cholesterol flocculation
CCPD	continuous cycle peritoneal dialysis
CCr	creatinine clearance
CCT	cranial computed tomography

continued ...

CCU	coronary care unit
CDC	calculated date (day) of confinement
CDH	congenital dislocation of the hip
CEA	carcinoembryonic antigen
CF	complete fixation; counting fingers; cystic fibrosis
C gl	with correction; with glasses
CGL	chronic granulomatous leukemia
Ch	cholesterol
CHB	complete heart block
CHD	coronary heart disease
CHF	congestive heart failure
CHO	carbohydrate
chol	cholesterol
chr	chronic
CI	coronary insufficiency
cib	food
CID	cytomegalic inclusion disease
CIE	counter immuno-electrophoresis
circ	circumcision
CIS	carcinoma in situ
CK	creatine kinase
ck	check
cl	clinic; chloride
CLD	chronic liver disease

continued ...

CLL	chronic lymphocytic leukemia
cl liq	clear liquid
cm	centimeter
CME	cystoid macular edema
CMG	cystometrogram
CML	chronic myelocytic leukemia
CMV	controlled mechanical ventilation; cystometrogram; cytomegalovirus
CNS	central nervous system; cutaneous nerve stimulation
c/o	complains of
Co	cobalt
CO	carbon monoxide
CO_2	carbon dioxide
COH	carbohydrate
COLD	chronic obstructive lung disease
comp	compound
cond	condition
contra	against
COPD	chronic obstructive pulmonary disease
CP	cardiopulmonary; cerebral palsy
CPA	carotid phonoangiograph
CPAP	continuous positive airway pressure
CPD	cephalopelvic disproportion
CPE	cytopathic effect

continued ...

CPK	creatine phosphokinase
CPN	chronic pyelonephritis
CPPB	continuous positive-pressure breathing
CPR	cardiopulmonary resuscitation
CPS	cycles per second
Cr	chromium
CRD	chronic respiratory disease
creat	creatinine
CR	conditioned reflex
CRF	chronic renal failure
Cs	cesium
CS	central supply; cesarean section; complete stroke; conditioned stimulus
C & S	culture and sensitivity
CSF	cerebrospinal fluid
CSR	central supply room; Cheyne-Stokes respiration
CT	computer tomography
CTCL	cutaneous T-cell lymphoma
CTZ	chemoreceptor trigger zone
cu	cubic
CUC	chronic ulcerative colitis
CUG	cystourethrogram
CV	cardiovascular
CVA	cardiovascular accident; cerebrovascular accident
CVD	cardiovascular disease

continued ...

CVP	central venous pressure; Cytoxan, vincristine, prednisone
CWP	childbirth without pain
cx	cervix
CXR	chest x-ray film
cysto	cystoscopic examination; cystoscopy

-D-	
D	diopter (lens strength)
d	day
DAT	diet as tolerated
db	decibel
D & C	dilatation and curettage dilation and curettage
D/C, DC	discontinue
DCC	direct current cardioversion
DCR	direct cortical response
D & E	dilatation and evacuation dilation and evacuation
del	delivery
DES	diethylstilbestrol
DGE	delayed gastric emptying
DHFS	dengue hemorrhagic fever shock syndrome
diag	diagnosis
DIC	diffuse intravascular coagulation
diff	differential
DIP	distal interphalangeal
disch	discharge
DJD	degenerative joint disease

continued ...

DL	danger list
DM	diabetes mellitus; diastolic murmur
DNA	deoxyribonucleic acid
DNR	do not resuscitate
DOA	dead on arrival
DOB	date of birth
DOE	dyspnea on exertion
DQ	developmental quotient
DPT	diphtheria-pertussis-tetanus
dr	dram; dressing
DR	digital radiography
DRG	diagnosis-related groupings
D/S	dextrose in saline
DSA	digital subtraction angiography
DSD	dry sterile dressing
DT	diphtheria and tetanus toxoids
DTP	diphtheria and tetanus toxoids and pertussis vaccine
DTs	delirium tremens
DTR	deep tendon reflex
DUB	dysfunctional uterine bleeding
DVA	distance visual acuity
DVI	digital vascular imaging
DW	distilled water
D/W	dextrose in water
Dx	diagnosis

-E-	
E	enema
EBL	estimated blood loss
EBP	epidural blood patch
EBV	Epstein-Barr virus
ECC	extracorporeal circulation
ECG	electrocardiogram; electrocardiograph
ECHO	echocardiogram
E. coli	Escherichia coli
ECT	electroconvulsive therapy
ED	effective dose
EDC	estimated date (day) of confinement
EDD	end-diastolic dimension
EDG	electrodynogram
EDV	end-diastolic volume
EEG	electroencephalogram; electroencephalography
EENT	eye, ear, nose, and throat
EFM	electronic fetal monitor
EHD	electrohemodynamics
EIB	exercise-induced bronchospasm
EIA	enzyme immunoassay
Ej	elbow jerk
EKG	electrocardiogram
ELISA	enzyme-linked immunoassay; enzyme-linked immunosorbent assay
elix	elixir

continued ...

EM	electron microscope; emmetropia
EMG	electromyogram; electromyograph
EMS	electromagnetic spectrum
ENG	electronystagmography
ENT	ear, nose, and throat
EOG	electro-oculogram
EOM	extraocular muscles; extraocular movement
eos, eosins	eosinophils
EP	ectopic pregnancy; evoked potential
EPF	exophthalmos-producing factor
EPO	erythropoietin
EPR	electron paramagnetic resonance
EPS	extrapyramidal symptoms; exophthalmos-producing substance
ER	emergency room
ERG	electroretinogram
ERPF	effective renal plasma flow
ERT	external radiation therapy
ERV	expiratory reserve volume
ESD	end-systolic dimension
ESR	erythrocyte sedimentation rate
EST	electric shock therapy
ESV	end-systolic volume
ET	esotropia
et	and

continued ...

ETF	eustachian tube function
etiol	etiology
ETOA	ethyl alcohol
EU	Ehrlich units
ex	excision
exam	examination
exp	expiration
ext	extract; external

-F-	
F	Fahrenheit
FA	fluorescent antibody
FB	foreign body
FBS	fasting blood sugar
FDP	fibrin-fibrinogen degradation products
Fe	iron
FECG	fetal electrocardiogram
FEF	forced expiratory flow
FEV	forced expiratory volume
FFA	free fatty acids
FH	family history
FHR	fetal heart rate
FHS	fetal heart sounds
FHT	fetal heart tones
FIA	fluorescent immunoassay; fluoroimmunoassay
FME	full mouth extraction
FR	fibrin-fibrinogen related
fr	French (catheter size)
FRC	functional residual capacity
FROM	full range of motion
FS	frozen section
FSP	fibrin-fibrinogen split products
FT	family therapy
FTA	fluorescent treponemal antibody
FTI	free thyroxine index
FTND	full term normal delivery
FTT	failure to thrive
FU	follow-up
FUO	fever of undetermined (unknown) origin
FX, Fx	fracture

-G-	
g	gram
ga	gallium
GA	gastric analysis: general anesthesia
GB	gallbladder
GBM	glomerular basement membrane
GBS	gallbladder series; Guillain-Barre syndrome
G-Cs	glucocorticoids
GC	gonorrhea
GDM	gestational diabetes
GFR	glomerular filtration rate
GG	gamma globulin
GGT	gamma glutamyl transferase
GH	growth hormone

continued ...

GI	gastrointestinal
GLTT	glucose tolerance test
gm	gram
GMP	guanosine monophosphate
GOT	glutamic oxaloacetic transaminase
GP	general practice
gr	grain
grav I	pregnancy one; primigravida
GS	general surgery
GSW	gunshot wound
GT	glucose tolerance
GTP	guanosine triphosphate
GTT	glucose tolerance test
gtt	drops
GU	genitourinary
GVH	graft-versus-host disease
GvH	graft versus host
GVHD	graft-versus-host disease
GxT	graded exercise test
GYN, Gyn	gynecology

-H-	
h	hour
H	hydrogen; hypodermic
H & H	hemoglobin and hematocrit
HAA	hepatitis associated antigen; hepatitis Australia antigen
HAI	hemagglutination-inhibition immunoassay

continued ...

HASHD	hypertensive arteriosclerotic heart disease
HAV	hepatitis A virus
HB	heart block
Hb	hemoglobin
HBE	His bundle electrocardiogram
HbF	fetal hemoglobin
HBP	high blood pressure
HbS	sickle cell hemoglobin
HBV	hepatitis B virus
HCD	heavy-chain disease
HCG	human chorionic gonadotropin
HCl	hydrochloric acid
HCL	hairy cell leukemia
hct	hematocrit
HCVD	hypertensive cardiovascular disease
HD	hearing distance; hemodialysis; hip disarticulation
HDL	high-density lipoprotein
He	helium
H & E	hematoxylin and eosin stains
HDN	hemolytic disease of the newborn
HDS	herniated disk syndrome
HE	hereditary elliptocytosis
HEENT	head, eyes, ears, nose, throat
Hg	mercury

continued ...

hgb	hemoglobin
HI	hemagglutination-inhibition
HIV	human immunodeficiency virus
H & L	heart and lungs
HLA	human leukocyte antigen
HLR	heart-lung resuscitation
HM	hand motion
HMD	hyaline membrane disease
HNP	herniated nucleus pulposus
HO	hyperbaric oxygen
HOB	head of bed
H & P	history and physical
HP	hemipelvectomy
HPL	human placental lactogen
HPN	hypertension
HPO	hypothalamic-pituitary-ovarian
hr	hour
hs	at bedtime; hour of sleep
HS	hereditary spherocytosis; herpes simplex
HSG	hysterosalpingogram
HSV	herpes simplex virus
H_2O	water
H_2O_2	hydrogen peroxide
ht	height; hematocrit
HV	hospital visit

continued ...

HVD	hypertensive vascular disease
Hx	history
hypo	hypodermic, hypodermically

-I-	
I	intensity of magnetism; iodine
IABP	intra-aortic balloon pump
IACP	intra-aortic counterpulsation
IADH	inappropriate antidiuretic hormone
IASD	interatrial septal defect
IBC	iron-binding capacity
IBD	inflammatory bowel disease
IC	inspiratory capacity
ICCU	intensive coronary care unit
ICF	intracellular fluid
ICP	intracranial pressure
ICS	intercostal space
ICT	insulin coma therapy; indirect Coombs' test
ict ind	icterus index
ICU	intensive care unit
I & D	incision and drainage
ID	infectious disease
IDD	insulin dependent diabetes
IDDM	insulin-dependent diabetes mellitus
IDK	internal derangement of the knee

continued ...

IDS	immunity deficiency state
I/E	inspiratory-expiratory ratio
IEMG	integrated electromyogram
Ig	immunoglobulin
IgA	immunoglobulin A
IgD	immunoglobulin D
IgG	immunoglobulin G
IgM	immunoglobulin M
IGT	impaired glucose tolerance
IH	infectious hepatitis
IHD	ischemic heart disease
IHSS	idiopathic hypertrophic subaortic stenosis
IM	infectious mononucleosis; intramuscular
IMAG	internal mammary artery graft
IMF	idiopathic myelofibrosis
IMV	intermittent mandatory ventilation
inf	inferior; infusion
I & O	intake and output
IO	intraocular
IOP	intraocular pressure
IPG	impedance plethysmography
IPPB	intermittent positive pressure breathing
IQ	intelligence quotient
irrig	irrigation
IS	intercostal space
ISG	immune serum globulin
isol	isolation

continued ...

ITP	idiopathic thrombocytopenic purpura
IU	international unit
IUD	intrauterine device
IUP	intrauterine pressure
IV	intravenously
IVC	interior vena cava
IVCP	inferior vena cava pressure
IVD	intervertebral disk
IVF	in vitro fertilization
IVP	intravenous pyelogram
IVSD	interventricular septal defect
IVU	intravenous urogram

-J-	
JOD	juvenile-onset diabetes
JRA	juvenile rheumatoid arthritis
jt	joint
JVP	jugular venous pulse

-K-	
K	potassium
KB	ketone bodies
KCG	kinetocardiogram
KCl	potassium chloride
KD	knee disarticulation
KE	kinetic energy
kg	kilogram

continued ...

kj	knee jerk
KO	keep open
KS	Kaposi's sarcoma
KUB	kidney, ureter, bladder
KVO	keep vein open

-L-	
l	liter
L & A	light and accommodation
LA	left atrium
lab	laboratory
lac	laceration
LAD	left anterior descending
LAP	leucine aminopeptidase
lap	laparotomy
lat.	lateral
lb	pound
LB	large bowel; low back
LBBB	left bundle branch block
LBW	low birth weight
LBBX	left breast biopsy and examination
LBP	low back pain
L & D	labor and delivery
LD	lactic dehydrogenase
LDD	light-dark discrimination
LDH	lactic dehydrogenase
LDL	low-density lipoprotein
LE	left eye; lupus erythematosus
LES	lower esophageal sphincter

continued ...

lg	large
LH	luteinizing hormone
LHBD	left-heart bypass device
LHF	left-sided heart failure
LHR	leukocyte histamine release test
lig	ligament
L K & S	liver, kidney and spleen
LLE	lower left extremity
LLL	left lower lobe
LLSB	left lower sternal border
LLQ	left lower quadrant
LMP	last menstrual period
LNMP	last normal menstrual period
LOM	limitation of motion; loss of motion
LP	light perception; lumbar puncture
LPS	lipase
LR	light reaction
LRDKT	living related donor kidney transplant
LSB	left sternal border
LSD	lysergic acid diethylamide
lt	left
LTB	laryngotracheobronchitis
LTH	luteotropic hormone
LUE	left upper extremity
LUL	left upper lobe
LUQ	left upper quadrant
LV	left ventricle

continued ...

LVH	left ventricle hypertrophy
lymphs	lymphocytes

-M-	
M	meter; murmur
m	minim
MAO	maximal acid output; monoamine oxidase
MBC	maximal breathing capacity
MBD	minimal brain damage
mc	millicurie
mcg	microgram
MCH	mean corpuscular hemoglobin
MCHC	mean corpuscular hemoglobin concentration
MCT	mean circulation time
MCV	mean corpuscular volume
MD	muscular dystrophy
ME	middle ear
MED	minimal effective dose; minimal erythema dose
mEq	milliequivalent
M & F	mother and father
MFT	muscle function test
mg	milligram
mgm	milligram
MH	marital history
MHA	microhemagglutination
MI	myocardial infarction

continued ...

MICU	medical intensive care unit; mobile intensive care unit
MIP	maximal inspiratory pressure
ml	milliliter
MLD	median lethal dose
mm	millimeter
MM	multiple myeloma
MND	motor neuron disease
MOM	milk of magnesia
mon	monocytes
MP	metacarpal-phalangeal
MPJ	metacarpophalangeal joint
MR	mental retardation; metabolic rate
MRD	medical record department
MRI	magnetic resonance imaging
MS	mitral stenosis; multiple sclerosis; musculoskeletal
MSL	midsternal line
MTD	right ear drum
MTS	left ear drum
MTX	methotrexate
MVP	mitral valve prolapse
MY	myopia
myel	myelogram
myop	myopia

-N-	
Na	sodium
NA	not applicable; numerical aperture
NaCl	sodium chloride
NAD	no acute disease; no apparent distress
NB	newborn
NBT	nitroblue tetrazolium
N/C	no complaints
NCV	nerve conduction velocity
NED	no evidence of disease
NEG	negative
neg	negative
neuro	neurology
NF	National Formulary; negro female
NG	nasogastric
NGU	nongonococcal urethritis
NHL	non-Hodgkin's lymphoma
NICU	neurological intensive care unit
NIDDM	non-insulin dependent diabetes mellitus
NLP	neuro-linguistic programming
No	number
noc, noct	night
NPC	no point of convergence
NPH	neutral protamine Hage-dorn
NPN	nonprotein nitrogen

continued ...

NPO	nothing by mouth
NR	no response
NREM	no rapid eye movements
NS	normal saline; not stated; not sufficient
NSR	normal sinus rhythm
NSU	nonspecific urethritis
Nt	neutralization
NTG	nitroglycerin
N & V	nausea and vomiting
NVA	near visual acuity
NVD	nausea, vomiting, and diarrhea; neck vein distension
NVS	neural vital signs
NYD	not yet diagnosed

-O-	
OB	obstetrics
OB-GYN	obstetrics and gynecology
obl.	oblique
OBS	organic brain syndrome
Obs	obstetrics
OC	office call; oral contraceptive
OCC	occasional
OCD	oral cholecystogram
OD	overdose; right eye
od	once a day
OGN	obstetric-gynecologic-neonatal

continued ...

OGTT	oral glucose tolerance test
oint	ointment
OM	otitis media
OMR	optic mark recognition
OOB	out of bed
O & P	ova and parasites
OP	outpatient
OPD	outpatient department
OPG	oculoplethysmography
Ophth	ophthalmic
OPT	outpatient
OPV	oral poliovirus vaccine
OR	operating room
Orth	orthopedics
OS	left eye
os	mouth
OT	occupational therapy; old tuberculin
Oto	otology
OU	each eye
O_2	oxygen
oz	ounce

-P-	
p	after
P	phosphorus; pulse
P & A	percussion and auscultation
PA	pernicious anemia; physician's assistant; posteroanterior; posterior-anterior; pulmonary artery

continued ...

PABA	paraaminobenzoic acid
PAC	premature atrial contraction
PADP	pulmonary artery diastolic pressure
PAMP	pulmonary arterial mean pressure
Pap	Papanicolaou
paren	parenterally
PASP	pulmonary artery systolic pressure
PAT	paroxysmal atrial tachycardia
Path	pathology
PBI	protein-bound iodine
PBP	progressive bulbar palsy
PBT_4	protein-bound thyroxine
pc	after meals
PCT	plasmacrit time
PCU	progressive care unit
PCV	packed cell volume
PD	interpupillary distance; Parkinson's disease
PDA	patent ductus arteriosus
PDL	periodontal ligament
PE	physical examination
Peds	pediatrics
PEEP	positive end-expiratory pressure
PEF	peak expiratory flow rate
PEG	pneumoencephalogram; pneumoencephalography

continued ...

PERLA	pupils equally reactive to light and accommodation
PERRLA	pupils equal, round, regular, react to light and accommodation
PET	positron emission tomography; preeclamptic toxemia
PFT	pulmonary function test
PG	pregnant; prostaglandin
PGH	pituitary growth hormone
PGL	persistent generalized lymphadenopathy
pH	acidity; hydrogen ion concentration
PH	past history; personal history; public health
PI	present illness
PICU	pulmonary intensive care unit
PID	pelvic inflammatory disease
PIF	peak inspiratory flow
PIP	proximal interphalangeal
PK	pyruvate kinase; pyruvate kinase deficiency
PKU	phenylketonuria
PL	light perception
PLS	primary lateral sclerosis
PM	physical medicine; postmortem
PMA	progressive muscular atrophy
PMH	past medical history

continued ...

PMI	point of maximal impulse
PMN	polymorphonuclear neutrophils
PMP	past menstrual period; previous menstrual period
PMR	physical medicine and rehabilitation
PMS	premenstrual syndrome
PMT	premenstrual tension
PND	paroxysmal nocturnal dyspnea; postnasal drip
PNH	paroxysmal nocturnal hemoglobinuria
PNS	peripheral nervous system
PO	by mouth; orally; phone order; postoperative
POC	products of conception
polys	polymorphonuclear leukocytes
pos	positive
post-op	postoperatively
PP	after meals; postpartum; postprandial; pulse pressure
PPA pos	phenylpyruvic acid positive
PPBS	postprandial blood sugar
PPD	purified protein derivative
PPLO	pleuropneumonia-like organisms
PPS	post perfusion syndrome
PPV	positive pressure ventilation

continued ...

PR	peripheral resistance; pulse rate
Pr	presbyopia; prism
PRA	plasma renin activity
PRBC	packed red blood cells
PRC	packed red cells
PRE	progressive restrictive exercise
preg	pregnant
preop	preoperative
prep	prepare
prn	as needed
proct	proctology
prog	prognosis
PROM	passive range of motion; premature rupture of membranes
pro time	prothrombin time
PRRE	pupils round, regular and equal
PSP	phenolsulfonphthalein
PSS	progressive systemic sclerosis; physiological saline solution
psy, psych	psychiatry
PT	paroxysmal tachycardia; physical therapy; prothrombin time
pt	patient; pint
PTA	plasma thromboplastin antecedent, factor XI
PPT	partial prothrombin time
PTB	patellar tendon bearing

continued ...

PTC	plasma thromboplastic component, factor XI
PTCA	percutaneous transluminal coronary angioplasty
PTD	permanent and total disability
PTE	parathyroid extract
PTH	parathyroid hormone
PTT	partial thromboplastin time; prothrombin time
PU	peptic ulcer; pregnancy urine; prostatic urethra
PUD	peptic ulcer disease; pulmonary disease
pul	pulmonary
PV	peripheral vascular; plasma volume; polycythemia vera
P & V	pyloroplasty and vagotomy
PVC	premature ventricular contraction
PVD	peripheral vascular disease
PVOD	peripheral vascular occlusive disease
PVT	paroxysmal ventricular tachycardia
pvt	private
PWB	partial weight-bearing
PWP	pulmonary wedge pressure
Px	prognosis

-Q-	
q	every

continued ...

qd	every day
qh	every hour
q 2 h	every two hours
QID, qid	four times a day
qm	every morning
qn	every night
qns	quantity not sufficient
qod	every other day
qoh	every other hour
qt	quart; quiet
q.q.	each
quad	quadrant

-R-	
R	rectal; respiration; right
RA	rheumatoid arthritis; right arm; right atrium
Ra	radium
rad, rem	radiation absorbed dose; roentgen-equivalent-man
RAF	rheumatoid arthritis factor
RAI	radioactive iodine
RAIU	radioactive iodine uptake determination
RAS	reticular activating system
RAST	radioallergosorbent
RAT	radiation therapy
RBBB	right bundle branch block
RBC	red blood count; red blood cell
RBCV	red blood cell volume
RBE	relative biological effects

continued ...

RCA	right coronary artery
RD	respiratory distress
RDA	recommended daily allowance
RDS	respiratory distress syndrome
reg	regular
rehab	rehabilitation
RE	right eye
REM	rapid eye movement
RER	renal excretion rate
RES	reticuloendothelial system
resp	respirations
RF	rheumatoid factor; rheumatic fever
RFS	renal function study
RH	right hand
Rh neg	Rhesus factor negative
Rh pos	Rhesus factor positive
RHD	rheumatic heart disease
RHS	right-sided heart failure
RIA	radioimmunoassay
RIF	right iliac fossa
RIST	radioimmunosorbent
RL	right leg
RLC	residual lung capacity
RLD	related living donor
RLE	right lower extremity
RLL	right lower lobe
RLQ	right lower quadrant
RM	respiratory movement

continued ...

RML	right mediolateral
RMSF	Rocky Mountain spotted fever
RNA	ribonucleic acid
RND	radical neck dissection
R/O	rule out
ROA	right occipitis anterior
ROM	range of motion rupture of membranes
ROP	right occipitis posterior
ROPS	roll over protection structures
ROS	review of systems
ROT	right occipitus transverse
RP	retrograde pyelogram
RPCF	Reiter protein complement fixation
RPF	renal plasma flow
RPG	retrograde pyelogram
rpm	revolutions per minute
RPO	right posterior oblique
RPR	rapid plasma reagin
RQ	respiratory quotient
R & R	rate and rhythm
RR	recovery room; respiratory rate
RSR	regular sinus rhythm
RSV	respiratory syncytial virus
rt	right; routine
RT	radiation therapy; respiratory therapy
RTA	renal tubular acidosis

continued ...

rt lat	right lateral
rtd	retarded
RUL	right upper lobe
RU	roentgen unit; routine urinalysis
RUE	right upper extremity
RUL	right upper lobe
RUQ	right upper quadrant
RV	residual volume; right ventricle
RVH	right ventricular hypertrophy
RVS	relative value schedule
RW	ragweed
Rx	prescription; take; therapy

-S-	
s	without
S-A	sinoatrial
S & A	sugar and acetone
SA	salicylic acid; sinoatrial
SAAT	serum aspartate aminotransferase
SACH	solid ankle cushion heel
SACP	serum acid phosphatase
SAFP	serum alpha-fetoprotein
SALD	serum aldolase
SALP	serum alkaline phosphatase
SAM	self-administered medication program
SB	stillbirth

continued ...

SBE	subacute bacterial endocarditis
sc	subcutaneous
SCA	sickle cell anemia
SCC	squamous cell carcinoma
SCD	sudden cardiac death
SCI	spinal cord injury
schiz	schizophrenia
SCID	severe combined immune deficiency
SCPK	serum creatine phosphokinase
SCT	sickle cell trait
SD	septal defect; shoulder disarticulation; spontaneous delivery; sudden death
SDAT	senile dementia of Alzheimer's type
SDM	standard deviation of the mean
SDS	sudden death syndrome
sec	second
SED	suberythema dose
sed rate	sedimentation rate
seg	segmented neutrophils
SEM	scanning electron microscopy
semi	half
seq	sequela; sequestrum
SES	subcutaneous electric stimulation
sev	sever; severed

continued ...

SF	scarlet fever; spinal fluid
SG	serum globulin; skin graft
SGA	small for gestational age
s gl	without correction; without glasses
SGGTP	serum gamma glutamyl transpeptidase
SGOT	serum glutamic oxaloacetic transaminase
SGPT	serum glutamic pyruvic transaminase
SH	serum hepatitis; sex hormone
sh	shoulder
SI	saturation index
SICU	surgical intensive care unit
SIDS	sudden infant death syndrome
SISI	short increment sensitivity index
SLAP	serum leucine aminopeptidase
SLE	St. Louis encephalitis; systemic lupus erythematosus
SLPS	serum lipase
SM	simple mastectomy
sm	small
SMAC	sequential multiple analysis computer
SMG	senile macular degeneration
SMR	submucous resection

continued ...

SMRR	submucous resection and rhinoplasty
SNR	signal-to-noise ratio
SNS	sympathetic nervous system
SO	salpingo-oophorectomy
SOB	shortness of breath
SOM	serous otitis media
SONO	sonography
SOP	standard operating procedure
sos	if necessary
SPBI	serum protein-bound iodine
SPE	serum protein electrophoresis
sp gr	specific gravity
SPHI	serum phosphohexisomerase
SPK	serum pyruvate kinase
SPP	suprapubic prostatectomy
SPR	scanned projection radiography
SR	sedimentation rate; stimulus response; system review
Sr	strontium
ss	half
SS	signs and symptoms; soap solution
SSE	soap suds enema
SSU	sterile supply unit
ST	esotropia
staph	staphylococcus
STAT, stat	immediately

continued ...

STD	sexually transmitted disease; skin test dose
STH	somatotropic hormone
STK	streptokinase
strep	streptococcus
STS	serologic test for syphilis
STSG	split thickness skin graft
subcu	subcutaneous
SUI	stress urinary incontinence
supp	suppository
surg	surgical; surgery
SVC	superior vena cava
SVD	spontaneous vaginal delivery
SVG	saphenous vein graft
SVN	small volume nebulizer
Sx	symptoms

-T-	
T	temperature
T_3	triiodothyronine
T_4	thyroxine
TA	therapeutic abortion
T & A	tonsillectomy and adenoidectomy
tab	tablet
TAH	total abdominal hysterectomy
TAO	thromboangiitis obliterans
TB	tuberculosis
TBD	total body density
TBF	total body fat

continued ...

TBG	thyroxine-binding globulin serum level
TBI	thyroxine-binding index
TBW	total body weight
Tc	Technetium
TCDB	turn, cough, deep breathe
TCP	time care profile
TD	total disability
TDM	therapeutic drug monitoring
TDT	tone decay test
temp	temperature
TEN	toxic epidermal necrolysis
TENS	transcutaneous electrical nerve stimulation
TES	treadmill exercise score
TF	tactile fremitus
TFS	thyroid function studies
TGA	transposition of great arteries
THR	total hip replacement
TIA	transient ischemic attack
TIA-IR	transient ischemic attack incomplete recovery
TIBC	total iron binding capacity
tid	times interval difference; three times a day
tinct	tincture
TKO	to keep open
TKR	total knee replacement
TLC	tender loving care; total lung capacity
TM	temporomandibular

continued ...

TMJ	temporomandibular joint
Tn	normal intraocular tension
TND	term normal delivery
TNI	total nodal irradiation
TNM	tumor, nodes and metastases
TO	telephone order
top	topically
TP	testosterone propionate; total protein
TPA	tissue plasminogen activator; treponema pallidum agglutination
TPBF	total pulmonary blood flow
TPI	Treponema pallidum immobilization
TPN	total parenteral nutrition
TPR	temperature, pulse, respiration
TPUR	transperineal urethral resection
tr	tincture
TR	tuberculin residue
trach	tracheostomy
TRBF	total renal blood flow
TRH	thyrotropin-releasing hormone
TSD	Tay-Sachs disease
TSH	thyroid stimulating hormone
TSP	total serum protein
TSS	toxic shock syndrome
TT	thrombin time

continued ...

TTH	thyrotropic hormone
TUR	transurethral resection
TV	tidal volume
TVH	total vaginal hysterectomy
TW	tap water
TWE	tap water enema
Tx	traction

-U-	
U	units
UA	urinalysis
UC	ulcerative colitis; uterine contractions
UCD	usual childhood diseases
UCG	urinary chorionic gonadotropin; uterine chorionic gonadotropin
UCR	unconditioned reflex
UE	upper extremity
UFR	uroflowmeter; uroflowmetry
UG	upper gastrointestinal; urogenital
UGI	upper gastrointestinal
UK	unknown
UL	upper lobe
ULQ	upper left quadrant
umb	umbilicus
UN	urea nitrogen
ung	ointment
UOQ	upper outer quadrant
UP	uroporphyrin

continued ...

UPP	urethral pressure profile
UR	upper respiratory
ur	urine
URD	upper respiratory disease
URI	upper respiratory infection
urol	urology
URQ	upper right quadrant
US	ultrasonic
USP	United States Pharmacopeia
UTI	urinary tract infection
UV	ultraviolet
UVJ	ureterovesical junction

-V-	
VA	vacuum aspiration; visual acuity
vag	vaginal
VB	viable birth
VBP	ventricular premature beat
VC	acuity of color vision; vena cava; vital capacity
VCG	vectorcardiogram
VCUG	voiding cystourethrogram
VD	venereal disease
VDG	venereal disease, gonorrhea
VDH	valvular disease of heart
VDRL	Venereal Disease Research Laboratory
VDS	venereal disease, syphilis
VE	visual efficiency
VEP	visual evoked potential

continued ...

VER	visual evoked response
VF	vocal fremitus
VG	ventricular gallop
VH	vaginal hysterectomy
VHD	valvular heart disease; ventricular heart disease
VI	volume index
vin	wine
vit cap	vital capacity
VLDL	very-low-density lipoprotein
VP	venipuncture; venous pressure
V & P	vagotomy and pyloroplasty
VPC	ventricular premature contraction
VPRC	volume of packed red cells
VS	vital signs
VSD	ventricular septal defect
VZV	varicella-zoster virus

-W-	
W	water
WA	while awake
WB	weight-bearing; whole blood
WBC	white blood cell; white blood count
W/C	wheelchair
wd	wound
WD	well-developed

continued ...

WDWN	well-developed well-nourished
wf	white female
w/n	well nourished
WNL	within normal limits
w/o	without
WR	Wassermann reaction
wt	weight
w/v	weight by volume

-X-	
x	multiplied by; times
XDP	xeroderma pigmentosum
XM	cross-match
XR	x-ray
XT	exotropia
XU	excretory urogram

-Y-	
YOB	year of birth
yr	year

-Z-	
Z	atomic number; no effect; zero

Flash Cards

INSTRUCTIONS

- Carefully remove the flashcard pages from the book.
- Cut the cards apart to create 126 flashcards.
- Use these cards to learn the word parts, to test yourself, and as a periodic review.
- By putting cards together, you can create terms just as you have done in the word building exercises.

A-	*AB-*
AD-	*ADIP/O*
AF-	*-ALGIA*
ANGI/O	*ANTE-*
ANTI-	*ARTERI/O*
ARTHR/O	*ATHER/O*
BRACHY-	*BRADY-*

away from

away from, negative, not, without

fat

toward, to, in direction of

pain, suffering

toward, to

before, toward

relating to blood or lymph vessels

artery

against, counter

plaque, fatty substance

joint

slow

short

BUCC/O	*CARCIN/O*
CARDI/O	*CAUD/O*
CEC/O	*-CENTESIS*
CEPHAL/O	*CERVIC/O*
CHOL/E	*CHONDR/O*
COL/O, COLON/O	*CORTIC/O*
COST/O	*CRANI/O*

cancerous

cheek

tail, lower part of body

heart

surgical puncture to remove fluid

cecum, blind gut

neck, cervix

head, relating to the head

cartilage

bile, gall

cortex, outer region

colon, large intestine

skull

rib

CUTANE/O	*CYAN/O*
CYST/O	*DACRY/O*
-DEMA	*-DESIS*
DERM/O, DERMAT/O	*DORSI, DORS/O*
DYS-	*-ECTOMY*
EF-	*-EMESIS*
-EMIA	*ENCEPHAL/O*

blue

skin

tear, tear duct, lacrimal duct

urinary bladder, cyst, sac of fluid

to bind, tie together

swelling (fluid)

back of body

skin

surgical removal, cutting out, excision

difficult, painful, bad

vomiting

out

brain

blood, blood condition

ENDO-	*ENTER/O*
EPI-	*ERYTHR/O*
-ESTHESIA	*GASTR/O*
GERONT/O	*GEST/O, GESTAT/O*
-GRAPHY	*GRAVID/O*
GYNEC/O	*HEMAT/O, HEM/O*
HEMI-	*HEPAT/O*

small intestine

within, in, inside

red

upon, above, on, upper

stomach, belly

sensation, feeling

bear, carry young or offspring

old age

pregnancy

writing, process of recording

blood, relating to blood

woman, female

liver

half

HYPER-	*HYPO-*
HYSTER/O	*ILI/O*
-ITIS	*KERAT/O*
LABI/O	*LARYNG/O*
LEUK/O	*LINGU/O*
LIP/O	*LITH/O*
LUTE/O	*-LYTIC*

under, below, decreased

over, above, increased, excessive

ilium, hip bone

uterus, womb

horny, hard, cornea

inflammation

larynx, voice box

lip

tongue

white

stone, calculus

fat, lipid

to reduce, destroy

yellow

MALAC/O, -MALACIA	*MAMM/O*
MEDULL/O	*MEGAL/O, -MEGALY*
MELAN/O	*MY/O*
MYC/E, MYC/O	*MYEL/O*
NAS/O	*NEPHR/O, NEPHRA-*
NEUR/I, NEUR/O	*OCUL/O, OCULO-*
OLIG/O	*-OLOGY*

breast	softening
large, great	medulla, middle, inner section
muscle	black, dark
spinal cord, bone marrow	fungus
kidney	nose
eye	nerve, pertaining to nerves
the science or study of	scanty, few

-OMA	*-OSIS*
-OSTOMY	*ONC/O*
OPT/I, OPT/O, OPTIC/O	*OR/O*
ORCH/O, ORCHI/O, ORCHID/O	*OSS/E, OSS/I, OSTE/O*
OT/O	*-OTOMY*
PART/O, -PARTUM	*-PATHY*
PEDI/A	*PERI-*

an abnormal condition	tumor, mass
tumor	to furnish with a mouth or outlet
the mouth	eye, vision
bone	testis, testes
cutting, incision	ear, hearing
disease, suffering, feeling, emotion	birth, labor
around, surrounding	child

PHLEB/O	*PHREN/O*
-PLASTY	*PNEUM/O, PNEUMON/O, PNEU-*
POD/O	*PROCT/O*
PULM/O, PULMON/O	*PY/O*
PYEL/O	*REN/O*
-RHAGE, -RRHAGE	*-RHAPHY, -RRHAPHY*
-RHEA, -RRHEA	*-RHEXIS, -RRHEXIS*

diaphragm, mind	vein
lung, air	surgical repair
anus and rectum	foot
pus	lung
kidney	renal pelvis, bowl of kidney
suture	bursting forth
rupture	to flow, discharge

-SCLEROSIS	*-SCOPY*
SEPS/O, SEPT/O	*-SPASM*
-STASIS	*SUB-*
SUPIN/O	*SUPRA-*
TACHY-	*THORAC/O*
THROMB/O	*UR/O*
VEN/O	*VENTR/O*

to see, visual examination

hardening

sudden contraction of muscles

infection

below

stopping, controlling

above, excessive

lying on the back

chest

fast, rapid

urine, urinary tract

clot

in front, belly side of body

vein

Index

B

C

D

E

F

G

H

I

M

N

O

P

Q

R

S

T

U

V